The Complete

Acne
Health & Diet Guide

Naturally Clear Skin
Without Antibiotics

Dr. Makoto Trotter
BSc (Hons), ND

For complete cataloguing information, see page 384.

Disclaimer

This book is a general guide only and should never be a substitute for the skill, knowledge and
experience of a qualified medical professional dealing with the facts, circumstances and symptoms
of a particular case.

The nutritional, medical and health information presented in this book is based on the research,
training and professional experience of the author, and is true and complete to the best of his
knowledge. However, this book is intended only as an informative guide for those wishing to know
more about health, nutrition and medicine; it is not intended to replace or countermand the advice given
by the reader's personal physician. Because each person and situation is unique, the author and the
publisher urge the reader to check with a qualified health-care professional before using any procedure
where there is a question as to its appropriateness. A physician should be consulted before beginning
any exercise program. The author and the publisher are not responsible for any adverse effects or
consequences resulting from the use of the information in this book. It is the responsibility of the reader
to consult a physician or other qualified health-care professional regarding his or her personal care.

This book contains references to products that may not be available everywhere. The intent
of the information provided is to be helpful; however, there is no guarantee of results associated
with the information provided. Use of brand names is for educational purposes only and does not
imply endorsement.

The recipes in this book have been carefully tested by our kitchen and our tasters. To the best of our
knowledge, they are safe and nutritious for ordinary use and users. For those people with food or other
allergies, or who have special food requirements or health issues, please read the suggested contents
of each recipe carefully and determine whether or not they may create a problem for you. All recipes
are used at the risk of the consumer. We cannot be responsible for any hazards, loss or damage that
may occur as a result of any recipe use. For those with special needs, allergies, requirements or health
problems, in the event of any doubt, please contact your medical adviser prior to the use of any recipe.

Design and Production: Kevin Cockburn/PageWave Graphics Inc.
Editors: Sue Sumeraj and Fina Scroppo
Copy editor: Kelly Jones
Proofreader: Gillian Watts
Indexer: Gillian Watts
Nutrient analysis: Magda Fahmy
Illustrations: Kveta/threeinabox.com

The publisher gratefully acknowledges the financial support of our publishing program by the
Government of Canada through the Canada Book Fund.

Published by Robert Rose Inc.
120 Eglinton Avenue East, Suite 800, Toronto, Ontario, Canada M4P 1E2
Tel: (416) 322-6552 Fax: (416) 322-6936
www.robertrose.ca

Printed and bound in Canada

1 2 3 4 5 6 7 8 9 FP 23 22 21 20 19 18 17 16 15

I dedicate this book to the love of my life:
my wife and the incredible mother
to my two young children.
Thank you for motivating me to
write this book and providing me
with encouragement along the way.
You have been so patient with me
through this journey, and I could
only have accomplished it with
your devotion and support.

Contents

Acknowledgments

To my patients, thank you for trusting me to help you, for being open to new concepts and for having the courage to take control of your health. You are my best teachers.

To Bob Dees, thank you for giving me a second opportunity to write for Robert Rose and for trusting my ideas and abilities through the book-writing process. Your experience and knowledge of book creation have been invaluable.

To the whole Robert Rose team, thank you for your tireless efforts with respect to editing, design, marketing and sales. You are a brilliant crew.

And most importantly, to my wife, daughter and infant son, thank you for your joyous souls, luminous energy and love. It is what keeps me going and moves me to be better.

Introduction

If you decided to pick up this book, you are likely frustrated: frustrated with the stubborn state of your skin; frustrated with how it affects your moods, your performance at work or school, your relationships and your self-esteem; and frustrated with the predictable pharmaceutical options you have been prescribed.

You likely also have hope: hope that there is a better way to treat your acne — an approach that works with your body and supports you internally in order to improve yourself externally.

Conventional Western medicine views your skin as an entity separate from your body. It uses a reductionist approach, meaning that the body and its systems are deconstructed and viewed as isolated components.

Applying harsh topical treatments is basically akin to using sandpaper to scrub blemishes off your skin. Though this may temporarily improve the appearance of your skin, it is not treating the cause of the problem, and acne typically recurs. In the same way, painting over water stains on your ceiling won't fix a hidden leaky pipe, and — consequently — the stains return.

Internal drug treatments permeate your whole body in an attempt to obliterate bacteria at the surface of the skin. They also suppress hormones or increase the turnover of skin cells. These approaches may or may not improve your acne and can cause side effects.

If you have consulted with a dermatologist, they more than likely have not directed you to a diet plan appropriate for acne. Though the mounting evidence that links diet to acne is hard to ignore, you may be told that there is no point to altering your diet.

In this book, I will review the published evidence that supports the connection between common dietary triggers and acne. I will investigate the lifestyle habits that may be contributing to your skin woes. I will also examine additional supportive nutrients that are most likely to assist you in your road to recovery from acne.

If you are also confused about your skin-care routine, you are not alone. We are exposed to a barrage of advertising that

> Applying harsh topical treatments is basically akin to using sandpaper to scrub blemishes off your skin. Though this may temporarily improve the appearance of your skin, it is not treating the cause of the problem, and acne typically recurs.

attempts to convince us that some new skin-care product is the final solution to curing acne. We know the claims are bogus, yet we succumb.

I will simplify what you really need to know about your skin-care routine. Which products are essential? Are there ingredients in cosmetics that may exacerbate your skin problems? Worse yet, are there ingredients in cosmetics that may compromise your long-term health? I will demystify the confusing and overwhelming world of cosmetics to determine what is and what isn't important.

The main goal of the treatment approach presented here is to work with your body and create an internal state that is less inflamed and more balanced. The approaches that are recommended in this book are designed to be gentle and supportive of your body. Normalizing the function of your hormones, your immune system and your digestion will cause your skin to follow suit.

You may feel that you need further assistance with assessing your skin and implementing lifestyle improvements, natural supplements and dietary changes. If this is the case, consult with a licensed naturopathic doctor or another qualified health-care provider who is experienced with treating acne.

On this journey, be easy on yourself. Don't beat yourself up if you deviate from the game plan, and don't expect that your acne will improve overnight. Anticipate a realistic timeline to achieve your goals and expect that your acne may move two steps forward and one step back as you walk along this path. Be persistent and in tune with the messages your body is giving you.

Find enjoyment in developing new, healthy habits and appreciate the other health benefits you will likely experience with your diet and lifestyle improvements. Find peace while cooking your own foods, comfort in knowing your ingredients, and pleasure when you savor your culinary creations.

This is not the easiest route to take, and I commend you for having the courage to be proactive with your health and making the effort to achieve your goals. I wish you best of luck on your journey to clear skin and becoming a healthier you!

> The approaches that are recommended in this book are designed to be gentle and supportive of your body. Normalizing the function of your hormones, your immune system and your digestion will cause your skin to follow suit.

Quick Guide to Managing Acne

Be aware of your stress levels and incorporate stress management techniques, regular exercise and adequate sleep into your daily life.

- Consult with a dermatologist to assess your skin and review all conventional treatment options with them.
- Consult with a naturopathic doctor specializing in acne to assess your skin from a holistic perspective; this will include evaluating the function of your hormones, digestive tract and immune system in addition to your diet, food sensitivities and stress tolerance.
- Eat a diet of whole foods, eliminating all processed foods and artificial ingredients.
- Your main meals will comprise naturally raised meats, wild-caught fish and legumes for protein, along with non-starchy vegetables, gluten-free whole grains and healthy oils.
- Your snacks will include one or a combination of low-sugar fruit, non-starchy vegetables, nuts and seeds.
- Your beverages will include water and herbal tea.
- Cut out all forms of sugar, whether natural or refined.
- Eliminate all flours, high-sugar fruits, dried fruit and starchy vegetables.
- Avoid foods that contain gluten, dairy or eggs.
- Eliminate all juices, soft drinks, caffeine and alcohol.
- Eat regularly, approximately every 3 hours, consuming small to moderate-sized meals with healthy snacks.
- The most important supplements are L-glutamine, probiotics, fish oils, zinc, vitamin D_3, calcium D-glucarate and indole-3-carbinol. Consult with your naturopathic doctor to determine which are the most appropriate for you.
- Be aware of your stress levels and incorporate stress management techniques, regular exercise and adequate sleep into your daily life.

PART 1

Understanding Acne

CHAPTER 1
What Is Acne?

CASE STUDY

Acne and Picking

When Georgia, 17, came to my office, she had had acne since she was 13 years old. It was mild to moderate acne and the intensity was not out of the ordinary for a teenager. She was mild-mannered and somewhat shy, making only occasional eye contact on the first visit.

She suffered from anxiety and had a tendency to pick at her skin. She would prod acne pimples as soon as they started to develop on her face. Her acne greatly affected her self-esteem, and she attempted to get rid of them as soon as they formed. She would pick at her skin, looking in the mirror, for an extended duration of time, sometimes without even being aware of it.

Georgia was embarrassed about the skin picking, but she realized it was important to be truthful so I could properly assess her skin. She made sure that I knew she was motivated to do whatever she could to improve her skin.

I am always careful to tread lightly around teenagers when it comes to the topic of diet. It may be challenging for teens to take full control of their diet, particularly in social situations, and because it is typically the first time they are making dietary choices on their own. Of course, teens have to be given proper context with respect to dietary limitations so they understand that this is not a "forever" thing — rather, this is an initial treatment to improve their skin and it will be followed by easier-to-follow goals around long-term eating.

The last thing we want to trigger at an early age is paranoia about eating or foods. There is a fine line between understanding how to eat a healthy diet and becoming fearful of eating. The goal is to always take a balanced approach and to appreciate eating and nourishment and, ultimately, do the best we can to make healthy choices.

In Georgia's case, I pointed out that picking at her skin meant that she was likely experiencing anxiety, and I asked her about any stresses she was experiencing. She revealed that she was being verbally bullied at school by some peers and that her parents were often fighting. I referred her to a child psychologist, so that she could fully express and cope with her emotions in a safe environment. A counselor could help her develop strategies to improve her self-confidence and better deal with external stressors.

I also explained that if we worked together, we could improve the physical presentation of her acne through diet and lifestyle modifications and, consequently, she would have less reason to pick. However, she still needed to address the underlying emotional components of her stress with a counselor.

Georgia was motivated and eager to get started.

On the surface, acne seems much different from psoriasis, eczema, seborrhea and other common skin conditions, since acne is easily recognized. It is seen as a rite of passage for adolescents and teenagers as they enter and go through puberty, with varying degrees of severity. Severe cases can lead to scarring, particularly if flare-ups continue for years.

Acne appears on areas of the skin where we have the heaviest concentration of sebaceous glands. The most common areas are the face, chest, upper back and shoulders.

The most psychologically damaging acne can be severe disfiguring acne in adolescent years or persistent acne that continues into adulthood. I see patients who are in their 20s, 30s, 40s and even 50s who are still struggling with acne, when it should be a distant memory. In other cases, I have patients who had relatively clear skin during their youth but have adult-onset acne that started years or even decades after puberty.

> Acne is seen as a rite of passage for adolescents and teenagers as they enter and go through puberty, with varying degrees of severity.

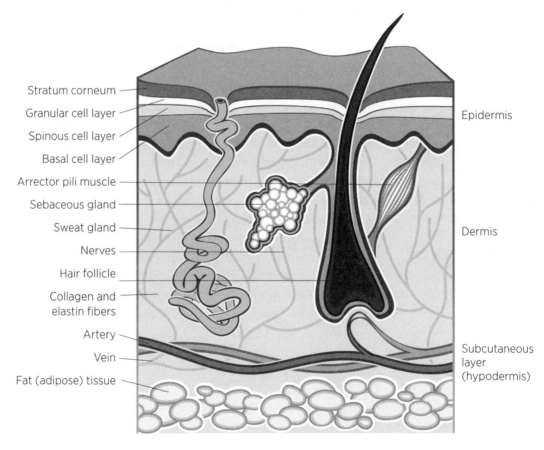

Stratum corneum
Granular cell layer
Spinous cell layer
Basal cell layer
Arrector pili muscle
Sebaceous gland
Sweat gland
Nerves
Hair follicle
Collagen and elastin fibers
Artery
Vein
Fat (adipose) tissue

Epidermis

Dermis

Subcutaneous layer (hypodermis)

Acne in a Nutshell

Acne is an inflammatory skin condition that affects the upper layers of skin. As a result of the inflammation, the skin may appear to have a reddened or pinkish base. The lesions that form are the result of blocked pores (sebaceous glands) that overproduce oily substances and can trap bacteria, creating small pockets of pus under the skin. This creates the classic whitehead pimple.

Degrees of Acne

- **Whiteheads:** Isolated small whiteheads are the most common. It is often hard to resist picking or popping these blocked pustules and squeezing out their contents. This creates an opening in the skin, which subsequently triggers the body to repair the skin and sometimes causes hyperpigmented (darkened) and scarred skin.
- **Severe acne:** When pimples appear at a faster rate and in a higher concentration, they can coalesce into much larger and more visible pustules that can be quite noticeable.
- **Cystic acne:** A severe form of acne, this occurs deeper in the skin and is slow to heal. The skin can be quite tender and painful, and the condition lasts for a longer period of time than classic acne. Because of its deeper penetration, cystic acne can create scarring as it heals, which can affect the texture of the skin and lead to cratering or pockmarks.
- **Blackheads:** Blackheads are opened pores that collect secretions of sebum (the oily substance secreted at the surface of your skin) and dead skin cells, and this causes them to appear as black dots on the skin. These can be extracted without breaking the surface of the skin, but they return because of their open nature, filling up again and eventually leading to blackheads.

Types of Acne

Acne may present as one type or as a mix of several types of pimples. The type of acne is categorized based on the kinds of lesions and their pathogenesis — that is, the cause of their development. Any type of acne can range in severity from mild to severe (based on the number of lesions and degree of damage to the skin).

Your family doctor or dermatologist may or may not have already told you what type of acne you have. If you were given a label for your acne, the descriptions below will help you understand why they named your acne the way they did. If you did not receive a label for your condition, the information below may help you understand in which category your acne fits.

Acne Vulgaris

This is the most recognized and most common type of acne. It is often a mixture of the various forms of skin lesions that can comprise acne, including pimples (whiteheads or blackheads), papules (small skin-colored bumps) and nodules (larger skin-colored bumps). This is the type of acne associated with hormonal changes related to puberty. It affects approximately 85% of the population between 12 and 24 years old. The intensity is usually mild, but it can become moderate to severe in 15% to 20% of those affected.

Acne Mechanica

This form of acne occurs in people who are acne-prone as a result of pressure, heat and sweat. As the name suggests, it is an aggravation of a mechanical nature; that is, it is prompted by some form of physical exertion and pressure. This typically occurs while exercising or playing sports, particularly when wearing tight synthetic clothing (for example, sports bras or compression wear). This causes pressure on specific areas, leading to heat and perspiration, which triggers a breakout.

Pityrosporum Folliculitis (Malassezia Folliculitis)

In this type of acne, there is a proliferation of yeast in hair follicles near the surface of the skin. The yeast, called malassezia, grows on everyone's skin, but in this condition, it leads to tiny raised lesions that are either pink or skin-colored and appear to make the skin bumpy. Typical areas include the face, neck, chest, shoulders and arms, and the lesions may be itchy or get worse with perspiration.

Any type of acne can range in severity from mild to severe (based on the number of lesions and degree of damage to the skin).

Severe Acne

The following four types of acne are classified as severe because they present with large, inflamed or disfiguring lesions, because of their resistance to treatment or because of severe sudden onset.

- **Acne conglobata:** This severe form of acne is related to elevated androgens (male hormones, such as testosterone). As a result, acne conglobata is more common in men than women. It consists of deeper lesions than in acne vulgaris, and may include nodules, abscesses and inflammation, which often start from blackheads. When abscesses are large and painful, they may require lancing and drainage by a physician. The lesions often leave scarring, which can sometimes be deep, ulcerated and disfiguring. The skin appears very inflamed and red.

- **Acne fulminans:** This rare and suddenly occurring severe form of acne is accompanied by a fever, joint inflammation and pain, typically in the hips and knees. Acne fulminans is very similar to acne conglobata, with nodules and abscesses on highly inflamed, damaged skin. The difference is in the timeline and the associated symptoms. Acne fulminans occurs suddenly and acutely and is associated with a febrile (feverish) state and joint pains, whereas acne conglobata is a persistent chronic condition that is not accompanied by a fever.

- **Gram-negative folliculitis:** The causative bacteria in this type of acne may be resistant to antibiotic treatment. Known as gram-negative bacteria, they proliferate typically after one or more courses of antibiotics.

- **Nodulocystic acne:** This form of acne, also commonly referred to as cystic acne, differs from typical acne vulgaris in that it consists of deeper lesions, called nodules and cysts. Nodules are hard lesions, whereas cysts are fluid-filled lesions; these can appear alone or in groupings and can be quite painful and slow to heal. When nodules and cysts manifest in close proximity, they can coalesce into larger lesions that can be deep under the skin and cause scarring that looks pitted.

Types of Pimples

Acne is characterized by several types of lesions. When you are looking at your skin during acne breakouts, you probably notice that there are different types of pimples. They can range from tiny, benign skin-colored bumps to large, deep, red and tender pimples. Alternatively, you may have the characteristic whiteheads and blackheads that come with acne.

The following descriptions will help you to better understand what you are seeing in the mirror.

Types of Acne

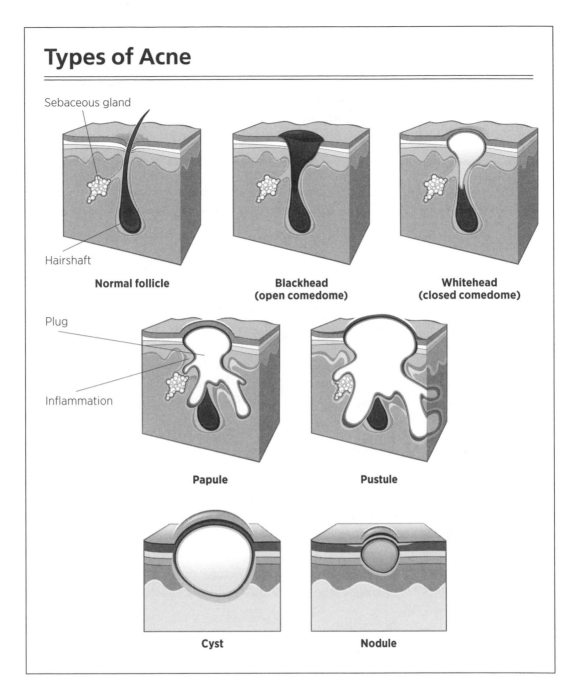

Sebaceous gland

Hairshaft

Normal follicle

**Blackhead
(open comedome)**

**Whitehead
(closed comedome)**

Plug

Inflammation

Papule

Pustule

Cyst

Nodule

Closed Comedomes

Closed comedomes are the well-known whiteheads that accompany acne. They are blocked oil (sebaceous) ducts that typically appear as small white pimples and they vary in size. They are called *closed* because they are enclosed by skin on their outer surface. Closed comedomes essentially have the same contents as blackheads (sebum and dead skin cells), but do not turn black because they are not exposed to air and, therefore, remain a lighter color.

Cysts

Cysts are pockets of cellular material, fluids or pus under the surface of the skin. The density of the contents can range from hard to soft to liquid, and the size can vary, too — from quite small to large. The distinguishing feature of cysts is that they are enclosed by a membranous sac. The material inside a cyst can feel like a tiny ball under the surface of the skin. Although cysts do not usually cause pain, they can sometimes become large and chronic. Cysts can be treated by sterile lancing and removal or by draining the contents.

Keratosis Pilaris

This bumpy skin condition is hereditary to some degree. It consists of small, hard lesions — plugs of a substance called keratin that become impacted and surface at hair follicles. The most common areas to be affected are the backs of the arms (triceps) or outer upper legs. Keratosis pilaris does not typically cause any pain or discomfort, but the bumps can become reddened and enlarged, making their appearance more obvious.

Milia

Milia are small plugs of keratin that get trapped under the skin. They are typically $\frac{1}{32}$ to $\frac{1}{8}$ inch (1 to 3 mm) in diameter and appear as tiny skin-colored or yellowish bumps that cluster on the face. They are not painful but are hard to the touch. Although milia are very common in infants (also known as baby acne) and resolve on their own, they can also appear in adults and be quite persistent.

Nodules

Nodules are bumps that form deeper under the surface of the skin. They are greater than $\frac{1}{4}$ inch (5 mm) in diameter and do not contain pus or fluids. They are similar to papules (see below).

Open Comedomes

Commonly referred to as blackheads, these pimples are termed *open* because they are open at the surface. Think of them as miniature pits that collect sebum — your natural protective skin oils — and dead skin cells.

Papules

Papules are small raised lesions that form just under the surface of the skin. They are less than $\frac{1}{4}$ inch (5 mm) in diameter. They do not fill with pus or fluid.

Pustules

These inflamed bumps under the surface of the skin are typically small in acne, but they can also become larger if they coalesce. They are tender and sometimes painful. Pustules have a characteristic white liquid (pus) that is visible under the skin, but they can also look red or pink because they are inflamed. They are enclosed, containing inflammatory immune cells and bacteria. In mild to moderate cases, it is recommended to leave pustules alone, rather than poking and prodding them, so that your immune system can "do its thing."

Types of Acne Scars

A major concern for people with acne is not just the current state of their skin, but the potential for long-lasting or sometimes permanent skin damage. Acne scars are any kind of scar tissue that develops as a result of acne. Scarring typically occurs when inflammatory acne lesions penetrate relatively deep into the skin, resulting in the trigger for scar tissue formation.

There are several classifications of scar tissues, based on the manner in which they impact the structure or color of the skin.

Depressed Scars

Depressed scars are acne scars that create a depression in the skin. Based on the way that the lesion and scar tissue develop, they can take on one of three different formations:

Boxcar lesions

Boxcar lesions are the result of inflammatory acne lesions that cause depressions in the skin. The name *boxcar* implies that the edges of the lesion drop straight down, with the bottom of the scar being flat; essentially, they have a squared-off appearance.

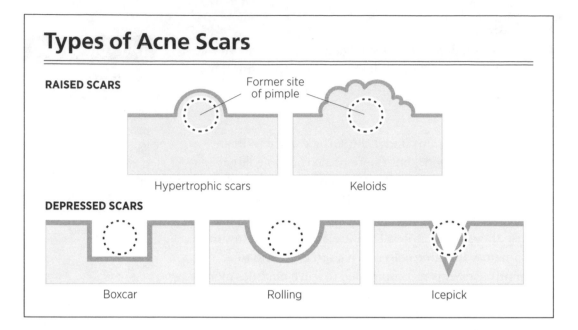

Types of Acne Scars

RAISED SCARS

Former site of pimple

Hypertrophic scars

Keloids

DEPRESSED SCARS

Boxcar

Rolling

Icepick

Icepick scars

Icepick scars are depressed scars that extend down from the normal surface of the skin in a chipped-out V-shaped depression. These depressed scars can be more difficult to treat because they can be fairly deep.

Rolling lesions

Rolling lesions are depressions caused by inflammatory acne lesions that leave a hollowed-out, round appearance. The edges of the lesions drop down from the surface of the skin in a curved, sloped manner, similar to the shape of a ski or snowboard half-pipe.

Raised Scars

Raised acne scars cause the skin structure to elevate above the normal surface level of the skin. There are two types of raised scars:

Keloid scars

Keloid scars are raised acne scars that extend outside of the boundaries that demarcated the previous acne lesion. In certain cases, they can be quite large and disfiguring, often extending beyond the circumference of the lesion.

Hypertrophic scars

Hypertrophic scars are raised acne scars that stay within the boundaries that demarcated the previous acne lesion.

Did You Know?

Rolling Scars
Rolling scars often appear in clusters and have the appearance of rolling hills.

Color Changes

Color changes at the former site of acne lesions can be marked by white, red or darkened areas of skin. They fit into one of three categories:

COLOR CHANGES

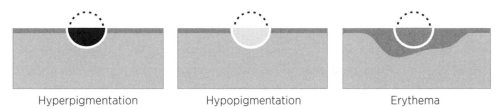

| Hyperpigmentation | Hypopigmentation | Erythema |

Erythema

The inflammation of acne can affect the distribution of small blood vessels (called capillaries) near the surface of the skin. The walls of the capillaries can be damaged and they can expand in size, which can cause reddening of the skin (*erythema* is the medical term for skin that is red). Erythema can occur while acne is active, but the concern is when it lasts long after acne has been treated.

Hyperpigmentation

Pigmentation changes can occur with or without actually changing the topography of the skin. Hyperpigmentation is the darkening of the skin and is related to the different amount of melanocytes (the cells that produce skin pigment, called melanin) in regenerating scar tissue. This becomes noticeable because of the contrast of skin color between the damaged and undamaged skin.

Hypopigmentation

Hypopigmentation is caused by the same process as hyperpigmentation, but it results in lightening of the skin.

> **Did You Know?**
>
> **Pigmentation in Acne**
>
> Melanocytes can be either overproduced or underproduced as a result of scar tissue and inflammation related to acne. This would result in hyperpigmentation or hypopigmentation, respectively.

The Psychology of Acne

One of the difficulties of having acne is that it primarily appears on the face, and is not something that can be hidden from friends, colleagues, family, romantic partners and strangers. For that reason, a person with acne is constantly aware of their condition and thinking about it. This has a snowball effect on their psyche and creates stress, which in turn can exacerbate hormone production and skin conditions, creating a vicious cycle.

Self-image needs to be addressed in patients with acne because it can actually stunt self-confidence, particularly if the acne has existed since the formative years. These damaging psychological effects can continue to have an impact long after the skin has healed.

The impact of acne can be pervasive. While patients with acne often feel a strong urgency to heal, it is important that they understand the expected prognosis and timeline, particularly when using natural approaches. The goal of using non-pharmaceutical approaches to treat acne is to treat a patient's internal health, which results in clear skin and is maintained for the long term.

Picking

Picking is, within itself, a psychological dilemma for those suffering from acne. That pustule staring at you in the mirror bothers you no end, and in your mind, it is blown up to volcanic proportions. It seems that everyone you encounter throughout the day is looking at that new breakout — it is all-consuming and you want to get rid of it at all costs.

Any encounter with a mirror (while you are using a bathroom or simply washing your hands) gives you another opportunity to take a look at that pimple and observe how close to the surface it is, sitting there, ready to be extracted. This time, maybe, it will come out cleanly, settle down quickly and heal by tomorrow. But that is hardly ever the case.

What is more likely to happen is that you notice this pustule fairly early in its development and, because you see it multiple times a day, you start to just touch it gently to see how it responds. You don't plan on prodding or picking at it, but next thing you know, you are in there with your fingernails, digging away at all sides of the pimple, trying to coax that pustule to come out cleanly and promptly. Instead, you are left with large indents at the edges of the pimple, highlighting its presence, along with a newly reddened and further inflamed pimple that may have some blood or fluid seeping out if you managed to break the skin.

The pimple pick becomes a futile mind game and it adds another layer to the psychology of acne, due to the continuous stress of trying to resist and ignore the urge to poke at your face.

FAQ

Q **Is there a way to break the vicious cycle of picking?**

A The best rule is to not touch. But it is easier said than done. Not picking the skin becomes an effort in self-discipline and compounds the stress of having acne in the first place. The catch-22 here is that stress can aggravate acne, so the more effort you make to resist picking, the more stress you experience, which can worsen breakouts.

The key to stop picking your skin is to accept your skin as it is and to reassure yourself that picking at it will not solve the problem but actually make it worse. Incorporate self-help techniques, such as breathing and meditation, when you feel the urge. Remind yourself of your other beautiful facial features, like your eyes, and shift your focus to these every time you look in the mirror. Remember that you are more fixated on your skin than anyone else is, and try to find the beauty in yourself that others see in you as well.

Doc Talk

Direct your energy away from obsessing in the mirror and focus on being proactive in addressing your acne. In order to be properly assessed, consult with a dermatologist for a conventional approach or a naturopathic doctor for a non-pharmaceutical approach. Weigh all the pros and cons of the treatments recommended and do what works best for you.

If the first treatment is not successful, find out why and keep persisting. You will eventually find a route to clear skin that works with your body and allows you to be content with your appearance so you can live your life with fewer distractions.

Why Do I Have Acne?

Making the Right Choice

Raoul was a pleasant 21-year-old man. He was in his second year of post-secondary education when he came to see me. He was frustrated with his acne, which had persisted since puberty and had worsened since he started college. He had read a lot of online blogs that provided an overwhelming amount of information regarding dietary changes and supplements that could help his skin. He was motivated to take control of his health and improve his acne.

A few weeks earlier, he had booked an appointment with a dermatologist and was excited to get some feedback and direction for treating his skin. Unfortunately, the dermatologist spent fewer than 5 minutes with him and gave him a prescription for Accutane. Raoul was quite disheartened because he was hoping for a non-pharmaceutical treatment plan, particularly since he had used prescription medication in high school that had offered him only temporary improvements. The dermatologist was also quickly dismissive when Raoul brought up the subject of diet, telling him that there was "no connection between diet and acne."

Raoul held fast to his goal of improving his skin naturally. He told me that he had just recently learned how to cook on his own and was trying out healthy recipes. He did not want to follow health advice off the Internet until he had consulted with a health professional for guidance.

It was clear to me that Raoul was ready and eager to benefit from diet and lifestyle changes, and we were both confident that we could improve his acne.

Predisposing Factors

Factors that may determine an individual's predisposition to acne include genetics, hormones, nutrients and hygiene.

Genetics

Research shows that there is a genetic component to acne, although specific acne genes have not yet been fully identified. Recent research is demonstrating that certain parts of the genome (our individual DNA makeup) can increase our susceptibility to hormone surges, inflammation and scarring in cases of severe acne — compared to people with clear skin.

Your parents' and siblings' experiences with acne can assist in predicting the course and potential trajectory of your own skin condition. Although your skin likely won't identically mirror that of your immediate relatives, knowing more about your family's history of acne may provide a plausible template of expectations and offer some ideas on ways to manage your skin.

Genetics play a role in how hormones manifest and in imbalances that may occur, and they may predict increased risk of hormone disorders. Certain genes can determine when hormone surges occur during puberty and when they level off. Acne is intimately connected to hormone surges and fluctuations in the body, and is therefore affected by the heredity of hormones.

Medical History

Providing your dermatologist or naturopathic doctor with answers to some of the following questions may be helpful in predicting prognosis and treatment of your own acne.

- At what age did your immediate family member have acne?
- At what age did it clear up?
- What type of acne was it?
- On which areas did it appear?
- What made it better?
- What aggravated it?
- Did they have any successful treatments for it?

Hormones

Acne is most commonly thought of as a teenager's problem. As teens or preteens transition into adulthood through puberty, they experience a surge of hormones that help with maturing the reproductive organs. This change in hormones is essential in transforming a child into an adult capable of reproducing. One of the (many) by-products of this increase is acne.

The hormone surges of testosterone and estrogen trigger increased production of sebum by the sebaceous glands and accelerated epidermis turnover. The combination of increased cells being made at the surface of the skin along with excess oil production leads to the perfect storm of clogged pores and hair follicles that harbor the bacteria responsible for acne, *Propionibacterium acnes*. This brewing concoction turns into a typical teenage acne pimple.

Hormone imbalances can be triggered by disease, genetics, medication, diet, lifestyle, smoking, stress or lack of sleep. In adult women with hormonal acne, commonly there are accompanying menstrual irregularities. In these cases, the skin typically becomes more sensitive or tends to break out in a predictable pattern associated with the woman's menstrual cycle. This is often related to estrogen levels being too high relative to progesterone, particularly in the second half of the menstrual cycle. The result is acne breakouts occurring before a woman's expected period. In other situations, women may have elevated levels of androgens (for example, testosterone, the most common), and this may trigger their acne, such as in polycystic ovarian syndrome (PCOS).

For men with hormonal acne, it is typically related to spikes in androgens, which may be related to an underlying overproduction by the testes or adrenal glands. Androgen levels may also be elevated by increased conversion from other hormones in the body. Excess testosterone may shunt hormone production to a more powerful androgen called dihydrotestosterone (DHT). In men, approximately 5% to 10% of testosterone typically converts to DHT, and DHT has twice the effect of testosterone in the body. As a result, increased levels of DHT are known to contribute to hair loss, prostate enlargement and also acne.

Cortisol is a hormone that is released when you are under stress. It is yet another hormone that, when elevated, is connected to an increased prevalence of acne.

Nutrient Deficiencies

Inadequate amounts of certain vitamins, minerals or other nutrients may affect the optimal functioning of our metabolic processes. These nutrients are often required to support the proper working of our enzymes (as cofactors), which are responsible for countless functions in the body,

Research Spotlight: A Diet Low in Nutrients

A 2014 Russian study showed that deficiencies in certain nutrients — vitamin A, vitamin D and zinc — correlated to an increased severity of acne. Two groups of participants between the ages of 15 and 25 were examined. The control group consisted of 90 subjects who were healthy and had no signs of inflammatory or noninflammatory skin lesions. The test group consisted of 90 subjects who had moderate to severe acne.

Their diets were assessed and compared according to calorie consumption, carbohydrate intake and nutrient content. The degree of severity and inflammation of acne were significantly linked to the following dietary traits: excess caloric intake and carbohydrate consumption and deficiency of intake of vitamin A, vitamin D and zinc.

Although this is a small study, its results are consistent with results from other studies that correlate acne to diet quality and nutrient intake.

Suboptimal Digestion

Conventional medicine views the digestive tract and skin as two distinct entities that should be assessed and treated separately — by a gastroenterologist and a dermatologist, respectively.

From a holistic perspective, the health and proper functioning of your digestive tract is critical to resolving skin concerns. Although the intestines and skin are not in direct proximity to one another, they are very closely linked in terms of their function. The skin is the barrier between our body and the external environment. Our intestinal tract, although located internally, is also a barrier that separates our body from the external environment (or the contents of your intestines, which are still "outside" of your body). Actually, the intestines are essentially the "skin" that covers the tube (our digestive tract) that runs from our mouth to our anus. As well, our intestines connect with our skin and are part of the same surface that envelops our body. When you think about it from this perspective, it becomes hard to imagine treating one without addressing the other.

In addition to these analogous roles, malfunctioning in the digestive tract can also commonly manifest on the skin. The digestive tract determines what is permitted or denied entry into the bloodstream, via the intestinal barrier. When the digestive system is not functioning properly, inflammatory particles — such as improperly digested molecules, fungi, bacteria, viruses — are mistakenly allowed to enter the bloodstream. These circulate through the vascular system and trigger an immune response, which leads to inflammation. The immune cells bind to the aggravating particle (the antigen) so they can be eliminated more efficiently. Skin has the largest surface area, so it makes sense that inflammatory reactions, such as acne, commonly develop here.

including repairing and regenerating tissues, controlling immune reactions and making or breaking down hormones. When nutrients are not abundant, some of these processes may be compromised and this may manifest as acne.

Although it is not fully understood how certain nutrient deficiencies can lead to an increased risk or severity of acne, the connection does exist. Nutrient deficiencies should be corrected in order to properly treat acne.

Hygiene

Proper hygiene is important to ensure that potential surface bacteria are kept under control, especially when you are more prone to acne, such as during puberty. When skin cell turnover is more rapid than normal, the likelihood of trapping and harvesting the growth of bacteria intensifies.

Skin care is not the solution or cure to acne, but it is helpful to keep it under control. Sloughing off skin cells (usually mechanically or chemically) can help prevent the development of clogged pores. Doing this in combination with daily cleansing limits the growth of new bacteria and allows the lesions to heal.

Think of it as like scraping your knee on a rock. To treat the injury, you first clean the area of dirt, debride it (remove damaged tissue) and then apply an antibacterial topical treatment to prevent infection. In the case of acne, the unnecessary tissues and cells need to be displaced and removed, and the growth of new bacteria limited.

Associated Conditions

It is important to rule out any potential underlying causes for your acne. If some of the symptoms of these conditions match your situation, talk to your doctor to determine if there is an underlying condition.

PCOS

Polycystic ovarian syndrome is a condition that affects women. Signs and symptoms include being overweight, depression, insulin resistance, increased testosterone, and cysts on the ovaries (contradictory to its name, there are not always ovarian cysts in PCOS). Women with PCOS often have irregular periods — they do not occur frequently enough or sometimes not at all. Their periods can be quite heavy and they may have problems conceiving. PCOS can also increase the risk of diabetes and heart disease.

As a result of the body's increased levels of insulin and the ovaries' increased testosterone secretion, acne often accompanies PCOS.

Congenital Adrenal Hyperplasia

Congenital adrenal hyperplasia is a hereditary genetic condition where certain enzymes in the adrenal glands are mutated and, subsequently, do not function properly in their role of producing hormones. This can affect various hormones, but most commonly it impairs the production of cortisol. As a result, there is a buildup of other hormones in the pathway, which typically leads to an overproduction of androgens. Acne, which is triggered by androgens, may be a manifestation of congenital adrenal hyperplasia.

This condition can manifest in different ways, with varying degrees of severity, based on the enzymes impacted. Symptoms may include genital abnormalities, early puberty (or no pubescent phase at all), menstrual irregularities, excess hair growth, infertility and vomiting.

FAQ

Q **Can certain medications trigger acne?**

A Yes, androgens, corticosteroids and lithium commonly promote acne.

- **Androgens,** such as testosterone, may be supplemented for a variety of reasons, including underproduction of testosterone (hypogonadism), gender transitioning (female to male), andropause (a term used to describe the decline of testosterone in men in their mid-40s to 50s) and to enhance sports performance (anabolic steroids). Because elevated androgens increase sebum production and turnover of the epidermis, acne can occur.
- **Corticosteroids** (commonly prescribed for inflammatory diseases) can lead to Cushing's syndrome when used for an extended time period. Acne is a potential side effect.
- **Lithium** acts as a mood stabilizer and has been used for decades, most commonly as a treatment for bipolar disorder. It also has uses in other psychiatric conditions. One of its common side effects is acne. It is not clear how lithium causes acne, but researchers believe that it can lead to increased white blood cells at the surface of the skin, which can increase the likelihood of an inflammatory reaction in the pores, triggering pimples.

Cushing's Syndrome

Cushing's syndrome occurs when the brain (the pituitary, specifically) signals the adrenal glands to overproduce cortisol. Cushing's syndrome describes the situation in which elevated cortisol levels in the body lead to certain physical manifestations in the body.

This syndrome may manifest as rapid central weight gain (mainly in the abdomen, torso and face), thinned skin, weakened bones, fat deposits at the back of the neck (described as a buffalo hump), depressed immunity, muscle breakdown, menstrual irregularities, infertility, facial hair growth, baldness, mania, depression and acne. Overexposure to cortisol leads to elevated blood sugar and increased androgens. Both of these situations contribute to acne.

Stress

We can experience stress in many different ways. When we say, "I am stressed," we usually imply that we are under mental or emotional stress — one of several ways that stress can affect our body. Psychological stress may be the most underestimated form of stress, but it may also be one of the most important determinants of our health outcomes.

Two other important broad categories of stress are physical and chemical. Physical stressors refer to a lack of basic physical necessities, such as exercise, sleep and proper nutrition. Chemical stressors refer to harmful stimuli, such as medication, cigarettes, alcohol, radiation and artificial/processed ingredients. These are chemicals (or things that trigger the production of unnatural chemicals in our body, as in the case of radiation) that disrupt the normal physiological chemistry in our body. Another term for chemical stress is oxidative stress.

Physical Stress

Physical stress describes the negative impact on our health of inadequate exercise, suboptimal sleep and an unhealthy diet. These variables are commonly overlooked and, as a society, we lack all three of these basic needs, which support our normal homeostatic and repair mechanisms. We often put emphasis on the fact that we can multitask and live such busy lives, require little sleep, eat on the run — and somehow we see this as an admirable quality. Even though

Overlapping Categories

There is a lot of overlap between each of these categories. Psychological stress, for example, will disrupt the normal balance of neurotransmitter molecules, which may be considered a chemical stress. Physical stresses, such as improper nutrition or lack of exercise, also affect the normal balance of hormones and metabolic chemicals, which describes chemical stress. Therefore, there is a lot of interplay between categories. The categorizations used here describe the main role of each of the stress triggers.

this has an impact on our well-being, we egg each other on to continue these unhealthy patterns.

Lack of sleep, irregular exercise and malnutrition are not good for our health in general; in particular, they set the groundwork for the development of acne. Inadequate sleep and a sedentary lifestyle contribute to suboptimal health and inflammatory states, and play a role in the development of acne.

Exercise

We have become more and more sedentary in correlation with advances in automation and technology that have led to a larger percentage of the population working at desk jobs that require little to no physical activity.

Exercise increases our sensitivity to insulin and improves our use of blood sugar. The development of acne may be related to the excess secretion of insulin in response to spikes in our blood sugar. Regular exercise helps stabilize insulin secretion and blood sugar levels.

Did You Know?

Regulating Cortisol
Regular physical exercise allows the body to both regulate sleep and normalize adrenal gland function. These play a role in stabilizing cortisol (our stress hormone) levels. Cortisol triggers the release of blood sugars — if its release is not adequately regulated, it can manifest as acne. Because exercise improves our normal daily fluctuations of cortisol, it may also help normalize the health of our skin.

Sleep

Sleep is a must. Americans slept on average 1 hour less per night in 2013 than in 1942, according to Gallup Poll survey data. As well, 40% of the American population reported that they sleep less than 6 hours, and 65% are not achieving the gold standard of 8 hours of sleep for adequate restorative rest. In general, the majority of us are functioning with mild to moderate sleep deprivation.

Of course, the risk of death (see Research Spotlight, opposite) is a big motivator for improving your sleep quality, but from an acne perspective, sleep is also crucial. Lack of sleep disrupts your normal diurnal rhythm (natural biological pattern based on a 24-hour day). The stress hormone cortisol fluctuates throughout the day, based on this cycle. In a healthy person with adequate sleep, cortisol starts out highest upon waking and gradually decreases throughout the day and night. By nighttime, it should be easy to fall asleep and have a restful sleep.

Lacking sleep — whether a result of a health condition or mood disorder or self-induced as a result of stress and overscheduling — will throw off your diurnal rhythm. Cortisol levels may be elevated before bed and bottom out during the day. The whole cortisol curve may actually be turned upside down, making you exhausted during the day

Typical Diurnal (24-Hour) Physiological Patterns

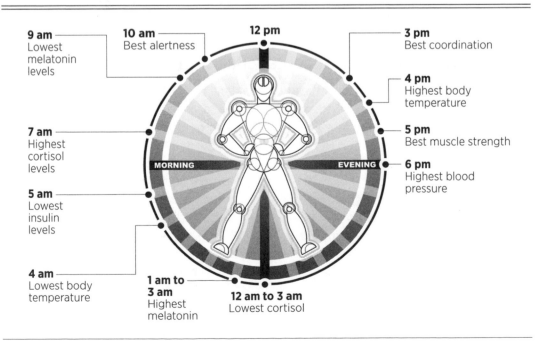

9 am Lowest melatonin levels

10 am Best alertness

12 pm

3 pm Best coordination

4 pm Highest body temperature

7 am Highest cortisol levels

5 pm Best muscle strength

MORNING

EVENING

6 pm Highest blood pressure

5 am Lowest insulin levels

4 am Lowest body temperature

1 am to 3 am Highest melatonin

12 am to 3 am Lowest cortisol

and restless at night. This effect perpetuates the whole unhealthy cycle, because you are not only tired but also wired and unable to get a good night's rest.

Chemical Stress

A more accurate descriptor for chemical stress is oxidative stress. Oxidative stress is what occurs when chemicals negatively impact our normal healthy physiology.

Oxidation is chemically balanced by enzymatic processes and antioxidants, which are compounds produced by our cells but that also naturally occur in many foods. We most often hear about antioxidants in terms of a food's nutritional benefit: they assist in neutralizing oxidation and the potential for disease, returning the body to a more balanced chemical state. If the body's supply of antioxidants is low, it will shift the balance to a place of oxidative stress.

Oxidative stress throughout the body can impact the concentration of chemically reactive molecules (reactive oxygen species, or ROS) in the sebum in our sebaceous

Did You Know?

Causes of Oxidative Stress
Oxidative stress may be triggered by a number of different external stimuli. It can be caused by air pollution, psychological stress, radiation, cigarette smoking, recreational drugs, alcohol and processed food ingredients.

FAQ

 What is oxidation?

Oxidation is a chemical process that normally occurs in cellular metabolism when molecules lose their electrons. If oxidation is not properly controlled (through a neutralizing chemical reaction called reduction), it damages normal cell function and can lead to the development of numerous diseases. The uncontrolled process of oxidation and how it affects the body is termed oxidative stress. Oxidative stress can cause harm to our cells' DNA, proteins, fats and enzyme constituents. Therefore, it is important to keep in check.

glands. Studies show that the sebum of patients with acne has higher levels of the inflammation-inducing ROS, as well as lower amounts of antioxidants. The levels of these oxidative markers were shown to correlate not just with the onset of acne but also with its severity.

The Cigarette Conundrum

Smoking is an aggravator of oxidative cellular damage to the body's cells. It is also a risk factor for a multitude of diseases. That being said, there are mixed results from studies that explore the connection between smoking and acne. Some studies indicate that smoking consistently increases the risk of acne, while others show a protective effect against acne, related to nicotine. There is definitely a connection between smoking and acne, but the mechanism that explains the opposing outcomes is still unclear.

It is possible that the nicotine in cigarettes may have a protective role in the development of acne. A similar protective effect of nicotine has been shown in two other inflammatory conditions: ulcerative colitis and Parkinson's disease.

The contrasting health-aggravating effects are likely the result of countless toxic chemical compounds (such as nitrosamines and polycyclic aromatic hydrocarbons) inhaled in tobacco smoke.

In any case, our goal is to reduce oxidative stress on the body, and smoking cigarettes regularly is a guaranteed way to increase that stress. The possible benefit to your skin from nicotine is debatable and is far outweighed by the long-term ill effects of smoking. Clearly, smoking should not be recommended as a treatment for acne, despite the mixed evidence.

The possible benefit to your skin from nicotine is debatable and is far outweighed by the long-term ill effects of smoking. Clearly, smoking should not be recommended as a treatment for acne, despite the mixed evidence.

Psychological Stress

Psychological stress is also an important trigger with acne. Many people notice that their skin breaks out during periods of mental and emotional stress; this is not simply coincidence. There is an associated link and there are physiological reasons to explain it.

Stress causes physiological changes, putting the body into a protective state at the expense of its normal functioning. This can impact inflammatory conditions, such as acne, in a few different ways:

- Stress may lead to abnormal functioning of the gut's filtering system.
- Stress influences hormone release, which increases blood sugar.
- Stress leads to increased sebum production.

Stress can negatively impact the permeability of the digestive tract, creating an abnormal state known as leaky gut syndrome. When this occurs, the digestive tract becomes more porous to particles that should normally be filtered out, such as bacteria, viruses, yeast, food molecules and toxic substances. When this abnormal functioning happens, any inflammatory process is prone to become

Normal Gut versus Hyperpermeable Gut

A. Normal, Healthy Gut Filter: Foreign particles are kept from being absorbed

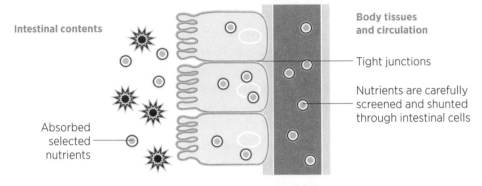

B. Hyperpermeable Gut Filter: Foreign particles pass through hyperpermeable, inflamed gut

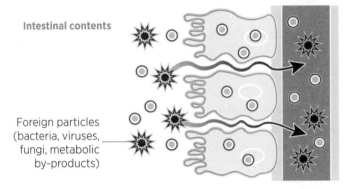

aggravated. In the case of acne, compromised intestinal permeability may be an important compounding factor. (For more information about this condition, refer to my book *The Complete Leaky Gut Health & Diet Guide*.)

Stress can influence hormone levels in the body. Under acute stress, your adrenal glands kick in and produce cortisol. Cortisol is the hormone responsible for our well-known stress reaction called the fight-or-flight response. This is the classic state we find ourselves in when we are suddenly startled: we either yell, curse and flail our limbs (fight) or we freeze or run away (flight).

Because the muscles are activated when fighting or fleeing, cortisol works by triggering an increase of sugar in the bloodstream. The sugar provides the muscles with energy for contracting, either to combat or to escape the stressful stimulus. However, neither response is typically carried out in our modern world.

Let's say you are facing a stressful situation — an exam or an important deadline to meet at school or work. In a professional environment, we do not have the option of beating up our boss or running out of the exam room. Therefore, the sugar in the bloodstream is not properly metabolized and the body has to then release insulin to reabsorb and store the sugar. Essentially, the stress response spikes blood sugar much like eating sugary foods, and thereby worsens acne.

Additionally, stress has also been shown to increase sebum production in the sebaceous glands, where pimples originate. The mechanism is not fully understood, but stress receptors have been identified in the sebaceous glands. With elevated sebum secretion, there is a higher likelihood that the sebaceous gland will become clogged and turn into an acne lesion.

Doc Talk

I always have a discussion with my patients about being very aware of their stress and the subconscious responses that may aggravate their acne. During stressful situations, you may resort to anxious habits to distract yourself from stress. If you are prone to chronic skin picking with acne, you will likely do this more often in stressful times. Skin picking intensifies acne lesions, leads to scarring and can perpetuate the cycle of acne by introducing more bacteria to the skin.

When you are stressed, you may also have less rational control over which foods you choose to eat. Typically, we gravitate toward carb-laden starchy foods, sweets or greasy, rich comfort foods. This emotional eating response can lead to short-term elevations in feel-good hormones, such as endorphins, serotonin and dopamine. Although they make us feel good momentarily, they will also trigger cycles in our body that are likely to lead to both increased acne formation and inflammation.

CHAPTER 3

Does Diet Play a Role?

CASE STUDY

Adult Acne

Cain, age 45, suffered from adult-onset acne, which had developed 20 years earlier and was not improving. He was self-conscious about his facial acne and rosacea (chronic redness of the skin). He came to his first visit with specific ideas of how his treatment plan should be developed. He described his diet as "very healthy" and seemed resistant to making any dietary adjustments. He suggested that I recommend supplements to help his skin.

I discussed the connections between the intake of dairy and sugar and the hormones that impact acne. He assured me that he didn't consume significant amounts of dairy or sugar.

Cain completed a detailed diet and symptom journal, which we reviewed together. I used a highlighter to emphasize meals, snacks and beverages that would contribute to his dairy and sugar load. The point was not to make Cain paranoid about foods but rather to convince him that his self-assessment was not as accurate as he believed. Dairy did, in fact, creep into his diet fairly regularly in the form of cream consumed in each of his three coffees, whey protein in his morning smoothies, and Greek low-fat fruit yogurt every afternoon. Sugar was hidden in his Greek low-fat fruit yogurt, in the orange juice he added to his smoothie, and in the seven-grain bread he used to make his lunch sandwich every day.

Cain started to see my point. I recommended a few basic support supplements but explained that the best results would come from adjusting his diet.

He committed to going full steam ahead with eliminating all dairy and sugar sources. He was extremely compliant with his new dietary program, and his acne and rosacea dramatically improved over the course of just 3 months. He also noted that he had improved focus at work and increased energy during workouts.

Cain was able to make some minor adjustments to keep his ongoing diet low in sugar and dairy for the long term. I typically suggest that patients eventually expand their diets and reintroduce foods, but Cain was happy to follow his healthier meal regimen indefinitely, as he thrived on structure and routine.

Diet plays a critical role in the health of your skin. It determines if nutrients are supplied at optimal levels. Making unhealthy food choices may lead to an inadequate supply of not only essential nutrients but also other beneficial compounds that support the health of your skin.

Sugar consumption is a prime contributor to acne. Our food supply is supersaturated with sugars in various forms. Sugar is incorporated into almost every packaged food product, and we add it as an ingredient to our cooking and as a flavor enhancer in our tea and coffee.

Even "healthier" forms of sugar deceive the consumer. We often believe we are getting something healthy when, in fact, we are still eating sugar disguised as a healthier, more wholesome alternative. In later chapters, we will explore in more detail the impact of sugar on our skin and how it can aggravate acne.

Over the past decade, convincing evidence in research literature has stated again and again that diet, particularly carbohydrates and high-glycemic foods, influences the prevalence and severity of acne. It is impossible to ignore the connection between acne and the consumption of sugar and carbohydrates (which turn to sugar).

Additionally, food sensitivities are becoming almost rampant in our society as a result of chronic overexposure to unnatural derivatives found in common foods. For example, dairy, gluten, eggs, soy and corn are common foods that can create a hypersensitive response via the immune system.

Did You Know?

Processed Foods
Typical diets are rife with processed ingredients, altered foods, artificial flavors, preservatives, texturizers, colors and sweeteners. When eaten regularly, these ingredients can contribute to inflammation and aggravate conditions such as acne.

Research Spotlight: Online Perception

A study in 2011 looked at the dissemination of information on YouTube about nutrition and its link to acne. Out of 87 videos examined, 85% of them indicated, at the least, a moderate correlation between acne and diet. Every year since, the number of instructional and testimonial videos about acne has increased exponentially.

I performed a quick search on YouTube in early 2015 for the term "acne treatment," resulting in 68,900 video recommendations. On Google alone, using the same keyword search resulted in 1.57 million hits for websites providing information about treating acne.

Although the Internet is rife with information that is not backed by rigorous science, it gives us a good measure of our collective experiences and successes with acne, and provides some degree of self-validation.

In my practice, the most common food sensitivity that I see correlated to patients with acne is to dairy and dairy products. Dairy and other food-sensitivity reactions can lead to or accentuate skin disorders, including psoriasis, eczema and acne. It is important to identify trigger foods by carefully reintroducing them after a period of elimination. Refer to the maintenance phase of the Vibrant Skin Diet plan (page 191) for more details.

Did You Know?

Dairy Dilemma

Dairy products have been shown to aggravate many inflammatory conditions, and their connection to the growing incidence and severity of acne is becoming stronger. Milk and dairy products have been shown to influence some of the hormonal factors that perpetuate the cycle and development of acne.

The Sugar Connection

Historically, our ancestors from more than 2,000 years ago would be able to consume pure sugar only if they encountered sugarcane plants and chewed on their hard stalks to extract the sweet liquid content, sugarcane juice.

It wasn't until the first few centuries CE that the process of crystallizing sugar was first developed. The cultivation and manufacturing of sugarcane crystals slowly improved during medieval times, but sugar did not become widely available until the 17th and 18th centuries.

Within the past 200 years, beet sugar and high-fructose corn syrup have been produced, and in the past 50 years, they have become exponentially ubiquitous. They have rapidly become commonplace in packaged food products as an ingredient. Sugar and all of its iterations persist in our food supply for a simple reason: they sell.

Refined man-made sugars are the same sugars found in whole foods, but they are super-concentrated, thereby increasing their effective dose. Think of sugar as rocks on a beach. Naturally occurring sugars found in whole foods would be analogous to a sandy beach with a few rocks scattered here and there. Walking across this type of beach would be comfortable, and stepping on a rock would not be

FAQ

Q Do we have an evolutionary need for sugar?

A On an evolutionary scale, very little time has passed since the introduction of refined sugar. Our bodies have not adapted to efficiently metabolize the continuous onslaught of sugar we consume.

    As a result, the compensatory mechanisms that assist us in processing sugar (for example, insulin shunting sugar out of our blood) eventually become overwhelmed, and our bodies experience unhealthy effects (diabetes, heart disease, obesity, hormone disorders and acne).

    We need sugar to survive, but our metabolism is designed to use *slow-release* sugars on an ongoing basis. Slow-release sugars are naturally available in whole food sources, providing us with the carbohydrates that allow our bodies to maintain a healthy equilibrium.

an issue thanks to the buffering effect of the surrounding soft sand. On the other hand, the effect of concentrated refined sugars on our physiology would be akin to the pain of walking across a rocky beach devoid of the balancing effect of sand.

Our bodies have an uncanny ability to adapt. Through adaptation we are able to survive, but this comes at a price. When we constantly create acute sugar influxes in our blood, non-life-threatening symptoms begin to appear that indicate something is not functioning properly. If the issue isn't addressed, symptoms can get worse to the point where they can affect our quality of life and eventually the outcome of our life itself.

For many people, acne may be a very early indicator that our body is not comfortable with the fuel it is being fed. Eating a healthy diet that is conducive to reducing sugar and insulin spikes will improve the skin in those who have a strong dietary component to their acne. By doing so, they are also reducing the risk of many additional chronic diseases that are linked to excess sugar and the body's corresponding insulin response.

Rapid developments in manufacturing systems have enabled us to produce mass supplies of refined sugars. Bleached isolates derived from sugarcane extracts became the white sugar we know today. High-fructose corn syrup is another inexpensive, highly processed and mass-produced sweetener.

Did You Know?

Refining Sugar

We concentrate sugars from plant sources by removing the natural components that slow our body's ability to access the sugars. We remove the outer coating (skins and husks) and the internal matrix in which the sugars are embedded (fibers, juices, bran, proteins and oil).

Q Why are we exposed to so much sugar?

A The problem is our taste buds. As a society, we love the taste of sweet foods — we are accustomed to sugar and we now expect our food to include a certain level of sweetness. As a result, packaged food products are developed with a certain degree of sweetness to appeal to the majority of the population. Although health-food products use less refined ingredients, they commonly also contain sugar. Because they represent a larger portion of the food market, they need to appeal to average taste buds. Often products will describe a sweetener as "natural," but don't be fooled: it is still a derivative of sugar.

Never in our existence have our bodies' metabolic processes had to deal with a constant and regular consumption of these concentrated sugar forms. These were not added to food products for health reasons; they were simply processed to make things taste better. Of course, if they tasted better, corporations could sell more products.

The seemingly improved taste experience has a threefold result:

1. Acutely, our sweet taste buds find this to be pleasurable. Historically, however, sweetness was never experienced at these concentrations, and it overwhelms our pleasure response centers to make us want more.
2. Insidiously, the effect on our brain physiology is akin to experiencing a sugar rush, a "high" that leads to endorphin release in our brain. This feel-good sensation becomes a psychologically addictive cycle.
3. After a blood-sugar spike, we experience a "crash" as our insulin levels overcompensate in an effort to bring our blood sugar below normal levels. Having low blood sugar (hypoglycemia) makes us feel tired and irritable, and we crave more sugar. The body develops a physical addiction whereby it periodically needs a quick blast of sugar in order to feel normal and function properly. A good example of this is the common mid-afternoon crash people experience at work, at which point they seek out sugary snacks to elevate their blood sugar.

It becomes apparent why sugar is added to almost every food product on the market. It has almost become a necessity

Did You Know?

Glycemic Index Measure

The glycemic index seems to be a reliable measure to weigh the effect of carbohydrate-rich foods on the severity of acne. Therefore, following a diet that includes foods with a low glycemic index is essential to treating acne successfully.

The Addictive Cycle of Sugar Consumption

"High"
"Feel-good" endorphins are released

"Pleasure"
Sweets stimulate our taste buds

"Crash"
Insulin secretion leads to low blood sugar

"Quick fix"
Sugar craving quickly improves our mood and energy

for a business to survive in the world of commercially prepared food products. However, the amount of sugar we consume, and the frequency at which we consume it, acts like an insidious poison in our body. It won't kill us right away, but it disrupts the functioning of different systems in the body. This affects our normal metabolic regulation and increases our risk of diabetes, heart disease, stroke, cancer and acne.

Considering the amount of evidence that supports the sugar–acne connection, it is surprising that many dermatologists do not provide dietary guidance to their acne patients before recommending pharmaceuticals.

Research Spotlight: Diet Triggers

A New York observational study in 2014 looked at the dietary intake of various foods of 248 subjects aged 18 to 25 years old. It compared the subjects' perceived severity of acne against their self-reported intake of certain foods. The results showed that those subjects with moderate to severe acne consumed more of the following foods (compared to those with mild acne or clear skin): foods with a higher glycemic index, added sugar, total sugar, milk, saturated fat and trans fat. The group with an increased severity of acne also consumed less fish compared to the other group. The results show that certain foods — specifically sugar, dairy and fish — may play a role in acne.

Top of Form

A 2014 review paper analyzed the results of several studies between 2009 and 2013 that investigated a link between diet and acne. The results point to a strong link between the consumption of carbohydrates and acne formation.

Puberty and the Skin

During puberty, the cells of the epidermis turn over faster than at other life stages. The combination of excess dead skin cells and excess oil can block the pores and hair follicles that are responsible for eliminating them. The blocked pores, in turn, become inflamed and harbor a bacteria called *Propionibacterium acnes*, which thrives in this mix of skin cells and oil under the surface of the skin, producing the pus you see when whitehead pimples are formed.

Nevertheless, the message is slowly being disseminated online and through word of mouth. It is crucial to understand the link and potential impact of refined carbohydrates in the diet and how they can impact the onset, severity and duration of acne.

Dietary sugar control is the first and most important step to successfully treating acne.

Sugar and Hormones

Sugar spikes directly affect the quality and regeneration of your skin tissue and also disrupt normal hormone metabolism, which consequently also affects the health of your skin. Elevated sugar levels trigger the release of two hormones: insulin and insulin-like growth factor (IGF). Both of these hormones can trigger the following responses, which contribute to the formation of acne:

- Increase inflammation
- Increase production of skin cells
- Promote sebum production (the oily substance produced in our skin's sebaceous glands)
- Increase production of testosterone and estrogen (from testes and ovaries)
- Increase the sensitivity of the skin to androgens (such as testosterone)
- Increase conversion of testosterone to the more acne-promoting androgen DHT

Research Spotlight: Carbohydrate Consumption

A study recruited 43 male acne patients between the ages of 15 and 25 years, who were monitored over 12 weeks. The control group ate carbohydrate-dense foods while the treatment group consumed a diet that emphasized proteins and low-glycemic carbs. The dermatological assessments were completed by investigators who were not told which patients belonged to which group.

Subjects in the treatment group experienced a decrease in weight, lower body mass index and improved insulin sensitivity over the course of the study. Those in the treatment group also showed an improvement in the severity of their acne: lesions decreased by approximately half compared to the control group.

The results demonstrate that carbohydrates may be a cause of acne, and that reducing carbohydrates and choosing lower-glycemic forms of carbohydrates may help in treating acne. This study also illustrates the likely link between increased insulin sensitization and improvement in acne.

There are many sebaceous glands in the skin and they respond to hormone signals in the body. Typical teen acne is a result of these glands responding to the new surge of hormones released by reproductive glands during puberty. This triggers the sebaceous glands on the face, back, neck and chest to release an oily substance called sebum at a higher than normal rate.

There are hormone-signaling pathways in the body that are known to be instigators of acne. These hormone signals communicate messages of action to the body via sensors in our cells. The typical Western diet can overstimulate one of our body's important cellular sensors, called mammalian target of rapamycin complex 1 (mTORC1).

An important protein complex, mTORC1 helps our cells determine when to make more building blocks or when to start limiting and rationing material based on the availability of nutrients in its environment. Because it determines whether your body exists in a healthy or a diseased state, it is critical that mTORC1 functions effectively.

When its activity is reduced, it can lead to wasting states, such as in age-related muscle loss, cancer, heart disease and chronic lung disease. When its activity is elevated, it can contribute to chronic inflammatory diseases, autoimmune conditions, metabolic disorders and neurodegenerative disease.

Increased mTORC1 activity increases androgen secretion, which leads to excess secretion from the sebaceous glands. As we know by now, this promotes acne.

By eating a healthier diet that is high in fruits and vegetables, with healthy sources of proteins, fats and carbohydrates, we can normalize mTORC1 activity and decrease the development of acne. The Vibrant Skin Diet Plan follows the same parameters. See page 160 for more information.

The concept that certain carbohydrates aggravate hormonal triggers for acne was further validated in a small 2008 Australian study that investigated hormone level changes based on glycemic load consumed. Eating a diet that has a high glycemic load led to increases in IGF-1 and androgens in subjects with acne as compared to the group eating a diet with a low glycemic load.

Did You Know?

The Western Diet

The Western diet typically involves the following:

- High caloric intake
- High glycemic load
- High consumption of dairy
- High intake of trans fats and mass-produced meat

Consuming too many of the foods that fall into these categories will overstimulate mTORC1, which can promote acne.

Research Spotlight: The Role of Insulin-Like Growth Factor 1

A 2011 study investigated the relationship between insulin-like growth factor 1 (IGF 1) and acne. It looked at the occurrence of acne in subjects with Laron syndrome, a congenital disorder in which IGF-1 is not produced in the body. It demonstrated that a deficiency of IGF-1 will prevent acne. When IGF-1 was administered to subjects at an initial high dose, presumably bringing their body's concentration of IGF-1 to a higher than normal level, they experienced symptoms of excess androgens (such as depleted menstruation) in addition to acne occurrence. Once these subjects received a lower dose of IGF-1, their acne consequently cleared.

Advanced Glycation End Products

Sugar acts on the skin in the same way sugar reacts in crème brûlée. Sugar can bind to proteins in the body and skin, changing their natural state and essentially crystallizing them. This produces compounds called advanced glycation end products (AGEs).

Your skin is designed to be a strong yet supple support material that contains and protects your tissues. It also functions as a permeable barrier that prevents unwanted material or microorganisms from entering the bloodstream. It is porous enough to allow the secretion of sweat (via sweat, or sudoriferous, glands) and sebum (via sebaceous glands), as well as to allow the absorption of substances through the skin and into circulation.

Our skin is flexible enough to allow it to move with our body and strong enough to act as a protective barrier against the normal forces of friction and pressure.

> Advanced glycation end products (AGEs) negatively affect our skin's appearance — by tightening, aging or weakening it. They essentially cause the collagen in our skin to brown like chicken skin baking in the oven.

When the skin is youthful and soft, it appears vibrant, smooth and glowing. Advanced glycation end products (AGEs) negatively affect our skin's appearance — by tightening, aging or weakening it. They essentially cause the collagen in our skin to brown like chicken skin baking in the oven. AGEs accumulate in skin through the aging process and are produced more quickly in situations of sugar dysregulation, such as diabetes.

This compromises the skin's natural ability to absorb and eliminate. Its capacity to hold moisture is inhibited, making skin dehydrated. Skin glycation plays a role in the aging response of the skin; that is, aged skin becomes less pliable and more dehydrated, and develops wrinkles. In the shorter term, glycation may also contribute to the development of acne.

This is just another chronic effect of the unhealthy intake of dietary sugars and carbohydrates. Glycemic control in the diets of diabetic subjects has been shown to decrease the glycation of collagen in the skin.

The Dairy Dilemma

Milk and Bone Health

There is much debate about the true value of consuming milk products and their purported role in improving the health and strength of our bones. The information is difficult to sort through because the dairy industry's powerful marketing campaigns promote milk's possible benefits. There is no doubt that concentrated levels of protein, calcium and phosphorus, along with other minerals and vitamins, are found in milk.

Here are some of the questions that remain unanswered:

- Does our body properly assimilate and use these nutrients in a way that necessitates its consumption for our bone health?
- Do the nutritional benefits of consuming milk regularly outweigh the potential adverse effects?
- Does obtaining the milk we drink from mass-produced grain-fed cows sacrifice its quality?
- Is cow's milk required as part of a healthy diet?
- Does pasteurization affect the health benefits of milk?

We do not have answers to all of these questions yet. However, there have been some recent studies (see Research Spotlight, page 48) that may shed some light on how bone health is influenced by milk intake.

We need to reexamine our dependence on milk for our bone health, particularly with the evidence compiled over the years. Many of us feel guilt if we don't consume enough dairy, because our outdated diet recommendations and culture continue to emphasize that its consumption is almost mandatory.

We have yet to fully understand why milk may not provide the presumed benefits to our bone health. It could be the result of modern mass overproduction sacrificing the quality of our supply and the type of feed we give to dairy cows. Or perhaps other forms of dairy (yogurt, kefir, cheeses) may provide more health benefits than milk.

Many of us feel guilt if we don't consume enough dairy, because our outdated diet recommendations and culture continue to emphasize that its consumption is almost mandatory.

Research Spotlight
Dairy Debate

In 2014, a Swedish study looked at the milk consumption patterns of 61,000 women and 45,000 men over a 20-year period. It showed that high milk intake (three or more 8-ounce/250 mL glasses of milk a day) substantially increased risk of mortality in both men and women, and increased risk of hip fractures in women. In subsets of these groups, it was also shown that blood levels of both inflammatory and oxidative stress markers were elevated in response to increased milk consumption. Furthermore, for each glass of milk consumed per day, mortality levels increased and there were no reductions seen in hip-fracture rates, contrary to public perception.

Another study, of 96,000 participants, investigated milk consumption in the teenage years and looked at how it affected the risk of fractures for the subjects in later years. It showed that increasing milk consumption (from less than two glasses per week to one, two, three or more glasses per day) in the subjects' teenage years did not reduce their hip-fracture risk as older adults. In fact, for men, each glass of milk consumed per day increased the risk of hip fracture by 9%.

Interestingly, the first study also found a strong link between intake of fruits and vegetables and decreased risk of hip fractures.

From the perspective of acne and inflammatory diseases, it seems that milk may be a detriment.

Dairy, Hormones and Acne

Cow's milk and other dairy products have been shown to promote the incidence of acne. Human breast milk is consumed in infancy as a natural food that promotes a period of rapid growth in the body. It increases insulin and IGF-1 in the bloodstream. But we know that both of these hormones trigger responses in the sebaceous glands that lead to the development of acne. Thus, consuming cow milk or other dairy products in adolescence or adulthood contributes to the cycle that triggers acne.

It has also been shown that milk raises our levels of dihydrotestosterone (DHT), a hormone that instigates acne formation. Eliminating or reducing dairy products, along with other foods that cause sensitivities, is an important step in resolving acne in the long term.

Consuming milk increases insulin and IGF-1 levels in our blood. This response mimics that of foods with a high glycemic index. These two hormones, along with androgens, are shown to be elevated in patients with acne, and levels

Did You Know?

The Milk Effect

Sugars and high-glycemic foods trigger hormonal responses in the body that set the stage for the development of acne. Milk has been shown to have a similar impact on the hormones.

correspond with the number of acne lesions and the amount of sebum secretion from the sebaceous glands.

Researchers theorize that persistent acne in adulthood accompanied by elevated levels of IGF-1 may even be an indicator for an elevated risk for cancer. These effects may be mitigated through dietary modifications that include limiting exposure to milk proteins and high-glycemic foods. Although milk has a relatively low glycemic index, it triggers similar hormonal responses in the body that can perpetuate the development of acne.

Insulin Resistance

Acne is a primary concern, understandably, for anyone reading this book. In any case, the ultimate goal is to improve your acne. Although acne is not a life-threatening condition, it does tremendously affect your quality of life and self-esteem. That being said, acne that results from dietary hormonal triggers may also be viewed as a type of risk indicator for insulin resistance and its associated conditions. Insulin resistance is related to increased body mass index (a measure that correlates body weight to height) and many modern-day chronic diseases, such as diabetes and heart disease.

The good news is that improving your acne through dietary and lifestyle intervention also subsequently benefits your future outcomes and risk of chronic illness.

Additional Perspectives on Diet

You will see that this book's recommended diet plan for treating acne is not just a straight elimination of dairy and sugar. Glycemic control and the elimination of dairy proteins is a priority, but this is an oversimplified approach to treating acne.

When the goal is to reduce inflammatory states in the body — acne, in this case – we need to ensure that whole, healthy, properly sourced ingredients and healthily prepared meals are incorporated into daily living. We also need to focus on eating adequate amounts of fruits and vegetables.

Food Sensitivities

Food sensitivities can include any of the following reactions:

- **Classic food allergies:** This is the well-known classic allergy presentation and it occurs immediately. Reactions include hives, swelling, itching, flushing, shortness of breath, wheezing, vomiting, diarrhea and/or severe anaphylaxis. This reaction is usually referred to as food allergy. This type of quick-acting hypersensitivity response is mediated by a class of antibodies in the immune system called immunoglobulin E (IgE).

- **Atypical food allergies:** This is the lesser-known allergy presentation and it does not occur immediately. Symptoms are more chronic, with a slower onset, and they can include conditions such as inflammatory skin reactions, mood changes, menstrual irregularities, digestive disorders, joint or muscle pain, and autoimmune conditions. This type of delayed food reaction is often referred to as a food sensitivity, despite the fact that it is actually a type of allergy. This type of delayed hypersensitivity response is mediated by a class of antibodies in the immune system called immunoglobulin G (IgG).

- **Food intolerances:** This is a general term that refers to various other forms of food reactions that do not involve the immune system. The most well-known example is lactose intolerance, which occurs when your body is deficient in lactase, the enzyme that digests the lactose sugar in milk and dairy products. When your body is not adequately producing a protein (in this case, lactase), it is termed a metabolic disorder. Symptoms of lactose intolerance become evident quickly (within 1 hour) and are typically gastrointestinal, such as bloating, gurgling, abdominal pain and diarrhea. Some people experience food intolerances to additives in food, such as MSG (monosodium glutamate), sulfites (in dried fruit and wine) and food coloring. These food intolerance reactions can vary in their presentation, from fatigue and insomnia to mood disorders and digestive complaints.

- **Pharmacologically active compounds:** These include ingredients that cause a physiological response. The most common example is caffeine, which stimulates the nervous system, leading to anxiety and feeling physically jittery. This is the normal action of caffeine in our bodies and, therefore, is not an individually variable food sensitivity.

Q **Why are atypical food allergies important considerations in reducing acne?**

A There is a growing awareness of delayed-onset food allergies and their effects on chronic health concerns. As a result, researchers are conducting more studies to delineate the relationship between IgG food allergies and their response in the body. It seems clear that IgG food reactions contribute to inflammation in the body and can aggravate chronic digestive symptoms and chronic skin conditions, such as eczema; they can also cause a number of additional symptoms.

Although acne and its connection to IgG food sensitivities has yet to be studied directly, there are a growing number of inflammatory conditions that are now attributed to leaky gut syndrome, which is then aggravated by the continued consumption of foods that trigger an IgG allergic response. In an inflammatory skin condition such as acne, I recommend eliminating foods that could potentially keep the cycle of inflammation going.

To minimize any potential sources of inflammation, the Vibrant Skin Diet Plan eliminates the most common food aggravators in the IgG food allergy category: dairy, eggs and gluten.

That being said, there may be individual differences in the degree of responsiveness to the same dose of caffeine, even though the pharmacological action of caffeine will still be the same.

Dietary Correlations

A Korean study in 2010 investigated specific foods in the diet of 783 subjects with acne and 502 subjects free of acne. Those in the group with clear skin ate more fish, leafy greens, yellow vegetables and cruciferous vegetables. The group with acne consumed higher amounts of junk food, instant noodles, soda, snacks, fried chicken, roast pork, nuts, processed cheese and seaweed. In addition to the types of food consumed, researchers also evaluated the timing of meals. The group with acne also skipped breakfast more often and did not eat meals as regularly as the control group.

With respect to the consumption of seaweed and nuts, which are both plentiful in nutrients and low on the glycemic scale, there are likely other reasons why they may have contributed to acne in the 2010 Korean study.

Seaweed is a popular ingredient in snack foods in Korea.

> There may be individual differences in the degree of responsiveness to the same dose of caffeine, even though the pharmacological action of caffeine will still be the same.

Research Spotlight
Food Triggers by Disease

A 2013 Chinese study showed that children with diseases of various origins experienced IgG allergy reactions to a higher number of foods if their condition involved more systems in the body.

Because disease can manifest with inflammation in the body, it seems to follow that there may be more food triggers that develop because of disease in the body. On the flip side, food allergies left untreated — in other words, continuing to consume these foods — may also contribute to the promotion of disease by perpetuating inflammation in the body. Many of these connections are being attributed to leaky gut syndrome. Leaky gut syndrome is a condition in which your digestive filter is compromised. This leads to foreign particles penetrating through the normally selective gut wall into circulation, which leads to the development or exacerbation of inflammatory conditions in the body. (For comprehensive information about leaky gut syndrome and its treatment, please refer to my book *The Complete Leaky Gut Health & Diet Guide*.)

The research supporting the hypothesis that iodine intake instigates acne is limited and old (mostly from the 1960s and before).

Processed snack items with seaweed may also contain sugar, MSG, refined vegetable oils and/or hydrogenated oils. This is consistent with the fact that the group consuming more seaweed also reported a higher intake of junk and snack foods. This would be a more likely scenario than the explanation the study authors proposed: that there is a link between the iodine in seaweed and acne. The research supporting the hypothesis that iodine intake instigates acne is limited and old (mostly from the 1960s and before). In addition, the dosages that were observed to cause acne-like eruptions were considerably higher than what would be ingested in a typical Korean diet. For example, 500 mg of potassium iodide pills (containing about 375 mg of iodine) were shown to trigger pustular eruptions in two patients, which improved upon cessation of the supplement. By comparison, a large sheet of dried seaweed (about 2.5 g) would contain about 37 mg of iodine — about one-tenth of the dose used in this study and others.

As for nuts, peanuts are a common "nut" ingredient in Korean snacks, even though peanuts are not actually nuts at all. Peanuts and peanut oils are high in omega-6 fatty acid oils, which aggravate inflammation and may contribute to inflammatory skin conditions such as acne. An even more likely confounding variable is the fact that most peanut and nut snacks typically contain sugar and other sweeteners, thereby increasing their glycemic index and making them more likely to promote acne.

A 2006 study in Jordan examined the perceptions of 166 subjects with acne to see what types of foods in their diet they believed correlated with acne breakouts. The foods they reported to most likely make their acne worse were (listed in descending order): nuts, chocolate, cakes and biscuits, oily food, fried food, eggs and dairy products.

The nut issue, again, is likely related to how they are incorporated into the diet. Pistachios and walnuts are commonly used in Jordanian cuisine in their desserts (for example, baklava, knafeh, ma'moul and um ali), and these foods often also include sugars. The same subjects also noted that increased fruit and vegetable intake improved their acne. Incidentally, a large percentage of subjects (86.1%) reported a very strong correlation between worsening acne and emotional stress and worry. Note also that dairy, listed as an aggravating factor for acne, was listed further down the list. This is likely because in Jordanian cuisine, dairy is mainly consumed in fermented forms, such as yogurt, which are less prone to trigger sensitivities.

A 2014 Italian study analyzed the dietary factors that were linked to the onset and severity of 563 subjects' acne. It showed that milk, dairy products, sweets, chocolate and cakes were instigators of acne. It also connected a low consumption of fish and inadequate intake of fruits and vegetables to moderate to severe acne.

Most peanut and nut snacks typically contain sugar and other sweeteners, thereby increasing their glycemic index and making them more likely to promote acne.

Research Spotlight: Daily Dairy

A large study in 2006 examined the dietary habits of 6,094 adolescent girls evaluated over a 3-year period. Their food journals were analyzed to monitor milk consumption, and their incidence of acne was recorded at the end of the study period. There was a clear indication that the occurrence of acne was elevated in those who consumed regular amounts of dairy. Those who consumed 2 or more daily servings of milk — as compared to the group who consumed less than 1 serving a week — showed a 20% increased incidence of acne.

Interestingly, when the fat content of milks was assessed, it showed that higher-fat milk did not impact acne. In fact, low-fat skim milk showed a slightly elevated incidence of acne compared to higher-fat whole milk. This is consistent with the theory that it is the dairy proteins in milk products, not the fat, that are the likely aggravators of acne.

Doc Talk

My patients are often concerned about calcium intake and bone health with a diet low in dairy products. Based on my research, I reassure them that it is not necessary to consume dairy to support our bone health. That being said, calcium is still an important mineral needed to support bone density and can be plentiful in a diet that also heals acne.

Eating a balanced diet containing leafy greens, fruits, beans, seaweed, fish, shellfish, tofu, tempeh, nuts and seeds provides a balanced portfolio of calcium sources. Grass-fed meats are one of the best sources of vitamin K_2, which directs calcium to be shunted from our blood into our bones. Remember also that bone health is not just dependent on dietary calcium intake, but also on weight-bearing physical activity that stimulates your bones to "request" calcium from your blood.

PART 2

Managing Acne

CHAPTER 4

Conventional Treatments

Rebound Acne after Stopping Birth Control

Evi, now 29, developed facial acne during puberty. It was initially moderate and typical in appearance for a young teenager. However, when she turned 19, her acne started to dramatically worsen. Her pimples increased in frequency and became larger, more painful and deeper. Because they were slow to heal, her skin was constantly bombarded with overlapping layers of lesions: some were just developing, some were fully mature whiteheads, and others were either recovering pimples or discolored acne spots. It was too much for Evi to bear. Her dermatologist put her on a testosterone-suppressing birth control pill designed to treat acne, called Diane-35. Her skin cleared up dramatically over a 6-month period, and Evi was happy with the improvement.

At 25 years of age, Evi decided she wanted to come off birth control pills. Three months later, her acne began to reappear with a vengeance. She tried to be patient, but after another 3 months of severe acne, she reluctantly chose to restart Diane-35, which again settled her skin. She was frustrated that she was forced to go back to using a prescription.

Evi came to see me 2 years later, when she was in a serious long-term relationship and preferred not to be on artificial hormones — particularly because she wanted to start a family within a couple of years. She was terrified that her skin would "freak out" as it had the last time.

I put her on a 3-month protocol that included the Vibrant Skin Diet Plan and supplements that would support and improve the metabolism and elimination of hormones. We worked to regulate her digestion, and I suggested she consume regular amounts of spearmint tea to lessen the rebound effect of testosterone after ceasing use of Diane-35.

Three months after being off birth control, Evi's skin developed some mild acne, and I reassured her that this was normal as her hormones normalized. The main goal was to dampen the testosterone spike that occurred the first time. By 6 months, her skin had settled down without any major flare-ups. Evi was relieved that she had managed to get through the transition without the aggravation she had experienced a couple of years earlier. We weaned her off the supplements that were supporting her hormones, and she maintained a low-sugar diet. Her skin had consistently stayed clear when I followed up with her a year later, and she and her partner were preparing to start a family that summer.

Conventional acne treatments address what may be contributing to acne, but not necessarily what is causing it. Your family doctor or dermatologist may prescribe medications, but they typically don't offer diet or lifestyle recommendations. Keep in mind that there may be side effects associated with prescriptions, and these can range from mild to severe depending on the treatment plan. Prescriptions include:

- Antibiotics (oral and topical)
- Birth control pills
- Isotretinoin (Accutane)
- Testosterone blockers
- Topical retinoids

There may be side effects associated with prescriptions, and these can range from mild to severe depending on the treatment plan.

Antibiotics (Oral and Topical)

Oral broad-spectrum antibiotics are ubiquitously recommended as a treatment for acne. Common examples of these are tetracycline, doxycycline and minocycline.

These are commonly recommended at a daily dosing schedule of between 6 weeks and 3 months. I have seen patients who have been recommended this protocol on an "as needed" basis, depending on acne recurrence. I have also seen a handful of patients who have been on a daily antibiotic regimen for a year. Unbelievably, one patient was on daily antibiotics for 7 years straight. This sort of continuous antibiotic regimen is overkill for treating acne, particularly when it can lead to other problems.

Keep in mind: the antibiotics are targeting bacteria in a relatively small surface area of the skin, so they must be dosed at a high enough concentration to be dispersed throughout the bloodstream and still be at adequate levels to kill acne-related bacteria. This means that a concentrated dose is penetrating every other part of the body that hosts trillions of beneficial microorganisms. These probiotic colonies make up an ecosystem that supports the defense mechanisms within our immune system. This ecosystem of symbiotic bacteria is called your microbiome.

Oral antibiotic therapy used for the treatment of acne vulgaris was shown to cause significant alterations in the microbial colonies in 33% of patients over a 4- to 5-month period.

With long-term or repetitive use of antibiotics, the healthy balance of your microbiome will be destroyed. This has been linked to many conditions, including allergies, asthma, recurrent infections, digestive issues, yeast infections and mood disorders.

With topical antibiotics, the skin is being treated locally. There is a much lower dose applied, which then reduces the likeliness of side effects occurring in other systems in the body. This also means, however, that it may not be as effective at treating the bacteria in the affected skin because it is applied to the surface and may not penetrate the lesions in the same way that an oral antibiotic would.

It has been shown that applying topical clindamycin did not lead to any significant changes in stool microbiota (bacterial colonization) after twice-daily applications over an 8-week period. This means that its safety profile is much better than that of oral antibiotics in terms of maintaining your good bacteria internally; however, its efficacy would also be reduced.

Topical antibiotics are also commonly commercially available in creams or gels that are mixed with other compounds, such as retinoids, to target acne.

FAQ

Are antibiotics effective in the treatment of acne?

Effectiveness of antibiotics for acne can range from no improvements to occasional longer-term improvements. Most commonly, results are temporary and acne recurs once treatment ceases.

Essentially, the antibiotics can temporarily provide relief because they eliminate the bacteria that are trapped within the pimples in acne, which consequently reduces their growth and intensity. However, the treatment does not solve the underlying problem that is causing the trapped sebaceous gland to be formed in the first place. This means that once the antibiotics are completed, the cycle will start all over again.

Birth Control Pills

Acne linked to hormone fluctuations that are related to a woman's menstrual cycle may be treated using birth control pills.

Birth control pills are a common recommendation because of their widespread use for contraception. They may also help regulate a woman's menstrual cycle if it is irregular, or support mitigating premenstrual symptoms, dysmenorrhea (menstrual cramping) or menorrhagia (heavy or prolonged menstrual flow). Because of the additional benefits, many women aren't dissuaded by the fact that birth control pills must be taken on a daily basis.

When a woman is looking to start a family in the near future, birth control pills can't be used because of their effects on fertility. Some women also choose to avoid birth control pills that contain synthetic hormones because of their associated increased risks of clotting and/or certain types of cancers (breast, cervical and liver).

Despite having tried various brands of birth control pills with different doses and combinations of estrogen and progesterone, some women experience intolerable side effects. They include nausea, dizziness, breast tenderness, mood changes, headaches, depressed libido, severe weight gain and irregular bleeding. In these cases, alternative treatment routes should be explored.

Birth control pills that contain androgen-suppressing medications can be effective in treating acne, but the

FAQ

Q Which birth control pills are used to treat acne? How do they work?

A Some pills have a greater affinity for acne due to their testosterone-lowering effects. These often contain norgestimate, which is a synthetic form of progesterone (contained in Ortho Tri-Cyclen, Estrostep and Yaz). Norgestimate leads to a decreased circulating level of testosterone.

Alternatively, there is Diane-35, which contains cyproterone acetate, a compound that suppresses androgens (male hormones, such as testosterone) and their action in the body. Diane-35 functions as a contraceptive but has an inherent — although rare — risk of blood clotting, so it is prescribed primarily for moderate to severe acne. It is not prescribed for contraception as a primary goal, but rather for conditions related to increased androgens, such as acne, hirsutism and polycystic ovarian syndrome.

These "combination oral contraceptives" with androgen-suppressing medications are successful in settling or resolving symptoms of acne in 59% to 70% of cases, at least for the duration of the treatment.

Side Effects of Isotretinoin

The potency of isotretinoin doesn't come without long-term side effects. Among them, patients may experience dry, burning skin, dry eyes, dry lips and dry mucous membranes in the respiratory tract and even the genitalia. It can also cause joint pain because of the erosive effects of isotretinoin on surface cells, which can include the protective coverings of joint articulations.

✳ Caution

Isotretinoin can cause serious birth defects, which is why it can't be taken during pregnancy, and you may be asked to do a pregnancy test before using it. For this reason, it is also recommended that oral contraceptives and other forms of contraception be used concurrently with isotretinoin.

catch-22 is the recurrence of acne after treatment stops — many times mild to moderate, but sometimes with a vengeance. Physiologically, if a hormone's action is suppressed for a long period of time and then it is permitted to act, the response of the body can be heightened and the hormone may be overproduced. Unfortunately, physicians don't typically explain this potential for acne relapse to patients before prescribing an androgen-limiting birth control pill.

Isotretinoin

Isotretinoin is the big gun of acne. It is more commonly known by its brand names, including Accutane, Absorica, Amnesteem, Claravis, Myorisan, Sotret and Zenatane. It is an oral retinoid (a derivative of vitamin A) that accelerates the speed of skin turnover. It is essentially the oral version of topical retinoids (see page 62). The big difference, however, is its potential side effects. In the same vein as oral antibiotics, isotretinoin must be dispersed at a high enough concentration throughout all the tissues in your body to target a small surface area of the skin.

Isotretinoin is typically dosed in daily regimens over 4- to 6-month intervals. The length of the regimen is determined by your dermatologist and is based on variables such as your weight, the concentration level and the dosage throughout the course of treatment.

Isotretinoin may be quite effective in controlling acne because of its powerful ability to increase cell turnover. On the other hand, just like most symptomatic treatments, the acne may recur at some point after treatment ends. It is not uncommon for patients to endure multiple courses of isotretinoin. Many patients who commit to isotretinoin can experience long-term success; however, I also see patients whose acne cleared long ago with isotretinoin use but who are still dealing with chronic conditions such as dry eyes and dry mouth decades later.

Isotretinoin is usually reserved for more severe forms of acne, such as cystic scarring acne, because of its intense side effects. It is usually prescribed after all other prescription options have been tried individually or in combination, with limited long-term effectiveness.

Isotretinoin has been shown to alter microbial flora in 75% of patients treated over a 4- to 5-month period. This was most prevalent in the nasal cavities, and antibiotic-resistant strains of pathogenic bacteria were also discovered.

During the course of treatments, patients will be asked to have blood tests every month to monitor the risk of liver damage and any effect on red and white blood cells.

Testosterone Blockers

Spironolactone is a medication from the late 1950s that was designed to suppress the androgens (such as testosterone and DHT) that can contribute to acne. It is also used to treat hypertension and acts as a diuretic because of its action on sodium absorption by the kidneys.

It may be used on its own or paired with a birth control pill to treat acne. It is typically not prescribed to men because of its testosterone-depressing effects.

As with oral contraceptives that suppress androgens, patients who stop using spironolactone may experience a rebound acne flare-up.

Acne may also be treated by decreasing the body's conversion of testosterone to dihydrotestosterone (DHT), a more powerful androgen. Medications that have this function impede the enzyme that mediates this conversion. The enzyme is called 5-alpha-reductase, and the medications that slow the action of this enzyme are termed 5-alpha-reductase inhibitors. This category of medication is used to treat acne as well as other health issues associated with excess androgens, such as hair loss and prostate enlargement. A study in 2007 looked at 12 women with alopecia (hair loss) or acne who were treated with finasteride, a 5-alpha-reductase inhibitor. Nine out of the 12 women benefited from the treatment for acne and hair growth.

Doc Talk

Unless there is a necessary medical reason for administering testosterone blockers, these are not something I would recommend solely for the treatment of acne. This is because they block the normal hormone pathways. As a result, their use may lead to other hormone-related problems, and it is likely that they may trigger a return of symptoms after you stop using them.

Topical Retinoids

Retinoids are also derivatives of vitamin A but are applied directly onto the skin. They assist in accelerating the cell turnover of the epidermis. If applied on a regular basis, the topical retinoid gradually starts to dissolve the upper layers of the skin, eroding the blocked pores that make up pimples. For this reason, topical retinoids may also be used to treat fine lines and wrinkles.

Retinoids increase production of the underlying newer layers of skin. This keeps your skin looking fresher and younger and prevents pimples from forming, but it comes with the side effects of skin burning, dryness, flakiness, tightness and sometimes redness. These symptoms are a result of retinoids on the skin surface.

Recently, retinoids are more likely to be prescribed in formats that are combined with other topical prescription products. The idea is that the effectiveness of the medication will be heightened with a multipronged approach to treatment.

Retinoids are usually prescribed in either cream or gel form. Creams may be more difficult to use for acne because they are emollients, meaning they contain oils that moisturize the skin. This slows their absorptive capabilities and may aggravate clogged pores that are a component of acne. Gels, on the other hand, penetrate into the skin, increasing their effectiveness and relative potency. However, gels may lead to worsened side effects.

Creams may be recommended for very sensitive skin, but gels are better suited for less sensitive skin when enhanced effectiveness is desired. Be sure to avoid sun exposure and use sun protection while on a course of retinoids, as they make your skin photosensitive.

FAQ

Q **What is the difference between topical retinoids and chemical exfoliators?**

A Topical retinoids are commonly viewed (mistakenly) as exfoliators. Much like chemical exfoliators, topical retinoids expose a renewed, smoother skin and can cause side effects such as irritated, flaking, burning or dry skin. However, topical retinoids do not cause the stratum corneum to be shed; rather, it relays a message to slow the growth of the stratum corneum and enhance the creation of new cells in the underlying skin.

Retinoids are well known as the powerful vitamin A derivatives used to treat acne both orally (for example, Accutane) and topically. Retinol is available in over-the-counter creams, but its use is unregulated. The other retinoid derivatives are available as prescription topical creams and gels.

Although there are three generations of retinoids, only the first and third are used in acne treatment:

- **First generation:** retinol, tretinoin (Retin-A), isotretinoin
- **Third generation:** adapalene, tazarotene

First- and third-generation retinoids vary depending on when they were developed and how they work. Based on variations in chemical structure, each topical retinoid offers different effects. All retinoids renew the skin; however, the third-generation retinoids have been shown to have anti-inflammatory effects on the skin.

Their effectiveness is also based on their concentration in the formula. They are typically available in three varying degrees of potency. Best known is tretinoin (brand name Retin-A), which has been in use for more than 30 years. Quickly taking its place among recommendations by dermatologists is the newer-generation adapalene (brand name Differin). Adapalene is preferred because it inhibits the development of keratinocyte cells (cells that produce the hard protein keratin in the skin), so it helps dissolve the hard plugs that lead to pimples.

Taken orally, retinoids may cause a number of possible side effects and toxicities. Topical retinoids are quite effective at preventing the formation of acne (comedogenesis). They may be useful in certain situations where acne is improving gradually but the patient is anxious for the appearance of the skin to improve quickly. It is not a long-term permanent solution to healing acne, but it can settle acne for the short term while you are concurrently working on internal changes to prevent acne formation.

Retinoids are notorious for causing irritation and burning of the skin, which may be more notable in the first few weeks and settle down thereafter. For some people, these effects may be too irritating to continue a regular regimen of retinoids. Fortunately, there are options of choosing a lower concentration of retinoids or decreasing their frequency of use.

Exfoliators: Chemical and Mechanical

Exfoliators are products or methods used to improve the cell turnover on the uppermost layers of the skin. Their purpose is to shed the thicker top layer of skin and reveal the smoother (but more sensitive) underlying components of the epidermis. This is useful for acne because it reduces the likelihood of clogged pores, which can lead to pimples. People also use higher-intensity exfoliating techniques to treat acne scars, increased pigmentation, fine lines and wrinkles.

Chemical Exfoliators

Hydroxy Acids

Most chemical exfoliators are types of compounds called hydroxy acids. Hydroxy acids are used in lower concentrations in over-the-counter chemical exfoliators that degrade the outermost layers of the epidermis (called the stratum corneum).

Hydroxy acids essentially cause the cells of the stratum corneum to "unstick" from each other by degrading the cementing material between the cells, which are then readily removed. This thereby increases the removal of dead skin cells (called sloughing of the cells) and allows for newer, fresher skin to be exposed at the surface. The goal is to reduce acne by limiting the potential for blocked, stressed pores.

The side effects of hydroxy acids may be redness, irritation, increased sensitivity, dryness, peeling or flaking at the site of application.

Hydroxy acids may also be used at much higher concentrations in dermatology clinics that offer chemical peels. Hydroxy acids are applied to the skin for a short duration and have a fast, aggressive approach to exposing deeper layers of the epidermis. This treatment is often used to treat not just acne but also scarring and wrinkles, and to smooth the skin. Chemical peels basically wound the skin in a controlled setting in order for it to reset with new skin formation.

Did You Know?

Outer Layer

The stratum corneum is made up of cells that are rapidly produced and cemented together. The characteristics of this outer layer of skin provide its waterproofing property and an additional, thicker outer layer of protection from the external environment and infection.

Hydroxy acids used for exfoliation include the following:

- Carbolic acid
- Citric acid
- Glycolic acid
- Lactic acid
- Malic acid
- Salicylic acid
- Trichloroacetic acid

Benzoyl Peroxide

Benzoyl peroxide is also used as a chemical exfoliator. It is well known thanks to a popular, highly marketed, celebrity-endorsed commercial about an acne skin-care line. Benzoyl peroxide is chemically different from hydroxy acids but essentially achieves the same goal — that is, to disrupt the integrity of the stratum corneum so it can be more easily shed to prevent and actively treat pimples and blackheads.

Benzoyl peroxide is also bactericidal (meaning it kills bacteria) to the bacteria connected to acne formation, *Propionibacterium acnes*. This is a secondary effect but one that gives it a role in improving acne.

Benzoyl peroxide may also be combined with antibiotics (clindamycin or erythromycin) or retinoids (adapalene) in topical prescription preparations to enhance its effectiveness in combating acne.

Mechanical Exfoliators (Laser, Abrasion)

Mechanical exfoliation involves physically encouraging the removal of the outermost layer of skin, the stratum corneum, using methods such as light abrasion and friction. Helping to ease off this layer slows and may prevent blocking of sebaceous pores.

Common home-care mechanical abrasion devices and substances include:

- Brushes
- Commercial electronic devices that use rotating or pulsating brushes
- Fragments of almond or apricot kernel shells
- Loofah sponges
- Micro-particles in cleansers
- Pumice
- Sea salt
- Sugar
- Textured cloths

Microdermabrasion

Microdermabrasion is a painless in-office mechanical exfoliation method. A device abrades the surface of the skin using vacuum suction and a fine abrasion head that uses

Did You Know?

Cancer Connection
Benzoyl peroxide produces free radicals (which have the opposite effect of cell-protective antioxidants), and its long-term safety has been questioned, based on some evidence of tumor promotion in animal studies. Because of the lack of concrete evidence that completely vindicates benzoyl peroxide from plausibly increasing the risk of cancer, certain countries outside of North America have limited the concentrations. Japan, for example, has yet to approve the use of benzoyl peroxide as an anti-acne medication.

crystals. Microdermabrasion may leave the skin slightly sensitive after the procedure.

This method targets only the surface layer, the stratum corneum. Like other exfoliating methods, the goal of microdermabrasion is to expose the newer underlying layer of the epidermis, thereby smoothing the skin and resetting the structure of the epidermis.

This procedure may be expensive and, in some cases, can trigger new acne breakouts, since calm skin may be aggravated by the stimulation. For some patients, microdermabrasion can make a big difference in reducing acne scars.

Laser Resurfacing

Laser resurfacing involves a pulsed beam of light that removes the upper layer of the epidermis. It is used to treat fine lines and wrinkles, and with acne is mainly used to treat scars.

The side effects of laser resurfacing are most commonly hyper- or hypopigmentation (darkened or lightened patches of skin), but can also include irritated skin, scarring and breakouts. It is important to find a qualified and experienced dermatologist to do this procedure. You may want to request a test patch on an inconspicuous area and suggest that the technician start with a light treatment.

The downside to laser resurfacing is that it can involve many treatments, which can be very expensive, and results are quite varied based on types of scars, variables in treatment and individual responsiveness. Be sure to discuss these options with your dermatologist before pursuing.

Doc Talk

Are these exfoliation processes necessary to treat acne? I would suggest that, in some cases, such as with severe acne scarring, more drastic measures — like chemical peels or resurfacing — may very well be warranted. Of course, ultimately, it is a personal decision.

In terms of regimented, less aggressive forms of exfoliation, I would say that these are definitely not going to solve your acne, but they may be helpful in controlling it. Think of these as periodically waxing your car versus just hosing it down with soap and water. Your car will quickly lose its waxy sheen, but it does control the dirt and enhance your car's appearance for a short time.

If the underlying issue is not addressed, the hormones controlling skin turnover will continue to act in the same manner. Exfoliation is a temporary solution that may be useful to maintain your skin while you are making the internal changes needed to address the root of the problem.

Sun Protection

Sun protection is an important part of preventing and treating hypopigmentation and hyperpigmentation (respectively, lightening or darkening of the skin, which accentuates old acne scars). Skin that has been disrupted because of acne initiates the process of healing at the site of each lesion. Different layers of skin contain different concentrations of melanin (the pigment in our skin that gives it color and is responsible for darkening with exposure to UV rays) and, therefore, will have a varied response to UV light exposure. Essentially, as your skin heals from a pimple, the underlying newer layers of skin are exposed, and they may "tan" differently than the surrounding areas. This leads to hypopigmentation or hyperpigmentation. Hyperpigmentation may be treated with laser therapy.

Avoidance

First and foremost, the best method to protect your skin from UV damage is to avoid the sun. This means limiting your exposure on moderate- to high-UV days as best as possible.

Covering the skin on your chest, shoulders and back is an easier task, since shirts and tops take care of the bulk of UV protection. However, it's important to limit your exposure to the sun even when you're wearing a layer of clothing — many fabrics, particularly those with a looser weave, allow some degree of UV penetration. Think of clothing as a good starting point to protect your skin from developing scars, but do not depend on it exclusively. As an additional precaution, consider UV-blocking clothes, now available, which have been developed to protect from the sun's UV rays.

Sunscreens

Commercial sunscreens use chemical ingredients to filter the UV rays and protect our skin from their harmful effects. Various chemicals are used to block UVA and UVB rays from reaching our skin. Common chemical UV filters include avobenzone, homosalate, octinoxate, octisalate, octocrylene and oxybenzone.

We do not yet fully understand all of the long-term implications of these chemicals. They may act as hormone disruptors and produce free radicals (as a result of absorbing UV rays), which can accelerate cellular damage.

Did You Know?

Acne Scarring versus Pigmentation

Acne-associated hyper- or hypopigmentation is quite different from other types of acne scarring that structurally alter the skin (see Types of Acne Scars, page 19). Structural scarring includes depressions or elevations in the normally uniform, even surface of the skin that are instigated by deep, damaging acne. This differs from pigmentation changes, which by themselves do not affect the elevation of the skin's surface.

Those with sensitive skin need to be particularly cautious about chemical sunscreens, since many sunscreens, which also include non-active ingredients, can be irritating to the skin. Of course, because sunscreen is used to protect against the cancer-causing effects of sun exposure, it makes good sense to apply it.

Research Spotlight
Infertility Risk

A U.S. study in 2014 followed 501 couples who were discontinuing the use of contraceptives and attempting to get pregnant. Success rates for pregnancy were monitored over the course of 1 year and compared to urinary levels of benzophenones (a chemical related to oxybenzone), a common ingredient in sunscreens that functions as a UV filter. The results showed that benzophenones may potentially have a negative impact on fertility. Elevated urine levels of 2,2',4,4'-tetrahydroxybenzophenone and 4-hydroxybenzophenone in male subjects correlated to an extended time before conceiving with their partners.

FAQ

Q Are there alternatives to chemical sunscreens?

A The alternative to chemical sunscreens is so-called natural sunscreens. They contain the ingredients titanium dioxide and zinc oxide, which function as physical barriers to reflect UV rays away from the skin. They are much safer ingredients because they do not penetrate tissues (as do chemical filters) and have not been found to disrupt hormones. The catch is that they often leave a shiny white-purplish residue on the skin. Depending on the quality of the non-active ingredients in sunscreens that use physical barriers, they could potentially aggravate acne by blocking pores.

Try various sunscreens (always relying on testers and samples first) to ensure that you find a sunscreen that works for your needs. It should provide you with protection against UV rays (to prevent skin cancer as well as hyperpigmentation) and limit your risk of potential long-term internal effects and skin irritation.

CHAPTER 5

Natural Skin Care

CASE STUDY

A New Skin-Care Routine

Hailey was a 23-year-old patient I had helped over the course of a year to improve her acne. She was an exuberant patient who was under a lot of stress as a result of her burgeoning career at a marketing agency.

Although we had achieved great results with the Vibrant Skin Diet Plan, she returned to my office 6 months later because her skin felt flaky and dry, and occasional new pimples were starting to emerge.

She was managing well on a long-term balanced diet that kept her sugar intake limited, with a treat once in a while. I did not feel that her diet was a concern at this point.

We reviewed several aspects of her lifestyle and diet and came to the conclusion that she might need to incorporate some new topical treatments to rehydrate her skin.

She had been following her previous skin-care routine, which consisted of an oil-free, dermatologist-approved cosmetic line. It had never aggravated her skin, but it did not improve her skin either. I reviewed the ingredients of her skin-care products, and they were (not surprisingly) rife with chemical ingredients. Although they helped cleanse her skin free of dirt, air pollutants, makeup and bacteria, they were stripping her skin of moisture. Because dehydrated skin can contribute to the development of acne, it seemed appropriate to recommend a new skin-care routine that was natural, non-aggravating and able to prevent dehydration.

I suggested she replace her current cleanser with a very gentle natural cleanser of liquid castile soap and to use the deep-cleaning-with-oil method (see page 78) every day for a couple of weeks, and continuing for three times a week thereafter. I also recommended that she apply a heavier natural hydrating cream after cleaning, to compensate for the harsh dry and cool weather we were experiencing.

She emailed me a couple of months later to tell me that she had immediately noted improvements in her skin's dryness and irritation with her new skin-care routine. Her breakouts also subsided after following this new regimen for a month.

The Oil-Free Myth

Oil-free skin-care products have been recommended in the dermatology community for decades to control acne. Cosmetic brands that are oil-free continue to be recommended by most dermatologists. The rationale seems logical and straightforward: skin with acne is oily; therefore, keep oil away from it.

However, there is a major flaw in this theory. Your skin overproduces oil because it is dehydrated. Eliminating oil from your skin-care routine only perpetuates this cycle of dehydration.

Among those suffering from acne, there is a big shift to moving toward skin-care products that contain natural oils. There are hundreds of online self-care videos demonstrating oil cleansing methods that replace the traditional recommendation of harsh, oil-stripping soaps. Many people with acne follow these regimens and they find that their skin is not only without aggravation but also clearer.

There seems to be a disconnect between the theories about how topical oil aggravates oily skin and how your skin really handles oil.

Using a natural oil that is gentle enough for your face to absorb and that offers an adequate amount of pH may provide enough hydration to prevent your skin from overproducing its own sebum. As a result, this prevents the clogging of pores and acne formation.

Test Patch for Sensitive Skin

The one caveat in using any topical product, whether commercial, natural, oil-free, prescription or natural, is that with sensitive skin, you should always do a test patch first to ensure that your skin does not react. I have seen enough patients with acne to know that even the most gentle, natural, hypoallergenic and noncomedogenic product won't work with everyone's skin type and acne presentation. Breakouts can occur for many different reasons, and these are related to individual sensitivities and differences in skin. Many products can aggravate not only acne but also the base of the skin, causing it to redden and flare up. Skin that is prone to acne is extremely sensitive.

I share this motto with my patients who have sensitive skin and acne: test before you invest.

Non-Aggravating Skin Care

Most of us are acutely aware that skin-care products won't make our acne go away, yet we somehow end up shelling out ridiculous amounts of money for the latest and greatest skin-care product.

Cosmetics will not improve our stress levels, normalize our hormones or stabilize our blood sugar. Nevertheless, there are some aspects of skin care that are important to implement on your path to clear skin. It is very unlikely that they will cure your acne, but they should help normalize your skin, hydrate your epidermis, minimize any possible long-term adverse effects and, most important, be gentle on your skin.

Our face is the area of our body that is least likely to be covered up by clothing and protected from the elements. Our facial skin goes through a lot of stress on a daily basis: makeup application and removal; exposure to air pollution; drastic climate and humidity changes outdoors and indoors; seasonal temperature changes; exposure to tears, saliva and nasal secretions; the constant undulation, wrinkling and unwrinkling associated with facial expressions and talking; and our tendency to regularly touch our face with our hands. It is, therefore, very important that we cleanse our skin to ensure that we remove any potential irritants.

Additionally, because acne is a condition most commonly associated with stressed and dehydrated skin, it is essential to keep skin properly hydrated, particularly after cleansing, and to use products that are gentle and, ideally, natural.

Hydration

Choose skin-care products that maintain hydration in the skin. This will prevent the loss of moisture to the environment via evaporation. This is particularly important in dry, windy and/or cold climates.

Emollients, more commonly known as moisturizers, are skin-care products that prevent water loss from the outer layer of the skin, the epidermis. Emollients help soften, hydrate and make the skin more pliable, thereby improving its ability to reach its ideal healthy state.

The type of emollient you choose depends on the level of protection your skin needs against dehydration, your skin type and the climate, along with personal choices, such as how it feels and appears on your skin. For instance, one person may choose to use a high-oil-content emollient only

Did You Know?

Emollient Types
There are several types of emollients, classified by their water-to-oil content. Lotions and creams have a higher water content and feel lighter and less greasy, but they do not offer as much barrier protection as an emollient with a higher oil content, such as an ointment or a salve.

at night because they don't want their skin to appear shiny during the day, and opt for a lighter product during the daytime. Someone with oilier skin may find an emollient with a higher oil content too thick on their skin and instead choose one with a higher water content, such as a lotion.

In order of increasing oil content, thickness and protectiveness, emollients are listed as follows:

1. **Lotion:** Approximately 80% water content, 20% oil ingredients; feels lighter on skin.
2. **Cream:** Approximately equal ratio of water to oil-based ingredients; this is the middle-ground option.
3. **Ointment:** Approximately 80% oil ingredients, 20% water content; thicker protection but heavier.
4. **Salve:** Devoid of water; contains a combination of oils, waxes and butters; very thick and protective; useful for dry, cold or windy environments and dry, dehydrated or flaking skin.

Another factor to consider is that the higher the water content, the more likely the product is prone to bacterial contamination. Bacteria require moisture for growth and reproduction. Because of this concern, almost all commercially available creams and lotions are likely to contain preservatives to prevent bacterial growth, thereby increasing their likelihood of irritating your skin (there are also unknown potential long-term risks of absorbing these preservatives through the skin). Essentially, products with a higher oil content are less likely to cause bacterial growth or contain preservatives.

What's in an Emollient?

Emollients function with the assistance of three different types of ingredients, each with a specific action:

1. An **occluder** provides an oil-based barrier that prevents the evaporation of moisture out of the skin.
2. A **humectant** draws in moisture from the surrounding air.
3. A **lubricant** decreases friction of the skin in cases where it rubs against other surfaces and materials, thereby preventing and protecting against potential irritation and aggravation.

Gentle Products

Gentle products may be synthetic or natural. Gentle products essentially have a low likelihood of aggravating or irritating your skin. Just the same, there are often reactions to even the gentlest of products. No product will be safe for every single person. Even the most hypoallergenic, well-researched synthetic chemical can irritate some people's acne, and likewise the gentlest natural products may cause reactions on sensitive skin in certain cases.

Patients are advised to use skin-care products that are tried, tested and true for their acne and skin type. Most people with acne have experimented with a vast array of skin-care products, different brands and acne-targeted product lines. Stick to a skin-care line that has been proven to be gentle and non-aggravating, even if it is synthetic, while you work on your internal health through nutrition and lifestyle changes.

Whether you use natural or synthetic products, the most important consideration is to ensure that they are fragrance-free. Synthetic fragrances are common skin irritants; however, natural fragrances are typically essential oils extracted from plants, which can also irritate the skin.

There are no hard-and-fast rules to help determine if a product is gentle — other than ensuring that it is fragrance-free and that it is tested and labeled as "gentle" or "hypoallergenic." This essentially means trusting that the company has done due diligence and has tested their product enough times to show a low likelihood of aggravation. Unfortunately, the terms are not regulated.

Further down the road, as your skin settles, it is recommended that you move toward a more natural skin-care regimen. This means that you would transition to using skin-care products that contain only naturally derived, and preferably organic, ingredients.

Cosmetic Ingredients to Avoid

The cosmetic industry is self-regulating, meaning there is no independent objective regulatory organization overseeing manufacturers. Many of the potentially harmful ingredients below can be found in the majority of bath products, lotions, shaving creams, shampoos and soaps.

Parabens
- The most common preservative; found in 75% to 90% of cosmetic products

> **Did You Know?**
>
> **Added Fragrance**
> The term *fragrance* refers to any synthetic ingredient that is used to "improve" a product's perceived smell. Fragrances are largely unregulated, and the term is general and not descriptive. Products are not required to reveal the name of the chemical(s) they use, and, therefore, products with fragrance should be avoided.

- Included in many "natural" or "organic" products
- Labeled as a paraben, or as ethyl-, methyl-, butyl-, propyl- or para-hydroxybenzoate
- Mimics estrogen, thereby disrupting hormones in the body
- Evidence shows that exposure leads to an increased risk of breast cancer

Imidazolidinyl/Diazolidinyl Urea
- The second most common preservative
- Disrupts hormones
- May trigger contact dermatitis (a red, itchy rash)
- Converts in the body to formaldehyde, which has shown links to cancer

Sodium Lauryl/Laureth Sulfate
- Ubiquitous foaming agent
- Used as an industrial engine degreaser and an industrial detergent
- A skin irritant; also converts to nitrosamines (a known carcinogen)
- Found in 90% of foaming soaps, toothpastes and even some natural supplements

Petroleum Jelly
- Additive to prevent moisture loss
- A semisolid mixture of hydrocarbons derived from oil
- An inexpensive ingredient
- Links to organ toxicity; an allergen to some

Propylene Glycol
- Surfactant, wetting agent, solvent
- Used in industry as a protein and cellular disrupter
- Links to organ toxicity in the brain, liver and kidneys

Ethanolamine/Diethanolamine
- An emulsifier and a foaming agent
- Links to cancer in animal studies

Isopropyl Alcohol
- A solvent and denaturant
- Can cause systemic and neurological toxicity
- Fatal if 1 oz (30 g) is ingested

Grapefruit Seed Extract (GSE)

- A "natural" preservative
- Some cosmetic-grade GSEs contain triclosan (antimicrobial), methylparaben (preservative) or benzethonium chloride (antiseptic)
- Main concerns are the potential additives to GSE and the lack of requirement to label these additional synthetic ingredients

Dyes (FD&C or D&C)

- Synthetic colors
- Dyes are federally approved for internal use in food, drugs and cosmetics (FD&C) or for external use in drugs and cosmetics (D&C)
- Derived from coal tar
- Studies have shown possible links to cancer

Fragrances

- Synthetic perfumes
- Thousands are available; not required to be specified on ingredients list; completely unregulated
- Can cause systemic toxicities; however, most toxicities are unknown because of lack of regulation
- Many are skin irritants and may trigger allergic reactions

The Basics of an Acne Skin-Care Regimen

A typical skin-care regimen usually consists of two to four of the following products:

- A gentle cleanser
- A hypoallergenic fragrance-free moisturizer
- A serum to further boost hydration of the skin (optional)
- Some form of exfoliator, whether chemical or mechanical (optional)

Let's look at each of these products individually and explore the criteria that are important in choosing an appropriate product.

Did You Know?

Gentle Action

Cleansers, just like soaps, are also antibacterial; however, they are designed to be gentler and more forgiving to the more supple nature of our facial skin. Cleansers are also less likely to strip away the skin's protective moisture and oils.

- **Cleansers** are meant to remove dirt, oil and makeup from the skin. A cleanser is only in contact with your skin for less than 2 minutes (on average) before you wash it off. It doesn't matter how much of an active ingredient is in any given cleanser; nothing will significantly cure acne. What a good cleanser will do is remove dirt, oil and makeup efficiently without irritating the skin, so that there is no buildup on your skin that can lead to clogged pores.
- **Moisturizers** can help soothe irritated skin and, depending on their ingredients, can help speed up the healing process of acne. Invest in a good basic cream that has no synthetic fragrances, colors, petroleum or other irritating ingredients.
- **Serums** are often formulated to contain a higher concentration of active ingredients. They are also lighter in consistency, which makes them feel more hydrating and as if they are penetrating more deeply.
- **Exfoliators** remove dead skin cells from the surface of the skin. See pages 64–66 for more information on several types of exfoliation.

Natural Products

Did You Know?

Irritating Essential Oils

Essential oil concentrates are often used in natural skin-care products because they provide a pleasing fragrance. But concentrated essential oils can irritate the skin. Exert caution even with natural skin-care products — if it has a strong scent, it may have a greater likelihood of causing a localized skin irritation.

Within the realm of the poorly regulated cosmetics industry, there is a lot of hype, marketing and misinformation. Chemical ingredients are not individually tested for long-term effects on the skin and the body.

Once acne has become manageable and skin inflammation has settled, consider moving toward more natural skin-care products for the long term. There is considerable evidence that shows that cosmetic products have a negative impact on our hormones. Several very common ingredients in skin-care products have also been linked to an increased risk of cancer and act as hormone disrupters. Ironically, most cases of acne are related to hormones and may actually be perpetuated by cosmetics typically used to treat acne in the first place. In order to discern if a "natural" cosmetic is actually natural, first ensure that it does not contain any of the ingredients in the Cosmetic Ingredients to Avoid list on pages 73–75.

With so much overexposure to xenoestrogens (foreign estrogens found in cosmetics, plastics, industrial chemicals and pesticides), it seems like an easy decision to avoid skin-care products that could contain toxic ingredients and to proactively choose skin-care products that are as natural as possible.

However, the caveat with natural products is twofold: quality of application and potential for skin irritation.

It is difficult to create a natural product that applies smoothly to the skin and absorbs adequately. The common problem with the majority of natural cosmetics is that their ease of use is subpar. Picture trying to apply a thick cream that just sits on the surface and gets smeared around, leaving a white coating on your skin that refuses to sink in. This may sound like an extreme example, but it is more common than you might suspect. The reason that synthetic ingredients are so widespread is that they make the cosmetic glide better, render it easier to absorb and feel smoother. For a skin-care manufacturer, it is a much easier route to take.

Natural products are absolutely a better option for your internal health, but they are not necessarily safe or gentle on your skin.

Good-quality natural cosmetic products should have a nice consistency when applied to the skin and should include as little essential oil as possible, particularly for sensitive skin on your face. Try a sample first to ensure it applies well and does not cause any aggravation.

> ✱ **Caution**
>
> Beware of natural skin-care products that have a high water content (creams and lotions) but do not contain any type of natural preservative. These products have shorter shelf lives and are at higher risk of having bacterial growth. Also, do not use any skin-care products (whether natural or synthetic) past their expiration date, as bacterial contamination may have compromised the contents.

FAQ

 What do the terms *natural* and *organic* mean on skin-care products?

The term *natural* is applied without regulation, is frequently misused and is essentially worthless.

A label stating that a product is "made with organic ingredients" means that it must contain a minimum of 70% organic ingredients, but these ingredients may be mixed with unwanted synthetic chemicals as well. An "organic" cosmetic product must contain at least 95% organic ingredients. A skin-care product labeled as "100% organic" must contain only organically raised agricultural ingredients. The higher the percentage of organic plant-product ingredients (generally speaking), the safer the product is and the less likely it will contribute to an increased risk of cancer.

Do-It-Yourself Natural Skin-Care Methods

There are countless recommendations online for do-it-yourself skin-care methods. Search any cosmetic blogs, vlogs and YouTube videos and you will be inundated with an overwhelming number of homemade natural skin-care recipes.

The volume of information is compounding exponentially online. The dilemma is not whether your question will be answered on the Internet, but rather how to determine which of the countless answers and methods have validity.

Deep-Cleaning Your Skin with Oil

To most acne sufferers, the thought of putting oil on their face is frightening. Old-school dermatology dogma has led us to believe that oil is the enemy and can actually cause acne. As mentioned before, acne is not caused by the topical application of oil.

> The application of certain oils can help soothe irritated and inflamed skin, ultimately healing the skin.

Hormones, stress, sugar imbalances, genetics, improper diet and many other factors lead to acne. In fact, the application of certain oils can help soothe irritated and inflamed skin, ultimately healing the skin.

Massaging your skin with oil is a deep-cleansing option that you can do once a week. You will need two types of oil: castor oil and your choice of a carrier oil (an oil that helps to dilute the thicker castor oil).

Initially, try for a 1:4 ratio (castor oil to carrier oil) and adjust according to your preference. The dryer your skin, the *less* castor oil you will use; the oilier your skin, the *more* castor oil you will use.

Castor oil has long been known as a purifying and detoxifying oil, mainly because it dissolves impurities and debris on the skin. The carrier oil's purpose is to dilute the stickiness of the castor oil to allow for a more fluid consistency for application. As well, the carrier oil itself provides its own unique benefits to your skin. I recommend using only high-quality organic, cold-pressed olive oil, rosehip oil, jojoba oil or sunflower oil. These oils are packed with vitamins and nutrients, such as essential fatty acids, that are beneficial to the health of your skin.

To deep-clean your skin, follow these simple instructions:

1. Combine castor oil and carrier oil in a clean sealable jar and invert it several times to thoroughly mix the two oils.
2. Pour a quarter-size amount of cleansing oil into your palm and distribute evenly over your entire face.

3. Use your fingertips to massage your face, using gentle circular motions; focus on areas that are especially problematic for you.
4. Relax and continue massaging your face for 5 to 15 minutes. You may even feel some blackheads release from their pores as you are massaging.
5. Wet a clean washcloth with warm water. Apply the washcloth to your face, and let its heat warm your face as you gently massage off the oil with the washcloth.
6. Repeat two or three times or until it feels like the oil is sufficiently removed.
7. Depending on how your skin feels, you can leave it as is or apply a few drops of the oil blend or a neutral moisturizer to your skin and massage it in.
8. If you store the leftover oil blend, be sure to label it with either the carrier or castor oil's listed expiry date (whichever one is earliest).

Easy Moisturizing Mask for Inflamed Skin

Both honey and extra virgin olive oil provide hydration to the skin. Honey contains several naturally occurring antibacterial compounds, while olive oil delivers skin-healing essential fatty acids.

1. Combine 1 tsp (5 mL) each liquid honey and extra virgin olive oil.
2. Massage into clean skin.
3. Relax and let the mask penetrate and soothe the skin for 10 minutes.
4. Rinse off gently with warm water (and a washcloth, if needed).

Gentle Exfoliating Scrub

Baking soda is a natural and gentle exfoliating agent. Honey is the medium that holds the baking soda, and it provides antibacterial protection to the pores, which are being disrupted by the exfoliation.

1. Combine 1 tsp (5 mL) baking soda and 1 tbsp (15 mL) liquid honey.
2. Gently massage into clean skin for 1 minute.
3. Rinse off with warm water.
4. Apply moisturizer.

Did You Know?

Boosting Hydration from Your Moisturizer

If you feel that your moisturizer isn't providing enough hydration, especially in colder and drier weather or if a health condition is dehydrating your skin, simply add a few drops of a good-quality organic, cold-pressed oil to your moisturizer. Olive oil, sunflower oil, jojoba oil and rosehip oil blend nicely with almost any moisturizer.

Soothing Oatmeal Mask

Oats help soothe irritated, itchy and inflamed skin because they contain colloidal proteins that hold water. Be sure you do not have an allergy to oats before using this mask.

1. In a food processor, blend 1 cup (250 mL) organic oats to a fine powder.
2. Transfer 2 tbsp (30 mL) of the oat powder to a clean bowl and slowly stir in enough warm water to make a smooth paste.
3. Apply to clean skin and leave on for 10 minutes.
4. Rinse off with warm water.
5. Apply moisturizer.
6. Store remaining powdered oats in an airtight container for future use.

Doc Talk

My patients have tried and experimented with almost every type of synthetic and natural skin-care method out there. The consensus with natural skin-care methods is that the more basic the ingredients, the more likely a product will support your skin and not aggravate it.

I have listed a few of the skin-care methods and tips that I recommend to patients with acne. They are simple to prepare and use in the comfort of your home, gentle on your skin and proven to be most successful for their intended purpose. They help with cleansing your skin, boosting hydration, moisturizing, exfoliating and soothing inflamed skin.

Dietary Triggers for Acne

CASE STUDY

Constipation and Acne

Keiko is a healthy and active 28-year-old female who first came to my office with moderate deep cystic acne lesions affecting her cheeks, jawline and forehead. Scarring was also noted in these areas due to years of continual cystic lesions. She also had a mild presentation of whiteheads and blackheads, which appeared on her upper back and shoulders. Her acne was noticeably aggravated approximately 10 days before her expected period. She began to develop acne in her early 20s, after starting her university studies away from home. Her skin was clear during her pubescent years.

We discussed her digestive health — she suffers from chronic bloating and gas, which accompany normal to hard bowel movements. She has a bowel movement every 3 to 4 days on average, and there is straining every time, even when they are of normal consistency. With hard stools, she sometimes experiences rectal pain, but there had been no occurrences of bleeding.

She has been following a pescetarian diet (consuming seafood but not meat) for 5 years, which she implemented for both health and ethical reasons. After reviewing her diet, it was clear that Keiko consumed a lot of beans, rice and sandwiches, along with daily cheese and yogurt, which she took to supplement her diet with protein and calcium. She also drank tropical fruit smoothies with leafy greens at least three times a week.

I recommended on the first visit that she eliminate all dairy products, breads and tropical fruits, and rice when having beans. I also started her on a simple magnesium supplement and a high-potency probiotic to improve her bowel regularity. Magnesium is useful in normalizing bowel movements because it improves water flow into the colon, thereby helping to hydrate and soften the stool. This is a much healthier approach compared to laxatives, which stimulate the nerves of the intestines and can lead to a dependency.

These simple suggestions led to daily, easy-to-pass, soft bowel movements. We confirmed through IgG food sensitivity testing that she had a major sensitivity to all dairy products, but goat and sheep cheeses were tolerable.

After two weeks, Keiko's skin redness settled and the intensity of the inflammation of her cystic lesions decreased.

continued on next page

We continued working on diet and a basic supportive nutritional supplement program that included probiotics, fish oils and zinc. I gave her a more comprehensive diet plan to follow for 6 to 8 weeks, and she was very motivated and compliant.

At a follow-up visit 3 months later, Keiko's skin had significantly improved, with only minor whiteheads remaining on the jawline. Her forehead, cheeks, back and shoulders were all clear of acne, and she experienced no aggravation of her skin premenstrually. Digestion continued to function normally and bowel movements were regular, and we eliminated her magnesium use with no relapse of constipation. We discussed reintroducing some of her restricted foods in moderation, while monitoring for reactions.

When I followed up with her at the 6-month mark, Keiko's skin on her face, back and shoulders remained clear, with only the scars from the cystic acne on the cheeks remaining. She had stopped all the over-the-counter acne skin-care products that she had been relying on for years, with only minimal improvements. Her skin care was now basic and non-medicated.

Keiko was thrilled that her acne was no longer something that she had to just accept and constantly worry about. Her self-esteem had improved dramatically, and she felt empowered that she could make changes to impact her skin and overall health.

Hidden Sugars

We are easily swayed by claims of "natural sweetening," but these products still spike our blood sugar in the same way as the vilified white stuff.

Sugar is the white crystalline substance we all know too well as a culprit that spikes our blood glucose levels. We are aware that it is not healthy for us when we dump spoonfuls of it into our coffee. Indeed, it is not found in nature in that form, concentration or color. While we hate it for its effects on our health and its addictive quality, we love it for its sweetness and its ability to stimulate pleasure receptors in our brain to give us a quick, albeit short-lived, pick-me-up.

There are many other forms of natural sweeteners, which are essentially sugar but disguised by different names. Think of a wolf in sheep's clothing. We are easily swayed by claims of "natural sweetening," but these products still spike our blood sugar in the same way as the vilified white stuff.

In either case, whether refined or natural, sugar is considered a simple carbohydrate, meaning that it is readily absorbed into our bloodstream, thereby quickly spiking our blood sugar.

Natural Sugars

These sweeteners are naturally derived but still affect the body's blood sugar in a similar way to refined sugar:

- Agave syrup
- Amazake (amasake)
- Arenga sugar
- Barley malt
- Beet sugar
- Brown rice syrup
- Brown sugar
- Cane juice
- Caramel
- Coconut sugar
- Corn syrup and corn syrup solids
- Date sugar
- Demerara sugar
- Fruit juice
- Golden syrup
- Honey
- Jaggery
- Malt syrup
- Maple syrup
- Molasses
- Muscovado sugar
- Palm sugar
- Panela
- Rapadura
- Raw cane sugar
- Sorghum syrup
- Sucanat
- Treacle
- Turbinado sugar

> ### Did You Know?
>
> **Another Name for Sugar**
> Think of natural sweeteners as sugars with a few minerals and vitamins thrown in. The fact is that they are all still sugars and affect blood-sugar levels in the body in the same way. Consequently, this means that they will also have the same inflammatory effects as refined sugar.

Flour Equals Sugar

With acne, a big part of healing the skin is to normalize sugar balance in the body.

There are the obvious sugary culprits — like candy, chocolate bars, ice cream and desserts — which most people realize are connected to raising blood sugar. This is typically known to aggravate health problems such as obesity, diabetes and a host of other medical issues associated with regularly consuming an excess of sugar. As noted earlier, sugar imbalances in the body are also a common trigger for acne.

While we all know that these common sweet foods are detrimental to our health, it may still be difficult to control sugar cravings or limit their consumption. However, it is not just those obvious sugar-laden foods that can aggravate acne.

The more insidious form of sugar spiking is not caused by sugary treats but by flours. Flour is another form of simple carbohydrate. When you think of flour, think sugar. You want to avoid anything farinaceous (a nerdy term that is sure to impress your friends, which means any food made from flour), such as baked goods, breads, pastas, noodles, pancakes, muffins, crackers, crêpes, pitas and flatbreads. If it is made out of a flour, or a flour is listed in the ingredients, remember to translate that into *sugar*.

Complex Carbohydrates

Flours are grains that are hulled, processed, defatted and ground to a fine powder and then incorporated into countless food products. Grains are complex carbohydrates.

Relying on Sugar

All carbohydrates are essentially just sugar molecules or chains of sugar molecules of varying length. Sugar is required for the body to survive; it produces cellular energy, provides structural support, supports the nervous system and digestive tract, and helps to regulate fat and protein metabolism. For all of these reasons, we need to have a regular intake of carbohydrates in order to survive — the dilemma is deciding which types of carbohydrates work best for our body.

A grain's final purpose is to be broken down into sugar to fuel the body. This is the same with any carbohydrate; a carbohydrate is defined as a macronutrient whose breakdown product is sugar. However, the *complex* part of a complex carbohydrate grain means that it is in a form that is less accessible to us. Because its delivery system (the grain kernel) has more components (such as a husk, bran and oil) that need to be penetrated and assimilated, our body's ability to digest the carbohydrate is slowed down. This results in a more gradual release of sugar into the bloodstream.

With a dampened increase in glucose, our body can more readily use the carbohydrates for normal bodily functions as they are being absorbed. Ill health can occur when we have exceeded the rate at which our body requires glucose and the body shunts the excess into unnecessary processes. This can include systemic issues or localized presentations, like acne.

When a grain is pulverized in the flour-making process, its natural glucose-retarding constituents are removed. This means that flour is much more readily digested than a whole grain. It is quickly metabolized into its component sugars, causing an elevated rate of glucose release into the bloodstream. It is not a stretch to think of foods made with flour in the same vein as sugars — a piece of bread can have a similar effect on your body and skin as a candy bar.

Breaking Down Sugars

To understand how certain foods will impact your blood sugar, think about how accessible that sugar is for your body to digest, expose, enzymatically decompose and assimilate. Here are the most important points to consider:

- Glucose and fructose are the basic simple single sugar molecules that our body uses for energy.
- Glucose is converted in our bodies into long-branched chain molecules called glycogen, primarily in the liver and muscles.
- Chronic excess glucose and/or fructose intake leads to insulin resistance.
- Sucrose is a simple two-sugar molecule made up of glucose and fructose, and it is readily split apart in the body.
- Plant starches are straight chains of glucose.
- Plant amylopectins are branched chains of glucose.
- Glycogen is the long, highly branched storage form of glucose in humans and animals.

FAQ

Q **How do different foods, in particular sugars and flours, affect our blood sugar?**

A Sugars are basic single molecules (monosaccharides) or double molecules (disaccharides). Monosaccharides include glucose, galactose and fructose. Disaccharides include lactose (galactose + glucose), maltose (glucose + glucose) and sucrose (fructose + glucose). Lactose is a sugar found in milk products; maltose can be formed with the caramelization of glucose and also occurs in grains (for example, barley malt); and sucrose is derived from sugarcane and sugar beets — also called table sugar.

Starches are chains of glucose molecules called polysaccharides. These can be straight chains, called amylose, and they occur in plant-based starches (for example, root vegetables). When these plant starch chains have branching side chains of glucose molecules, the polysaccharide is then termed amylopectin. In humans and animals, these polysaccharides are termed glycogen, which is the storage form of glucose. Glycogen is more highly branched than amylopectin and is stored in the muscles and the cells of the liver. It is a secondary backup energy source (fats being the primary storage form of energy).

With straight chains of polysaccharides (amylose), the sugar molecules are cleaved off into two- and three-glucose pieces (disaccharides and trisaccharides, respectively) by an enzyme called amylase. Amylase is found in our saliva, thereby starting the digestion of carbohydrates in our mouth. The pancreas also secretes amylase, which further breaks down carbohydrates in the small intestines. The two- and three-glucose sugar units are then broken down by enzymes called maltase and alpha-glucosidase.

The branching in polysaccharides is an important feature that helps us to understand how different foods affect our blood sugar. The body requires special enzymes (debranching enzymes) to break the branches off; this slows down the release of sugar into the bloodstream. These enzymes are needed for the breakdown of both glycogen and amylopectin. Therefore, foods that contain longer-branched chains of carbohydrates release sugar in slower, more metabolically manageable components. This means that sugar spikes will be prevented and acne won't be aggravated.

- The more branched the polysaccharide, the more slowly it is broken down.
- If a grain is ground into a flour, its starches are much more easily digested.
- If a grain is an intact whole grain (a complex carbohydrate), your body must exert more effort to mechanically break it down to access and digest the starches.

Other Hidden Sugars

A less obvious source of sugar is fruits and vegetables. Fruits and vegetables are important sources of concentrated fiber, nutrients and antioxidants, all helpful for acne; however, certain types can lead to large sugar spikes and are best limited initially, while acne is being targeted.

Vegetables that are high in starches are termed starchy vegetables. Their starches are also readily converted into sugar in the body, which can aggravate acne. Starchy vegetables include root vegetables and tubers, along with a few others. These are explored in more detail in Chapter 10.

Although fruit contains a large amount of fiber, it is still a concentrated source of the fruit sugar fructose. Whole fruits are preferable in terms of glycemic control, compared to fruit juices. However, certain fruits have higher concentrations of sugar and are best avoided until acne has settled. These fruits are termed high-sugar fruits. Several tropical fruits as well as a few others are included in this category. For more information, see Chapter 10.

Dairy, Egg and Gluten Sensitivities

Dairy, egg and gluten are the three most common food sensitivities (between the immediate and delayed types of allergies). Dairy has been directly studied in its role as a contributor to acne. Evidence-based research is suggesting a possible connection (see page 47).

Eggs are a common food sensitivity, particularly with the delayed type of food allergy. In a 2013 Chinese study investigating the presence of IgG food allergies in children and adolescents, dairy proved to cause the highest level of sensitivity in infants. In school-age children, dairy was still the most common sensitivity, followed by eggs. In adolescents, however, eggs actually surpassed dairy for the most common food sensitivity.

Gluten and Acne

The health of the digestive tract is important to consider when treating inflammatory skin conditions, including acne. Because those with gluten sensitivities have symptoms related to the gastrointestinal tract, it is recommended

---

Did You Know?

Gluten-Free Health Myth

Gluten-free products are not a better option with respect to blood sugar's impact on your acne. People often assume incorrectly that gluten-free breads, for example, are healthier in every respect. Gluten-free products are a necessity for those who have an intolerance to gluten or a gluten sensitivity. From a sugar-spiking perspective, gluten-free grain flours are virtually identical to any other flours in how they affect blood sugar.

Research Spotlight: Eggs and Acne

Eggs have been connected to the aggravation of acne in three separate studies that spanned more than a century. In one study from 2006, 42% of subjects with acne reported that eggs worsened their skin. An older study from 1940 correlated links between acne and diet and incriminated eggs as one of the contributors to acne vulgaris. A doctor reported in 1912 that "eggs are a frequent cause of acne." This same doctor outlined that the consumption of two to three eggs may be followed by an acne breakout within 36 hours. This description fits the timeline of a food sensitivity's symptoms (particularly with the delayed type of food sensitivity).

to eliminate foods that contain gluten during acne treatment. The diet plan in this book does not include wheat flour, so exposure to gluten is already limited. Many foods that contain gluten, such as the majority of conventional baked goods and pasta, act as "double damage" for acne. The flour they contain is typically derived from wheat (the main source of gluten), which not only spikes blood sugar but also represents a potential food sensitivity.

Gluten should be avoided because of its likelihood to cause a food sensitivity. Celiac disease is one potentially severe form of an autoimmune condition that manifests as a permanent gluten intolerance; it is well known, but still underdiagnosed. People with celiac disease have to avoid foods containing gluten. But there is a growing awareness and acknowledgment in the medical community of another gluten sensitivity, termed non-celiac gluten sensitivity (NCGS). Those who have this condition function and feel better on a gluten-restrictive diet even though they have not been diagnosed with celiac disease.

Overexposure

Frequently ingesting dairy, eggs and gluten (or highly processed versions of them) effectively increases their concentration and essentially makes their action more potent, increasing the likelihood that our immune system will develop a hypersensitivity. Some of these food sensitivities can lead to irritation of the digestive tract, which thereby leads to an increased permeability of the intestinal wall. This allows particles to permeate the bloodstream and potentially trigger various inflammatory and autoimmune responses. This state of increased gut permeability is known as leaky gut syndrome.

Did You Know?

Non-celiac Gluten Sensitivity

Non-celiac gluten hypersensitivity (NCGS) is mainly characterized by symptoms in the digestive symptom and other body systems that benefit from gluten avoidance. In one recent study, 25% of patients with NCGS experienced gastrointestinal malabsorption, including weight loss, diarrhea and nutrient deficiencies. Another study showed that approximately 13% of the population self-reported a gluten sensitivity, and that they had an increased likelihood of presenting with symptoms of irritable bowel syndrome.

FAQ

Q **How have dairy, eggs and gluten become such common food sensitivities?**

A Part of the equation likely has to do with overexposure. It is not a surprise that the three most common food sensitivities are also some of the most widely consumed foods in the North American diet. For example, a common breakfast sandwich contains a couple slices of buttered bread or bagel, an egg or two, and a couple slices of cheese. This one meal alone contains ample amounts of egg, gluten and dairy, and these foods are also part of other meals in varying degrees of frequency and quantity throughout the day. These three ingredients are ubiquitous food items, so we are chronically exposed to them.

In the United States, 90% of all food allergies comprise only eight foods. Of these eight allergenic foods, three of them are milk, wheat (gluten) and eggs.

The second issue may have to do with being overexposed to the derivatives of these foods. Egg derivatives (for example, ovalbumin and ovomucoid) are commonly added to packaged prepared foods — often for their binding or texturizing properties. There are also multiple proteins extracted from egg whites that are used as ingredients in food products. Several dairy derivatives (for example, whey and casein) are also commonly used as texture and flavor enhancers in food products. Gluten (namely, any conventional flour, including white bleached flour) is used in almost every prepared food.

Genetically Engineered Foods and Glyphosate

Genetically engineered foods are created to be resistant to the herbicide glyphosate. Glyphosate is sprayed on fields of genetically engineered produce crops to control weed growth but doesn't kill the crop plants. Its use has become widespread and has increased exponentially since its commercial application started in the mid-1990s. It is mainly used on genetically engineered crops. Glyphosate use and penetration into the food supply has been linked to toxic effects in the body.

Mass Production

Eggs and dairy are produced on large-scale farms, and the feed of the animals is different from in nature. This may affect the nutrients in the eggs and milk that they produce. For example, there is a nutritional difference between the milk from grass-fed cows and the milk from grain-fed cows.

Grass-fed cows, which are a rarity in mass-produced dairy, produce vitamin K_2, while their grain-fed counterparts do not. Vitamin K_2 has been shown to decrease the risk of both heart disease and osteoporosis.

What's Responsible for Inflammation?

A study in 2014 investigated the link between a sequence of events that triggers an inflammatory reaction and disease by way of a food reaction. In this case, it was a unique examination of how depression was triggered by an inflammatory reaction related to the consumption of a common food component in wheat. Gliadin, a protein in wheat products, was examined as a culprit in promoting the leaky gut state. This state allows food molecules to pass into the bloodstream, activating an immune response that then induces IgG food allergies.

The cascade of events would unfold as follows:

1. Consume a food to which you are sensitive (such as gliadin)
2. Food sensitivity triggers gut irritation (by activating a protein in the gut wall called zonulin, which regulates intestinal permeability)
3. Irritation leads to increased gut permeability (leaky gut syndrome)
4. Food particles transfer across the gut wall
5. Immune response leads to development of IgG food sensitivities
6. Inflammatory reaction
7. Disease state (in this study, depression was examined)

> Grass-fed cows, which are a rarity in mass-produced dairy, produce vitamin K_2, while their grain-fed counterparts do not. Vitamin K_2 has been shown to decrease the risk of both heart disease and osteoporosis.

It was not the depression that was of most interest in this study, but rather the pathway that led to the disease state. It is likely we will discover that numerous other diseases follow the same series of events by way of the gut and food-sensitivity triggers. Acne may be another presentation of the inflammatory condition that is triggered by food sensitivities. This is a possible mechanism for how gluten, dairy and eggs may contribute to acne. This is also why it is recommended to avoid them while treating acne.

Ingredients That Contain or Are Derived from Dairy, Egg and Gluten

- **Dairy:** casein, lactose, lactalbumin, lactalbumin phosphate, modified milk ingredients, potassium caseinate, sodium caseinate, whey
- **Eggs:** albumin, binder, coagulant, emulsifier, globulin, lecithin, lysozyme, ovalbumin, ovomucin, ovomucoid, ovovitellin, vitellin
- **Gluten:** barley, couscous, durum flour, Kamut, oats, malt, rye, spelt, triticale, wheat, wheat berries, white flour, whole wheat flour

Doc Talk

In my practice — having administered the IgG food allergy test on many patients suffering from acne, irritable bowel syndrome, eczema, inflammatory bowel disease and menstrual irregularities — these results are consistent. Dairy and eggs (and gluten in third place) are by far the most common food sensitivities of the IgG category of food sensitivities in patients with digestive disorders and dermatological conditions.

In patients with acne, dairy and egg food sensitivities appear at a similar frequency. Clinically speaking, I have seen several patients with acne improve when they eliminate dairy and eggs and then noticeably break out when they reintroduce these foods in the early stages of treatment. (Note that the goal in the long term is to improve their tolerance to the foods to which they have sensitivities, thereby allowing them to reintroduce these foods without re-aggravating their acne.)

Healthy Diets That May Worsen Your Acne

Vegetarian Diet

People turn to vegetarianism for a number of reasons, including ethical considerations, health matters or a general distaste for meat. Vegetarian diets have an aura of being associated with good health.

However, eliminating meat in the diet may be done haphazardly without a lot of research into balancing nutrition and preventing vitamin or mineral deficiencies. First, it is important to ensure adequate sources of B_{12} and iron to prevent anemia. Second, carbohydrate consumption can get out of control after eliminating high-protein, low-carb meat options from your diet. And, as discussed earlier, excess carbohydrate consumption is a major trigger for acne.

One of the key issues in a vegetarian diet is the challenge of getting adequate protein. An easy substitute is dairy. Dairy products such as cheese, yogurt and milk are often consumed regularly to make up for a lack of meat protein. With a high intake of dairy, a common food sensitivity for those with acne, this becomes a potential problem.

There is such a large gap in the knowledge that exists between a healthy vegetarian diet and an unhealthy vegetarian diet. It makes sense to research ways to eat healthily as a vegetarian before you adopt the practice.

Processed foods — such as boxed macaroni and cheese, peanut butter and jelly sandwiches, cream cheese bagels and processed soy meats — are examples of easily accessible but unhealthy options for recently converted vegetarians, particularly if these foods are consumed on a regular basis. It not uncommon for vegetarians who make these food choices to see their skin worsen or develop other health concerns.

> One of the key issues in a vegetarian diet is the challenge of getting adequate protein. An easy substitute is dairy. With a high intake of dairy, a common food sensitivity for those with acne, this becomes a potential problem.

Raw Vegan Diet

Well, you can't get much healthier than this diet, right? It would appear that if someone follows a raw vegan diet and has acne, it is not diet that is the issue.

Think about it — raw vegans don't eat dairy, eggs or meats, and primarily eat whole foods. They are usually very knowledgeable about nutrition and balance and ensure that

FAQ

Q I've recently switched to a vegetarian diet. What foods won't aggravate my acne?

A Many people wrongly presume that animal protein and saturated fat are the main aggravators of their acne. Eating mainly grain and dairy products as a vegetarian is not a healthy approach. A healthy vegetarian diet is not just about what you are avoiding (meat); it should also focus on what you are including (plenty of vegetables) — case in point: the derivative root of *vegetarian* is the same as *vegetable*.

To eat a healthy vegetarian diet that supports your skin health and limits acne aggravation, follow these guidelines:

- Choose nondairy protein sources at each meal.
- Limit your refined carbohydrate intake.
- Balance your protein and carbohydrates.
- Incorporate plant-based foods that are high in iron and B_{12}.
- Eat 6 to 8 servings of vegetables per day.
- Eat 2 to 3 servings of fruit a day.
- Incorporate nuts and seeds as nondairy protein boosters in your meals and/or snacks.

Did You Know?

Sugar in Fruits and Vegetables

There may be one issue that contributes to acne in raw vegan diets: sugar control. The source of glucose spikes is not the obvious food sources; rather, the spikes may come from overconsumption of fruits and starchy vegetables.

they are getting enough protein from non-animal sources. Because their lifestyle and diet choices typically originate from a place of both ethics and health, they also usually avoid junk food, refined sugars, fast foods and processed foods, even if they are animal-free.

Raw vegans are very keen on fresh, nutrient-dense organic produce. This makes perfect sense any way you look at it, to nourish the body and protect against chronic disease. However, fruits and/or starchy vegetables make up a big part of the diet, particularly if a person is juicing regularly. Consuming juiced fruit and starchy vegetables (a common one is beets, which contain a concentrated amount of naturally occurring sugars) quickly adds many sugars to the body — and in a form that is readily absorbed. Juicing removes the fibers and bulk that would normally stall the assimilation of the sugars through the digestive tract into the bloodstream.

If you are prone to acne, your skin is very sensitive to sugar spikes. As a result, the raw vegan diet can deceptively contribute to acne unless sugar intake is carefully monitored, particularly if juicing.

Paleo Diet

Paleolithic, or paleo, diets are helpful to many people and help improve numerous health concerns. A big reason for this is the focus on quality basic foods that are high in protein and good fats, as well as reduced carbohydrate intake, thanks to the avoidance of all grain products and legumes.

The paleo diet generally consists of the following:

- Eggs
- Ethically raised grass-fed meats and pastured chicken
- Fats, such as nuts, seeds, coconut oil, butter from grass-fed cows, olive oil and avocados
- Seasonal fruits and vegetables
- Wild-caught fish

There are many interpretations of the paleo diet, but some suggest that certain forms of dairy are acceptable, including fermented sources like yogurt, kefir and aged cheeses. Eggs are consumed regularly and often in relatively high amounts (for example, 2 to 3 eggs a day is not unusual).

The carbohydrate intake and glycemic control portion of the paleo diet are exceptional. The main problem is that two of the more common food sensitivities are included: eggs and dairy. Many people following a paleo diet end up consuming large amounts of eggs and derivatives of dairy. These two food sensitivities typically follow right behind carbohydrates in the hierarchy of dietary triggers for acne.

Additionally, diets that are very low in carbohydrates can lead to increased levels of cortisol (the stress hormone), which can ultimately increase blood sugar. It seems counterproductive to follow a low-carb diet for the long haul when the whole point of restricting carbohydrates to such an extreme degree is to prevent your blood sugar from spiking. This is why maintaining small portions of grains and legumes in your diet is acceptable and may actually be beneficial for acne treatment and prevention in the long run.

Doc Talk

In order to effectively heal acne, it is best to not just control carbohydrates but also to avoid egg and dairy products for the duration of the program. It is also important to maintain optimal digestive and bowel function by keeping limited amounts of grains and legumes in your diet.

CHAPTER 7

Normalizing the Gut and Hormones

CASE STUDY

Hormonal Acne

Amaya is a 32-year-old female with mild acne that started at puberty, initially on her forehead and around her mouth. It increased in intensity when she moved away to university. The pimples became more severe and pustular and took several weeks to heal. They also moved to the jawline and upper neck. They tended to suddenly crop up about 1 week before her period and settle down the week after her period. The frustrating aspect was that there was no relief because the premenstrual breakouts did not have time to settle down before the next round of pimples started. Amaya's acne compounded constantly and was unrelenting.

After meeting with Amaya, I started her on a zinc and calcium D-glucarate supplement to support proper hormone metabolism and increase the elimination of excess estrogens (the timing of her premenstrual acne flare-ups points to an excess of estrogen relative to progesterone). I also started her on probiotics and fish oils to support digestion and reduce skin inflammation. We discussed the Vibrant Skin Diet Plan and what she could expect in terms of prognosis. She was eager to start right away.

We followed up after 1 month. Amaya's acne and inflammation had noticeably calmed down. She reported that her last premenstrual breakout had been much less intense than previous ones. Taking all factors into consideration, her acne already appeared to have improved by approximately 20% to 25%, which was promising.

By the 3-month mark, Amaya's acne had cleared up considerably, although she was getting occasional small whiteheads on her cheeks, unrelated to her menstrual cycle. Her jawline and neck had almost cleared, and her acne scars were starting to heal. She noted that her other menstrual symptoms — cramping, irritability and breast tenderness — had also substantially improved. This is a common added benefit that occurs when addressing hormonal acne. With her progress, we discussed a plan to cautiously reintroduce restricted foods back into her diet.

At 6 months, Amaya's skin was clear and she was very happy with her progress. She reported a very occasional "random small pimple that healed within a couple of days," but otherwise her skin was free of acne. Her diet had expanded and become manageable. Her skin did not break out even with occasional "cheats." We gradually phased out her hormonal supplements and probiotics without consequence.

From a holistic perspective, the health of your digestive tract is intimately connected to the health of your skin.

Anatomically speaking, our skin is continuous with our digestive tract. The skin on our face extends to our lips and continues with the mucous membranes that make up our mouth. Our mouth leads to our esophagus, stomach, small and large intestines and rectum. Our rectum opens at our anus, and again the epidermis envelops our buttocks and the rest of our body. Both our intestinal tract and our skin are our outer coverings that structurally hold us together.

From a histological perspective (the anatomy of cells and tissues), the skin and lining of the digestive tract are made up of various types of cells that help with different roles in the body. The epidermis is tauter and stronger and holds less moisture than the lining of the digestive tract. The digestive tract is in a moister, more protected environment than your skin; it is termed a mucous membrane.

Your skin is incredible because it has the ability to eliminate and absorb substances, yet it also functions as a mainly impermeable shield that protects us from temperature changes, sunlight and wind, as well as a water barrier that holds in our bodily fluids and prevents them from penetrating to the outside. It is able to absorb substances to a certain degree, mainly if they are fat-soluble compounds; these can seep through the thick outer layers of our skin (the stratum corneum and the translucent layer right below it, called the stratum lucidum) to gradually reach the lower layers of the epidermis, and then the dermis and the capillaries of our blood system.

Physiologically speaking, the digestive tract is the internal barrier that separates our body — including our blood, organs and tissues — from the external environment (the contents of your intestines). Both the skin and the digestive tract function as filters, with differing degrees of selectivity that allow us to both eliminate and absorb.

The skin and our intestines are inherently similar in structure and function, and, as a result, optimizing the health of our digestive tract is important. If we neglect to address digestion when trying to prevent and treat acne, we are missing a key component.

> **Did You Know?**
>
> **Permeable Lining**
> Mucous membranes, such as our digestive tract, are much more permeable than our skin, since their main role is to control the absorption of nutrients and the elimination of by-products and waste.

Resolving Constipation

From a holistic — or even just a more rational — perspective, bowel movements should actually occur on a daily basis at a bare minimum. Two to three bowel movements a day is considered healthy, and arguably even optimal.

Constipation is a digestive concern that leads to decreased elimination of metabolic by-products and toxins.

The definition of constipation is related to a few different abnormal symptoms of digestive function. Constipation typically refers to a decreased frequency of bowel movements, defined as three bowel movements or less a week. From a holistic — or even just a more rational — perspective, bowel movements should actually occur on a daily basis at a bare minimum. Two to three bowel movements a day is considered healthy, and arguably even optimal. In this case, that means an even larger segment of the population suffers from mild constipation.

States of Constipation

Other characteristics are used to determine constipation, such as stool consistency, the effort required for a bowel movement and the completeness of evacuation. Constipation can be any of the following:

- If the stool is hard and dehydrated, or pellet-like
- If there is straining when passing the stool, even if it is normal or soft in consistency
- If the stool feels incompletely evacuated
- If bowel movements are infrequent, defined as fewer than 3 occurrences a week
- Combinations of any of the previous three symptoms

Each of these situations may be experienced with either normal frequency of bowel movements or infrequent bowel movements.

FAQ

Q How does constipation relate to acne?

A Improper elimination through the digestive tract essentially leads to a backup throughout the system. Hormones and metabolic by-products are not efficiently excreted and can potentially reabsorb into circulation if they are not properly eliminated on a regular basis. This can affect the ideal balance of hormones in the body and cause inflammation. The skin has the largest surface area where blood circulates, and recirculating by-products can therefore trigger inflammation at this site. For patients prone to acne, constipation is likely to contribute to a continuing cycle of inflammation.

In a clinical setting, when patients have both acne and constipation, treating the constipation almost always leads to some relief from acne. I often observe some degree of improvement in breakout intensity and/or frequency after correcting constipation as the first step in the treatment plan.

Secrets to Resolving Constipation

We all know about increasing fiber to improve bowel regularity. The problem is that your bowel doesn't always respond the way it should, even when fiber intake levels exceed the recommended daily amounts.

In these cases, a food sensitivity may be complicating the picture and keeping your digestion functioning at a slower than normal state. However, it takes a few weeks to test for food sensitivities and eliminate them from your diet and for your body to adjust. This is the best long-term solution to resolving constipation, but in most cases, you want relief from constipation as soon as possible, particularly if it is playing a role in your acne.

Magnesium

One of the most reliable and safest ways to treat constipation is magnesium. I don't recommend the typical commercially available milk of magnesia, which often includes ingredients such as various sugars (sucrose, dextrose, maltodextrin, starches), food dyes and artificial sweeteners. It may help your constipation, but these ingredients are far from supportive of your skin health.

I recommend to my patients that they use a basic magnesium-citrate supplement, either in capsule or

> **Did You Know?**
>
> **How Magnesium Works**
>
> Magnesium works by osmosis, the passive movement of water from an area of lower concentration to a place of higher concentration. With a high concentration of magnesium in your colon, water follows it because of the osmotic effect, and thereby adds more water to your stool. The higher water content of the stool makes it easier to pass, with less straining and more complete evacuation.

powder form. Typical doses for capsules range from 150 mg to 200 mg. I recommend starting with one capsule before bed and increasing the dose by one capsule each day until a dose is achieved that leads to normal well-formed, easy-to-pass and complete bowel movements.

Magnesium's mode of action is gentler and safer than that of a laxative because it does not stimulate the nerves of the digestive tract. Pharmaceutical and herbal laxatives both target the nervous system to improve constipation; however, this leads to dependency on them, and often a rebound effect occurs, where constipation worsens after ceasing the use of laxatives.

As we incorporate diet changes that take into account food sensitivities and healthier food selection, the goal is to encourage the colon to function normally over time and to gradually eliminate magnesium from the patient's regimen.

> Treating acne effectively requires awareness of your emotional health and psychosocial stresses,
> and finding ways to improve them.

The Gut-Brain-Skin Connection

The gut-brain-skin axis is important to consider when treating acne effectively. Rather than just focusing on the state of the skin, it's equally important to address a patient's psychological health and digestive health. In other words, treating acne effectively requires awareness of your emotional health and psychosocial stresses, and finding ways to improve them. Additionally, the way you process and absorb your food, the health of your intestines, the quality of your bowel movements and any gastrointestinal symptoms may provide more clues to improving the health of your skin for the long term.

Brain–Skin Connection

Researchers have studied a connection between stress and inflammation of the skin. In 2008, a study on mice determined that this connection was brought on by a component of the nervous system. Allergic dermatitis, an allergic inflammatory disease of the skin, was shown to be exacerbated by stress. A small protein called substance P mediates the response from the nervous system to present as inflammation on the skin. This connection is known as the brain–skin connection.

Gut–Brain Connection

Studies have already confirmed a gut–brain connection. This gut–brain axis has been shown to have bidirectional nerve communication, which means that there is back-and-forth communication between the brain and the nervous system of the gut (the enteric nervous system, often termed the "second brain"). The brain assists in directing the function and coordination of our digestive function. More intriguing is the communication of our gut to our brain, which can influence our motivation, moods and cognitive abilities, even shaping our decision-making abilities.

The gut microbiome (the collection of bacteria in our digestive tract) also plays an important role in the gut–brain axis. Supporting the gut microbiome with probiotic supplementation has been shown to improve the symptoms of irritable bowel syndrome. The makeup of our intestinal bacterial flora plays a role in our digestive health by affecting the immune system and nervous system.

Research Spotlight
A Unifying Theory

If there are gut–brain, gut–skin and brain–skin axes, could there potentially be a gut-brain-skin relationship?

The concept of a gut-brain-skin axis was first proposed in a study 85 years ago. The authors, Dr. John Stokes and Dr. Donald Pillsbury, proposed that emotions and psychological abnormalities impacted the skin and that there was likely a mechanism involved that originated in the digestive tract. Therefore, the brain, the gut and the skin influenced the health of one another in an intimate cyclical relationship. Only recently has this relationship been further clarified.

A rat study in 2010 investigated the stress response triggering both skin inflammation and the inhibition of hair growth. This stress response was known to be triggered by a neurogenic pathway (mediated by the nervous system, or brain). Interestingly, when these rats were fed a strain of lactobacillus — a type of normal gut bacteria — the bacteria actually dampened the stress response of inflamed skin and inhibited hair growth.

By improving the health of the gut microbiome (the important gut ecosystem comprised of trillions of bacteria), the nervous system and, therefore, the skin were impacted. There was a connection between the gut, the brain and the skin. The authors of this study proposed that more research should be conducted on the gut-brain-skin axis.

Gut–Skin Connection

There is also a link between the gut and the skin.

A study in 2013 showed that incorporating probiotics into an antibiotic acne protocol improved acne in subjects. There is encouraging information to support the use of prebiotics (specific types of dietary fibers that are the "food" for your good bacteria) and probiotics in the treatment of inflammatory dermatological disorders, including acne. These results show that by improving the health of the gut, we also improve the health of the skin.

As a naturopathic practitioner, I believe optimizing the health of the digestive tract is key in treating skin conditions.

Balancing Hormones

Hormones are important regulators in our body that help keep us in a healthy state of flux. They respond to and compensate for deficiencies in other aspects of our health, with the main goal of helping us function and stay alive. But when they are elevated or reduced (beyond normal levels) as a compensatory mechanism over a sustained period of time, we may experience adverse effects.

The best-known example is diabetes. Our blood must maintain a safe margin of sugar levels. When we do not eat regularly and we consume excess sugars — or foods that turn into sugar — our blood sugar spikes. In response, insulin is released, which brings the amount of sugar in the blood back down to an acceptable range. When our body stops responding to constant surges of sugars and, hence, insulin, we develop diabetes. When diabetes develops and our hormones struggle to maintain an equilibrium (keeping blood sugar stable), we may experience a multitude of symptoms, signs and other health conditions, as well as compensatory reactions.

Insulin and IGF (Insulin-Like Growth Factor)

These hormones are linked to comedogenesis (the development of acne pimples), and their release into the bloodstream is closely linked to diet. The Vibrant Skin Diet Plan (see Chapter 10, page 134) was designed to first normalize blood sugar and, subsequently, to reduce the insulin and IGF response in the body. Refer to the Vibrant Skin Diet Plan for a detailed explanation of how foods can normalize excessive insulin and IGF secretion.

Cortisol and Melatonin

Cortisol is a stress hormone secreted by your adrenal glands in response to stress. Melatonin is a hormone produced by your brain's pineal gland to help promote and sustain sleep. Excess cortisol levels stimulate acne (see Chapter 2) and may be the result of various types of stress, underlying disease or the use of corticosteroid medication.

Cortisol has a relationship with melatonin in the body. When cortisol levels are high, they suppress the output of melatonin. In a 1992 study from Italy, human subjects exercised just before midnight. The physical stress (exercise) increased the secretion of cortisol, which was then followed by a suppression of melatonin.

Doc Talk

There is a vicious cycle of chronic stress and insufficient sleep, which feed into one another. This is an unhealthy scenario that I see all too often in my practice. Because elevated cortisol is associated with acne, stress and poor sleeping patterns need to be addressed in order to properly improve acne. Reducing cortisol and improving melatonin levels can be achieved by addressing physical and psychological stress (see Chapter 8). The impact of these hormones on acne is often overlooked and underestimated.

Relative Blood Concentrations of Melatonin and Cortisol Diurnal Fluctuations

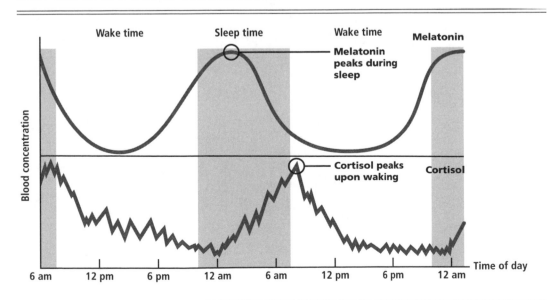

Progesterone and Estrogen

Progesterone and estrogen hormones related to acne are connected to the timing of a woman's menstrual cycle. In the second half of the menstrual cycle — the interval leading up to the start of menstruation — both progesterone and estrogen spike. This interval is also when a woman experiences premenstrual symptoms, the severity and duration of which can vary greatly from one person to another. Common symptoms experienced in the time preceding a period may include some of the following: acne, mood changes, bloating, diarrhea or constipation, headaches, cramping, breast tenderness and back pain.

When estrogen levels are high relative to progesterone levels, the number and severity of premenstrual symptoms are likely to increase. The measure for quantifying this relationship is the estrogen-to-progesterone ratio.

Progesterone and Estrogen Fluctuations During Menstrual Cycle

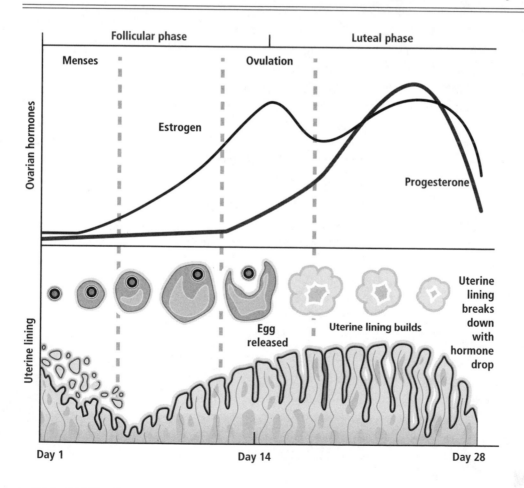

Research Spotlight: PMS Link

A case-control study in 1984 examined patients with premenstrual syndrome (PMS) against participants without any premenstrual symptoms. It showed that there was an altered estrogen-to-progesterone ratio in 7 out of 12 subjects with severe PMS.

A 1981 study from England showed that in the 4 days preceding menses, estrogen levels were higher in subjects with PMS as compared to the control group. Additionally, from 5 to 9 days preceding a period, progesterone levels were lower in those with PMS.

FAQ

 Q What can we do to decrease the estrogen-to-progesterone ratio?

A The first step is to decrease exposure to foreign estrogens. You can do this by decreasing your exposure to plastics, pesticides, commercial skin-care products and pollutants. Start by choosing glass, stainless steel or ceramic food and beverage containers in place of plastics. Select organic produce and meats to limit your exposure to pesticides. Choose skin-care products with natural ingredients. Pollutants may be more difficult to avoid, particularly related to outdoor air quality, but at home, you can use an air purifier in addition to a host of indoor plants to help process airborne chemicals.

The next step is to consume more phytoestrogenic foods (which act as "weak" estrogens in the body) to decrease your net dose of estrogen internally. Doing so buffers against the effects of "strong" foreign estrogens. Organic tofu, tempeh and miso soup can be used to reduce your body's estrogen burden. They do this by displacing the "strong" foreign estrogens (found in plastics, pesticides, commercial skin-care products and pollutants), such that they can be eliminated by the body.

Finally, eat more cruciferous vegetables, such as cabbage, cauliflower, broccoli, kale, Brussels sprouts and rapini. These contain certain natural compounds — for example, calcium D-glucarate and indole-3-carbinol — that support the elimination of excess estrogenic compounds from the liver.

Testosterone and Dihydrotestosterone

Androgens are closely connected to the development of acne. They stimulate the secretion of sebum from the sebaceous glands, as well as hyperkeratinization, a process that increases the production of a protein in the skin that congests pores. This combination leads to blocked sebaceous glands and the formation of acne.

Research Spotlight: Androgens and Acne

A 1995 study compared the hormone levels of 33 men with acne and 33 men who were acne-free (control group). The acne patients had a higher median level of measured androgens (testosterone, androstenedione and free androgen index) compared to the control group. This indicates that there are likely elevations in androgens for men with acne compared to those without acne.

Androgens include testosterone and several of its metabolic derivatives. This category of hormones controls the development and maintenance of male traits. When they surge in the body — during puberty or with anabolic steroid use — one of the characteristic adverse effects is acne. When acne appears years after puberty, a hormonal component related to excess androgen may be involved. There may be an excess of testosterone in either male or female patients.

Testing Levels

Testing blood serum testosterone levels may not provide enough information to determine if your results are actually high relative to someone who is acne-free. Androgen levels may still fall within the normal range (the range of androgen levels in normal, healthy individuals) when measured in the laboratory.

Saliva hormone testing — which measures bioavailable hormone, or hormone that is being used by your tissues — may provide you with more insight than standard blood hormone tests. Saliva hormone tests also often provide tighter normal-range values and, as a result, can provide you with a measuring point. For example, your testosterone may fall in the normal range for a healthy individual, but it may be flagged because it falls at the high end of the normal range. This indicates that elevated testosterone may be contributing to your acne.

Testosterone can convert into another, more potent androgen called dihydrotestosterone (DHT). Approximately 5% to 10% of testosterone typically converts into DHT in the body. DHT has twice the effect of testosterone on androgen receptors, so an equivalent amount of DHT may have twice the power to trigger acne, compared to testosterone. Elevated levels of DHT are connected to prostate cancer, benign enlargement of the prostate, male pattern baldness and acne.

Natural Inhibitors of 5-Alpha Reductase

The enzyme 5-alpha reductase dictates the conversion of testosterone to DHT. The following herbs, foods and nutrients can inhibit the levels of 5-alpha reductase enzyme in your body, and therefore the production of DHT:

- *Ganoderma lucidum* **(reishi mushroom):** Compounds in ganoderma called triterpenoids were shown to inhibit 5-alpha reductase activity.
- **Green tea:** The leaves contain epigallocatechin gallate (EGCG), which inhibits the formation of DHT.
- **Polyunsaturated fatty acids:** Specifically, gamma linolenic acid (found in borage oil, evening primrose oil and black currant oil) inhibits the production of 5-alpha reductase.
- **Riboflavin:** Vitamin B_2 (found in tempeh, tofu, spinach, beet greens, mushrooms and almonds) inhibits the production of 5-alpha reductase.
- *Serenoa repens* **(saw palmetto):** An extract of this herb was shown to reduce DHT.
- **Zinc:** Shown to specifically inhibit 5-alpha reductase.

CHAPTER 8
Stress Management

Stress Acne

Jacob, a 28-year-old male, had clear skin in his teenage years but developed moderate acne in his early 20s. It appeared on his cheeks, around his nose and on his forehead.

He was well researched in nutrition and had already made many healthy improvements to his diet a couple of years before meeting with me. I helped Jacob fine-tune some aspects of his diet and conducted a food sensitivity test, which determined some individual intolerances.

Jacob had studied law and was now articling at a big law firm. As a result, he was under intense pressure and worked long hours, with little time to exercise or sleep. His lunches and dinners were catered by the firm, and although he tried to choose the healthiest options available, they were not always ideal.

We implemented the Vibrant Skin Diet Plan, and I encouraged him to make sleep a priority as much as he could within his schedule. We also ran a saliva hormone panel that measured his levels of cortisol (stress hormone) throughout the day — morning, noon, evening and bedtime — along with testosterone. His results showed that his cortisol levels were high when they shouldn't be (bedtime) and low in the first half of the day (when they should be at their highest). This was not surprising, based on his chronic stress. His testosterone level was also at the high end of the normal range for his age.

The combination of these results indicated that Jacob's highly stressful lifestyle and lack of sleep were playing major roles in the perpetuation of his acne. We worked together to make a priorities list and figured out compromises in his weekly routine so that he could manage to get adequate sleep.

After 3 months, we followed up. Jacob had been able to end his dependence on caffeine and subsequently improve his focus, sleep quality and energy. Because he was more efficient at work, he was able to get more done during his time at the office and get a much needed extra hour of sleep every night.

His acne had improved dramatically by the 3-month mark, by approximately 75%. And at future visits, we noted that his skin continued to improve with his healthier routine and diet.

With his body more rested, we also discovered that Jacob was much more tolerant of foods in his diet that had previously triggered acne breakouts. His immune system was better regulated, and his tolerance threshold to allergenic foods increased as a result of the improved quality and duration of his sleep.

Physical Stress

Physical stresses are stressors that prevent our body from functioning at its optimum. The three most underestimated physical stressors — ones that have dramatically changed over the past century — include lack of exercise, lack of sleep and poor nutrition.

Exercise, sleep and proper nutrition are basic and fundamental aspects of our health that are sorely overlooked in modern society. Exercise is the process by which our body maintains, optimizes and strengthens itself. Sleep is our body's time to recuperate and heal. Nutrition is the fuel that allows us to function, and the quality of the nutrition determines how well we thrive. These all need to be optimal for us to be well and feel well, and also for our skin to be healthy.

Our body is a complicated machine, but with a huge added bonus: it is highly adaptable. We adapt to stresses that are not beneficial to our health and that may even be harmful to our body. Our body adjusts, adapts, resets its new "norm" and continues on its way. This adaptation process to harmful stimuli is called maladaptation. We have a built-in tolerance buffer that makes it seem as if everything is okay — even when sacrifices are being made by our repair systems and metabolic pathways. These sacrifices may not show up as distinct symptoms immediately, but over time, physical manifestations can develop.

The optimal diet and nutrition plan that is best suited for the treatment of acne is explained in more detail in Chapter 10.

Exercise

Exercise was a part of daily life a few centuries ago. But automation, transportation and mass production have

> **Did You Know?**
>
> **Achieving Exercise Goals**
> Talk to a registered kinesiologist or experienced certified personal trainer to help you design a safe exercise regimen that works toward achieving your personal fitness goals.

Research Spotlight: Sweat It

A study in 2008 investigated the effects of exercising on acne. Researchers compared three groups: one group didn't exercise; one group exercised, then showered immediately; and one exercised, then showered several hours later. There were no significant differences in acne presentation between or within any of these groups after the 2-week study. The study showed that perspiring when exercising does not aggravate acne.

changed that, and our need to exercise has quickly depleted and continues to do so. The vast majority of occupations involve sitting down at a desk and staring at a computer. If we need something to eat, there is no need to forage, harvest or hunt; we simply drive to a grocery store or restaurant.

Benefits of Exercise

We need to incorporate exercise to benefit our overall health, but exercising may specifically help with acne in the following ways:

- Normalizing hormones that are out of balance
- Helping you manage stress
- Improving immune function
- Decreasing inflammation in the body
- Improving insulin sensitivity

Sometimes people avoid exercise because they believe that it may aggravate acne because of sweating, but this is not the case for the majority of people with acne. The only form of acne that might be aggravated by exercise is acne mechanica. Acne mechanica is aggravated by heat and pressure, but by taking preventive measures, such as wearing loose clothes that allow heat to radiate away from the skin (certain synthetic materials or pure cotton), exercise can be done safely without directly instigating acne.

> Acne mechanica is aggravated by heat and pressure, but by taking preventive measures, such as wearing loose clothes that allow heat to radiate away from the skin (certain synthetic materials or pure cotton), exercise can be done safely without directly instigating acne.

Exercise Tips

Start slowly, making sure to exercise according to your fitness level, and gradually increase the intensity of your exercise regimen.

- Find exercises that you enjoy (at the gym or home, or by joining group sports).
- Always start slowly and gradually increase your intensity.
- Choose an exercise buddy to keep you company and make you feel accountable to your routine.
- Record your progress and incorporate incremental fitness goals you can work toward.
- Schedule time for your exercise.
- Make exercise a priority; encourage it to become a habit.
- Stay hydrated — replenish lost hydration by consuming 4 cups (1 L) of fluids for every 1 hour of moderately intense physical exercise.

- Work up to a goal of 45 to 60 minutes of regular moderate to intense physical exercise three to four times a week after 3 months.
- If you have physical limitations, consult with your doctor or physiotherapist to determine which exercises are appropriate for you.
- Consult with an experienced certified personal trainer or registered kinesiologist to design a program that is safe and works best for you.

Sleep

Sleep is one part of the triad of crucial requirements for your body, in addition to regular exercise and a healthy diet. Assess your sleep patterns to determine if inadequate sleep is affecting your quality of life and triggering your acne. Try to determine your sleep duration, quality and regularity and how these are impacting your waking life. Once you have a better picture of your sleep patterns, you can determine what may have been disrupting your sleep and how to improve it.

If you need more assistance, consult with a health professional. Try to avoid a prescription sedative unless you have exhausted all other options.

Start by improving your sleep hygiene (your bedtime routine) and ensure that you address stress levels, anxiety and depression. See Sleep Tips, on page 110, for additional support in getting a good night's sleep.

Most important, make sleep a priority. It is critical for the health of your skin, as well as your mind and body.

> Assess your sleep patterns to determine if inadequate sleep is affecting your quality of life and triggering your acne. Try to determine your sleep duration, quality and regularity and how these are impacting your waking life.

Sleep Journal

Keep a sleep journal over a couple of weeks and record answers to the following questions:

- What is your bedtime routine?
- Did you use light-emitting electronic devices before bed or in bed?
- Did you use alcohol, cannabis or other substances to assist with your sleep?
- What time did you get in bed?
- Approximately how long did it take you to fall asleep?
- How many times did you wake up at night?
- What time did you wake up for the day?
- Did you use the snooze function on your alarm clock?

- How many hours did you sleep?
- Did you feel rested in the morning?
- How was the quality of your sleep?
- What prevented you from sleeping?
- Did you feel anxiety before bed or in the middle of the night?
- Did you nap during the day?

Sleep Tips

- Follow a routine every night, such as taking a relaxing bath or reading a printed book.
- Wear comfortable sleep clothes.
- When you wake at night, no matter what, do not look at the time. Looking at the time can create anxiety and prevent you from returning to sleep.
- Shut down all light-emitting electronic devices 90 minutes before bed.
- Make sure your room is adequately dark. If, for whatever reason, it can't be, use a sleep mask.
- Consider a white noise machine to drown out background noise.
- Wear earplugs to reduce external sounds that are beyond your control.
- Eliminate caffeine, alcohol and other substances that stimulate or sedate the nervous system.
- If you worry about your alarm not sounding, set more than one alarm. This way, you can trust that you won't miss your alarm ringing and you'll sleep more peacefully.
- Do not use the snooze button. Snoozing wastes time during which you could have continued to sleep. Set the alarm once and get up at that time. Your body will accommodate.
- Do not fool yourself that "catching up" on sleep (for example, on the weekend) works. Undersleeping and oversleeping both affect health outcomes. Find a way to even out your sleep hours throughout the week, instead of playing catch-up.
- Invest in a high-quality mattress and pillow. Physical and postural discomforts are common factors that cause insomnia.
- Ask your doctor for a referral to a sleep clinic to rule out any underlying medical conditions, such as sleep apnea.
- Ask your naturopath about melatonin or other natural sleep remedies that can be safely used.
- If you have anxiety about day-to-day responsibilities, write a to-do list in the evening. This can prevent your mind

Do not fool yourself that "catching up" on sleep (for example, on the weekend) works. Undersleeping and oversleeping both affect health outcomes. Find a way to even out your sleep hours throughout the week, instead of playing catch-up.

from inflating the stresses right before bed or in the middle of the night.

- Go to bed at the same time every night.
- Keep lights dimmed in your home for 2 hours before your bedtime.
- Ensure that you are properly managing your stress levels. Talk to a therapist if you feel overwhelmed by stresses.

Chemical Stress

Smoking

Smoking exacerbates numerous health conditions, and acne is included in the list. Inhaling the combustible by-products in cigarette smoke creates reactive chemicals called free radicals, and these damage tissue and disrupt normal cell function, intercellular communication and proper circulation.

There are some studies that show the opposite effect, that nicotine may have a protective effect on acne. Nevertheless, cigarette smoking is never something that should be recommended in the treatment of acne. It increases the risk of a multitude of serious chronic health concerns — lung disease, heart disease, stroke and cancer, to name just a few — which automatically outweighs any potential (but yet unconfirmed) benefit that smoking may have for improving acne. Even if nicotine were shown to improve acne, there are a few compelling reasons to avoid it as a treatment approach. First, it is an addictive substance; second, it does not treat the cause of the acne. Most important, nicotine would not be a healthy long-term solution for treating acne.

The toxic compounds in cigarette smoke stress our skin cells, thereby creating abnormal reactions, such as the well-known response of accelerated skin aging and wrinkling. Smoking also likely accelerates and intensifies the development of acne.

> The toxic compounds in cigarette smoke stress our skin cells, thereby creating abnormal reactions, such as the well-known response of accelerated skin aging and wrinkling. Smoking also likely accelerates and intensifies the development of acne.

Research Spotlight: Smoke Damage

Cigarette smokers have been shown to have higher levels of the cell messengers (cytokines) that promote inflammation. Specifically, a cytokine called interleukin-1 alpha was found to be higher in a 2014 study of subjects with acne lesions. These cytokines may contribute to perpetuating the cycle of acne by creating oxidative damage within the sebaceous glands.

Did You Know?

Scoring Substance Abuse

If you are using alcohol and/or recreational drugs on a regular basis and they are impacting your social relationships and physical health, you may have a substance abuse problem. Acne may be a manifestation of alcohol and drug use, but there may be more crucial psychological disturbances that need to be addressed. If addiction is part of the picture, speak with a therapist specializing in substance abuse.

Alcohol and Recreational Drugs

Excessive alcohol intake and regular cannabis use have both been shown to increase the likelihood of developing acne. Regular use of any illicit or recreational drug is likely to exacerbate oxidative damage in the body, which would thereby increase the risk of acne. Besides the active constituents that trigger damaging intracellular oxidation reactions, the combustible chemicals released from smoking recreational drugs will also vastly increase any potential oxidative stress in the body and skin.

Although alcohol is theoretically safe to consume in small amounts in the long term and may even offer some antioxidant protection (for example, in the case of wine), it should be removed from the diet in the short term when treating acne. Alcohol contains easily assimilated carbohydrates, which can worsen acne. Furthermore, alcohol is added to sugary liquids (soft drinks and juice, sometimes with artificial ingredients), and these also likely perpetuate the inflammatory cycle. The yeast in any fermented alcohol — beer, wine, cider, sake — causes a common food sensitivity that may also potentially aggravate acne.

Monitor Substance Use

Be aware of your substance-use pattern (alcohol and/or recreational drugs). Assess your frequency of use and how it impacts your life. If you answer yes to any of the following questions, you may have a substance abuse problem. Talk to your naturopath or therapist for guidance.

- Is stress a trigger for you to consume alcohol and/or use recreational drugs?
- Do you think about using these substances more than a few times per week?
- Is your dependency affecting work, family, friends or relationships?
- Has anyone ever commented that you have a substance abuse problem?
- Is substance use affecting your sleep, energy, motivation or tendency to get sick?
- Do you feel that you can't live without alcohol and/or recreational drugs?

Reducing Oxidative Stress

The first step in addressing your body's total oxidative stress is to reduce or eliminate obvious triggers, such as smoking, recreational drugs, alcohol, exposure to pollutants, radiation and unhealthy foods. The second step is to incorporate antioxidant foods in your diet.

1. Reducing Triggers

Reduce your exposure to plastics, cleaning products, bacterial/viral/fungal infections, commercial skin-care products (see Cosmetic Ingredients to Avoid, page 73), chlorinated or fluoridated water, fire retardants and any other modern toxic chemical that you may be exposed to on a daily basis. Being dehydrated can also be a trigger for oxidative stress.

- **Radiation:** Radiation comes in the form of wireless communication, to which we are now chronically exposed. Reduce your exposure as much as possible. Constant exposure to radiation may disrupt the normal chemistry in our cells and tissues, presumably by triggering the formation of chemicals called reactive oxygen species, which lead to oxidative cellular damage.
- **Pollutants:** Pollutants in our air, water and food supply are ubiquitous and, as a result, persist in our bodies and environment. Chemicals such as phthalates — chemicals in plastics that make them flexible — are in products we use many times throughout a typical day. Phthalates are even found in the majority of people's blood and tissues, despite the fact that this is a relatively new chemical group that we have been exposed to only in recent decades.

  There are endless additional pollutants to which we have a risk of chronic exposure: mercury (in water and seafood), carbon monoxide (air pollutant), cadmium (exhaust fumes), pesticides (fruits and vegetables), polychlorinated biphenyls (coolants), perfluorooctanoic acid and polytetrafluoroethylene (nonstick products, including Teflon), polycyclic aromatic hydrocarbons (fossil fuels) and dioxins (pulp and paper mills), just to name a few.
- **Unhealthy foods:** Unhealthy foods and food ingredients that can trigger oxidative stress should also be avoided, including hydrogenated or partially hydrogenated oils, preservatives, artificial flavors and colors, heat-processed oils, sugar, alcohol, charred meats and rancid oils. Foods sprayed with pesticides are also detrimental to our health. Avoid foods and liquids that have been stored for a long time in plastic or metal (for example, bottled water and canned tuna), as these materials can leach into the food and be ingested.

> Constant exposure to radiation may disrupt the normal chemistry in our cells and tissues, presumably by triggering the formation of chemicals called reactive oxygen species, which lead to oxidative cellular damage.

2. Incorporating Antioxidants

The second step is to regularly consume foods that contain powerful healthy antioxidants. People get caught up in the newest health craze reported to have the "most" antioxidants — they consume this food item for a few weeks and then fall off the wagon. Choose a few common antioxidants that you can find at your local grocery store and incorporate them into your cooking on a daily basis. Go for things that are accessible and work with your style of cooking and eating.

Doc Talk

I tell patients that antioxidant foods, as a very general rule, can stain your clothes. Antioxidant chemicals naturally reflect light. So, if a food has a lot of color in it, you can safely assume that it is chock-full of healthy antioxidants. Think of these foods as good examples: turmeric, blueberries, pomegranates, beets, tomatoes and dark leafy greens.

This general rule, however, does not mean that the opposite is also true. Many foods that don't have a lot of color can still be plentiful in antioxidants: fish, nuts, garlic, cauliflower and beans.

For the record: this is just a rule of thumb and absolutely does not apply to cola products and artificial colors!

Mental-Emotional Stress

When you experience a perceived threat, your heart rate increases, stress hormones (such as cortisol) release, and your sympathetic nervous system (fight-or-flight response) is activated. Cortisol tells your body to dump glucose into your bloodstream so that muscles have access to it if you need to fight or run away from the negative stimulus. Of course, if you are in a meeting at work, fighting and running away are likely not professionally acceptable options. As a result, your body does not use the sugar in a physically active way and the blood-sugar release is not consumed by muscle tissue as it should be. In response, your body releases insulin to normalize your sugar level.

You may recognize similarities to what happens when you eat foods that elevate blood sugar. Think of your stress response as eating a chocolate bar. Understanding the similarity of these reactions helps you make the connection between stress and acne. You must be able to manage mental-emotional stress and strengthen your stress tolerance in order to have clear skin for the long term.

A Balancing Act

A very important concept for patients suffering from acne is the role of cumulative stress.

It can be mind-numbing to determine why a reintroduced food is sometimes tolerated without a breakout, yet at other times a variation of the same food may lead to a major acne flare-up. Rather than losing sleep overanalyzing your diet and wondering why one form or amount of food may or may not trigger a relapse of acne, it is more important to step back and examine potential stressors other than just the dietary ones.

If, for example, you are currently experiencing a great deal of stress at work, with many looming deadlines and pressures, and, as a result, are sleeping inadequately, you need to understand that this is a multipronged stress in itself. When you take these stressors into consideration, you may notice that, during this time period, your tolerance to certain foods declines.

FAQ

Do you have some strategies to help me manage my acne during stressful periods?

Once your skin becomes stable and clear, always be aware of your total burden of stress. Here are two strategies for maintaining your healthy skin and managing your diet:

1. During periods of high stress that are beyond your control, your threshold tolerance to dietary triggers may be depressed, so go back to a more stringent diet by following the guidelines of the Vibrant Skin Diet Plan.
2. When external stresses settle down and acne is under control, you can once again allow for more flexibility. Carefully reintroduce foods that may have triggered a skin flare-up; your body will be more tolerant.

Remember, your skin responds to stress from all realms — mental, physical and emotional. It is a delicate balancing act, and when some of these aspects of our health are compromised, we have to compensate for it by focusing our attention on improving other areas (like diet).

Picture a canoe being stocked with supplies. It can hold a moderate amount of items and its function isn't greatly affected. Even with a relatively full load, if handled carefully, the canoe can be steered and guided safely. However, when the supplies are stacked too high and are too heavy, it is easy for the canoe to tip over.

Likewise, the more weight and stress your body carries, the easier it is for your body to "tip over" and succumb to a physical manifestation like acne.

Dealing with Stress

It is not uncommon to hear "Yes, I deal with my stress by exercising" or "I have a drink after work to de-stress." These strategies help distract you from the stress you experienced earlier in the day, but are they actually helping you to better deal with stress in the moment?

The answer is no. The two examples are coping mechanisms that help balance out your stress levels in the short term, and they may be useful to help you get through the day. Of course, some of these coping strategies are much healthier than others, but they are not retraining you to change how you experience stress in the first place.

Two people may perceive a potentially threatening situation completely differently. What one person considers a high-level acute stress may just be a passing moment to someone else. These triggers and our reactions to them are based on our experiences, our genetics, our personality and the environment in which we were raised.

The most challenging part of our human experience is to improve our innate reactions and to rewire our established patterns of negativity in response to stressful stimuli. If we can achieve these improvements, we can objectively and calmly react to stressful situations so they don't aggravate

Did You Know?

Changing the Stress Response

Improving our reactions to stress can take a lifetime, and we need measures that can start us on the right path. If we adopt new, constructive habits that help us settle our stress response, we will slowly view situations more objectively and react more rationally and less emotionally.

FAQ

Q **What can we do about stressful situations?**

A The pragmatic solution to dealing with a stress stimulus is one of two things:

1. Get rid of the stress.
2. Find ways to better manage your response to the stress.

us and perpetuate the instigating trigger. In this way, we neutralize the inherent potential energy in the initial stimulus and, in essence, defuse an emotional grenade.

Work and School

If stress comes from work or school, as it commonly does, you are not likely to stop either activity; you have bills to pay and knowledge to gain. However, in certain situations where the stress is insurmountable, you may need to take a step back and reexamine your choices. It may mean finding new opportunities or even changing your line of work in order to function within your own stress tolerance levels and to improve your quality of life. Keep in mind that, although stress can manifest as acne, stress can also contribute to chronic disease.

Relationships, Family and Friends

When the stress originates from your family, friends or partner, things are more complicated. A relationship, whether a friendship or a love interest, may be broken off if it becomes too toxic and leads to chronic stress. You might choose to put more effort and communication into a relationship to salvage it, but if your actions are not reciprocated, you may need to sever the relationship to protect yourself.

Family is a little trickier. Your family is always your family, and that relationship is nonnegotiable. That being said, you may need to distance yourself at some point from a family member who is a source of chronic negativity. Because familial and blood ties are deep, it can be one of the most difficult choices to make. You may even need to seek professional help to guide you on further communication or on the difficult decision to stop communication completely in order to protect yourself.

Stress-Release Exercise

This simple technique will help you reset both emotionally and physiologically in the midst of a stressful situation. This relaxation process can be done within a few minutes, and practice can help you feel calm even after a few seconds. While it is a calming method, it also serves as a reminder to your endocrine and nervous systems that you are initiating different pathways than you normally take. You can perform this exercise alone or inconspicuously when surrounded by other people, whether at work, with friends or family, or in a public place.

1. **Figure out where your happy place is.** Your happy place does not have to be the cliché of lying on a white sandy beach on a sunny, perfect day, with calm waves lapping the shore. It can be this image, but it does not have to be. A happy place can be envisioning your child's laughter, your wedding day or your dog sleeping in the crook of your arm. It could be the feeling you get when you are relaxing in the sun in your backyard or running through a ravine on a clear day. For some people, it may be cooking an incredible meal, writing a creative story, painting a vibrant canvas or taking a hot bubble bath.

   Your happy place should be an image of a memory or an experience that gives you that indescribable feeling of sincere, unadulterated joy and one that causes you to smile uncontrollably.

2. **Visualize your happy place.** Fully immerse yourself in that memory and notice how it makes you feel content, comfortable and calm. To start out, practice this exercise while you are in a relaxed state, preferably seated in a comfortable chair or lying down. This usually works best with your eyes closed. The more often you practice this technique, the easier it will be to reach a similar state of positive emotions and physical feelings. When you are able to do this successfully, not only will your psycho-emotional state recollect those positive feelings, but the hormones (endorphins, dopamine, serotonin) associated with them will also be engaged. This means that you are truly reliving that experience, emotionally and chemically.

   Practice this every day for 10 to 15 minutes. You can make it part of your morning routine, your lunch break or your bedtime routine as you settle down to sleep at night.

3. **Practice deep, slow breathing.** This simple method helps to oxygenate your tissues and helps you de-stress. Breathe in through your nose slowly, deeply and fully, feeling your lungs expand with air. At the top of your breath, when your lungs are as full as they can be, hold your breath and slowly count to three. Gradually exhale through your mouth. Expel as much air as you can from your lungs, until you can't release anymore. At the bottom of this breath, hold and slowly count to three again. Slowly breathe in again, as you did initially, and repeat

Deep, slow breathing helps to oxygenate your tissues and helps you de-stress.

the process. Inhale and exhale in this manner throughout your calming visualization. It will become second nature.

As you become comfortable with this breathing method, you can increase the hold at the top and bottom of your breath. Hold for 4 seconds each, then 5.

4. **Integrate breathing and calming techniques into everyday situations.** Methods like meditation and breathing are useful to center yourself and give you insight, but they are typically carried out in a calm, comfortable setting. The challenge is to incorporate and implement relaxation techniques in stressful environments.

Start with small situations, such as a car cutting in front of you on the road, a salesperson providing poor customer service, or accidentally dropping your soup on the floor. These are small events that can often quickly trigger frustration, anger or even rage. Breathe and find your happy place, and do this for a full minute or two, until you feel ready to reassess the situation realistically and from a calmer perspective.

Use the same methods when dealing with pressing deadlines at work, when you encounter a manipulative colleague or when you have an argument with a friend or family member. This technique gives you a bit of space to approach the situation in a calmer, clearer state of mind.

> Small events can often quickly trigger frustration, anger or even rage. Breathe and find your happy place, and do this for a full minute or two, until you feel ready to reassess the situation realistically and from a calmer perspective.

Assessing a Stressful Situation

Situation: A driver cuts you off on the highway, which makes you see red. Your temperature rises, you quickly become enraged and you automatically react: "How dare he startle me and make me slam on my brakes? That awful human being made me lose my spot in the lane. I am going to speed up to him, honk my horn, look him in the eyes and shake my fist at him to teach him a lesson. He'll be sorry!"

Alternative Response: Alternatively, you may realize beforehand that driving tends to cause you stress and that you often become short-tempered behind the wheel and experience road rage. When a driver cuts you off, you instinctively get angry, but you tell yourself: "I'm feeling angry again — I want to teach that guy a lesson. But really it's futile to do that because nothing positive ever comes out of it. In the end, it just makes my stress even worse. Really, I'm just stressing myself out and wasting my own time.

And that guy could be my father. Or maybe he is exhausted and stressed out himself. Anyhow, maybe it's just a reminder to me to drive more cautiously."

Strategies to Better Manage Stress

- **Meditation:** Work to calm your mind through the practice of meditation. You may be able to find local meditation workshops that are offered for free at hospitals, community centers or private clinics.

- **Counseling:** If self-help strategies are just not cutting it, you may need the help of a professional. Licensed psychologists and psychotherapists are trained to assist you with implementing behavioral strategies to repattern your reactions to stresses. They can also lend a caring ear to help you deal with your inner stresses, and be an objective guide to help you communicate in a healthier way.

- **Journaling:** Get a pen and paper and start writing down the things that are stressing you out the most. Elaborate on how these stressors are making you feel. If you are angry, write it down. Don't hold back. Be sure to brainstorm on strategies you can use to improve the origins of your stresses. Journaling can be one of the best uninhibited outlets for you to express your deepest thoughts and feelings. Your journal is for your eyes only. If you are concerned about confidentiality, shred the pages after you are done with them.

- **Creative outlets:** Find ways to release your stresses creatively. It can be creative writing, painting on canvas, knitting, cooking — do something that you truly enjoy, and let your creative juices flow. It may not sort out your actual stresses, but it can provide you with physiological responses that help you to have a better perspective.

- **Exercise:** Moving around and getting physically active can improve your stress tolerance by increasing the release of healthy neurotransmitters, such as dopamine and serotonin.

- **Deep breathing:** Deep breathing can even be incorporated into a stressful situation to help you refocus and gain clarity on the situation (see Stress-Release Exercise, page 117, for more information).

- **Music:** Listen to music you love. Crank up your favorite tunes, the ones that make you feel good. Sing along and belt them out (even if you don't know the lyrics). Music can match your mood and help you feel better. On the other hand, it can just provide you with good old-fashioned stress release.

- **Laughter:** It is the best medicine, so find a way to release your inner happiness. Laughing will help you feel better. Watch a funny movie, listen to your favorite comedian, read a hilarious blog or call a friend who makes you laugh.

- **Socializing:** Connect with friends, family and loved ones to vent and get a fresh perspective on your stresses.

When you can see a stressful situation for what it is, it allows you to distance yourself from it so that you can reset your thinking and react in a more neutral way. This conserves your energy, prevents you from stressing out and allows you to better enjoy your life.

Of course, this exercise ties back to acne because it limits your response to perceived stressors in your life, thereby preventing your skin from breaking out.

Doc Talk

Practicing strategies to manage stress is so essential because chronic stress is the insidious aggravator of many of our modern-day health problems. Flare-ups in our stress hormones perpetuate unhealthy physiological responses that lead to and aggravate acne. Prioritize stress reduction — it may be one of the missing keys to solving your acne.

CHAPTER 9
Acne and Emotions

CASE STUDY

Anger/Self-Criticism

Brock, a 25-year-old patient, has had problematic and persistent acne for 12 years, starting at puberty. His pimples tend to be very slow to heal, have a red inflamed base and turn into pustular whiteheads. They appear in clusters on his cheeks and neck.

His acne has bothered him no end. When he came to see me, he expressed that these constant breakouts angered him because it felt like "My body is turning on me and I have lost control." It also made him feel ashamed and embarrassed. He felt that people judged him because of his acne, and saw him as "unclean" and "unreliable." I found these comments to be quite intense — a theme pervasive to his experience of acne.

We worked on improving Brock's diet and lifestyle to help settle his skin, but there were obvious emotional issues that could not be ignored. Addressing deep-seated anger and self-esteem issues was critical to improving his psychological health, especially because they were likely a metaphysical contributor to his acne.

When I brought this up with Brock, he was open to working on his emotions and understood that they might play a role in his acne. We did exercises to help Brock focus on the positive aspects of his appearance and discussed realistic assessment of how others perceived him. Using a mirror so he could be involved, I gave Brock an honest dermatological assessment of his skin. Yes, the lesions were moderate in intensity, but they were localized and relatively small in size. He told me that he appreciated having an objective assessment of his acne so he could see it for how it really was rather than how he had "blown it up" in his head.

When we discussed the timing of the onset of his acne in his adolescence, he recalled that it was initially quite minor but suddenly "exploded" one year. I asked him if there had been any stressful incidents that year, and he revealed that his parents had been constantly arguing and yelling and that they finally agreed to separate that same year. This was extremely traumatic for Brock, and he recalled becoming very angry and withdrawn during this time. He began blaming himself for his parents' failed relationship and felt his self-confidence wither.

I told him that what he was telling me about his emotions over his parents' relationship mirrored the conflict he had with his skin — he was angry and blamed himself for both. This was a revelation for Brock, and he fully understood this connection; he told me he was ready to let go of his anger and guilt.

I referred him to a psychologist so he could work on resolving these long-standing suppressed emotions about his parents that had manifested on his skin. I gave Brock some basic dietary advice as well as suggestions for nutritional support for his skin; I did not want to overwhelm him with major dietary changes while he was initiating therapy.

We followed up 8 weeks later, and Brock's attitude was much different. He seemed more calm and self-assured. He had achieved major breakthroughs with regular visits to his psychologist and told me that he felt like a weight had been taken off his shoulders.

Upon reassessment, his skin had vastly improved. There were only small pimples remaining on his cheeks, his neck had cleared and there were no visible whiteheads. The redness had also settled down substantially. Brock was happy with his skin's progress, but said it was not a concern for him anymore. He felt that he was finally able to stop using it as a scapegoat for his emotional baggage.

We understand that there is a physiological link between the health of our skin and the health of our emotional states. The brain and skin are intimately connected. Therefore, being aware of our emotional states is just as important as addressing the quality of our diet and lifestyle.

A dermatologist named Dr. Robert Griesemer developed the Griesemer Index in the late 1970s. It correlates emotional stressors to the presentation of various skin diseases. In his research of acne, he concluded that approximately 55% of patients with acne were affected by emotional stress. He also determined that it takes approximately 2 days for a stress trigger to affect the skin, potentially leading to the development of a pimple.

The following sections discuss the emotions linked to the development of acne and strategies for managing these negative emotions. The two most relevant emotions affecting acne are anger and self-criticism.

> It takes approximately 2 days for a stress trigger to affect the skin, potentially leading to the development of a pimple.

Anger

When anger is not expressed properly, it becomes pent up and suppressed. This suppressed anger can manifest in a multitude of ways in the body.

The cycle of negative emotions and acne is similar to the cycle of the chicken and the egg. Acne likely triggers anger in people. You may think: "I am so angry that I have to look this way!" "Why do I have to deal with this constantly?" "This is so embarrassing for me, and I can't stand it!"

Subsequently, anger promotes the stress response, which releases hormones in the body. Testosterone, which is closely linked to the development of acne, was shown to be increased in subjects when they experienced anger. More testosterone release during episodes of anger can promote acne.

Let's review the basics: acne commonly appears as a reddened, tender, pus-filled, localized and enclosed bump. It is inflamed and often takes time to settle down. The pus is the body's way of dealing with an enveloped infection — in this area of conflict, the body's immune cells are fighting off the targeted bacteria. This slurry, which contains the remains of your cells and the bacteria responsible for the infection, pushes up under the skin and raises it into a pimple, with inflammation and redness in the surrounding tissue.

If you consider this reaction from a metaphysical perspective, it describes unresolved, trapped conflict (pus-filled pimple) and anger (inflamed, reddened skin). Anger is an important emotion to address in the treatment of acne, particularly when it is not properly expressed.

Although anger is a natural, healthy response, in our complicated social interactions, we may decide that showing our anger is negative — that it would be disruptive or petty, or that we would be judged by others. Instead, we may decide to play along as though everything were fine, we may use

Research Spotlight
Emotional Causes

The relationship between anger and acne was examined in a study in the *British Journal of Dermatology*. Subjects with acne were surveyed to measure their acne treatment satisfaction, overall quality of life and skin-related quality of life. It was shown that these three criteria were all related to their innate disposition to anger. The authors of this study recommended that anger and other chronic emotional states be addressed in the proper care of patients with acne.

In a 2012 study from India, anger was shown to play a role in adult females with acne. These subjects experienced social and emotional challenges because of the anger and physical discomfort they felt in relation to their acne.

In 2006, a dermatology practice in Australia also noted that anger played a prominent role in the degree of symptoms experienced by their patients with acne. Some of these patients felt that their acne had "affected their personalities permanently and adversely."

passive-aggressive behavior to unhealthily communicate our feelings, or we may retreat and leave the situation quietly. All of these compensatory responses to feelings of anger are ineffective ways of communicating. When our feelings do not align with our behavior, we may start to experience psychological problems.

A stressful stimulus should be followed by an equally weighted response. Unfortunately, much of the time, the expression of the response is not properly balanced, and therefore is repressed. Energy and mass are intrinsically connected and proportionally equivalent ($E=mc^2$). So when an energetic response is not fully released, such as in healthy communication of anger, it may manifest physically.

The first step in monitoring our anger is to be aware of how often we feel angered, and to understand our individual triggers. One situational trigger may elicit extreme rage in one person yet be of such little consequence to the next person that it does not even compute as a stressor. In order to improve your negative responses, you have to first understand them better.

> When our feelings do not align with our behavior, we may start to experience psychological problems.

Anger Awareness Log

For the next week, keep a log of your anger responses. Use the following steps to guide you:

1. Keep a small journal with you (or track your responses on your smartphone).
2. Be acutely aware of your emotions throughout the day.
3. Make notes anytime you experience even a twinge of anger.
4. Record the time you felt angry.
5. Rate your anger experience on a scale of 0 to 5 (0 = you feel minimal displeasure; 5 = makes your blood boil).
6. Explain the trigger that made you feel that way (it may be something concrete in the moment or it could be a memory of a traumatic event).
7. Describe how you expressed your anger. Also indicate if you didn't do anything about it (you suppressed the feeling).
8. Give a rough estimate of how long you felt angry.
9. Rate your expression of anger on a scale of 0 to 5:
   0 = complete suppression: No one would know that you were angry; you even overcompensated by acting overly nice, despite the fact that you did not feel comfortable.

1 = passive-aggressive: You felt angry, pretending that everything was okay, but you threw in a sideways comment or gave the cold shoulder.

2 = anger with a side of guilt: You said something to express your discomfort but added a nice comment to immediately attempt to take the edge off.

3 = healthy expression of anger: You communicated your discomfort with the situation calmly and rationally, without using hurtful words.

4 = angry words: You expressed your displeasure with a raised voice and used some words that were not necessary, ones that could be construed as hurtful.

5 = lashing out: You were irate; you felt physical symptoms, such as flushing or an elevated heartbeat. You may have yelled, cursed or used words that were deliberately intended to hurt another person's feelings. You may even have hit or thrown things in your rage.

At the end of the week, look back and assess your instances of feeling angry and how you expressed your feelings and displeasure.

What's Your Rating?

Review your ratings for how you expressed your anger with each episode in your log. Did you consistently express your anger healthfully? How many 2s or 4s did you indicate? How many 1s or 5s did you score?

If you experienced episodes of anger and you can honestly say that they all fit into category 3, kudos to you. You are a paradigm of healthy expression, and you have both a good measure of self-protection and an aura of calm about you — either that or you are not being honest with your self-analysis!

On the other hand, if you rated any communication of anger as a 1, 2, 4 or 5, your communication style may be a t risk of affecting your overall health and the quality of your skin. Work with a professional therapist to help you formulate healthy responses for situations that overstep your boundaries and make you feel uncomfortable.

Understanding Triggers

Try to understand your triggers for anger, and why they affect you. There is always a reason for why certain stimuli affect

If you experienced episodes of anger and you can honestly say that they all fit into category 3, kudos to you. You are a paradigm of healthy expression, and you have both a good measure of self-protection and an aura of calm about you.

Anger Frequency

Look at the frequency of your angry episodes, the intensity of your anger and how long the episodes lasted.

- Were they so frequent, so severe or so long that they disrupted your day-to-day life?
- Is this a common pattern for you?
- Do these feelings sway your moods to such a degree that it is hard to feel happy on a regular basis?
- Do they prevent you from feeling motivated to take care of yourself?
- Do you feel less apt to socialize with friends?

If you answered yes to any of these questions, anger is playing much too large a role in your life. Try calming techniques such as meditation, exercise, yoga, deep breathing or the stress-release technique described on page 117.

If these methods do not provide you with enough support, you should strongly consider talking to a therapist or psychologist about the triggers for your anger.

you personally. Often you feel angry because of similar past experiences or unhealthy communication patterns you have with friends, family or relationships. Maybe you have been under stress and your tolerance is lowered. Commonly, the things that make us feel angry are reflections of the things we are unhappy about in ourselves. Consider all of these issues when assessing your triggers.

Self-Criticism

Another common psychological presentation that coincides with acne is low self-esteem and, consequently, self-criticism.

Acne has been shown to have deep psychological ramifications for patients. It negatively affects self-esteem and is correlated with depression. In adolescents and adults, acne has been shown to impact many facets of emotional well-being.

Acne negatively impacts quality of life at every age, distorts body image and reduces self-esteem. It can even result in discrimination at work or in a social environment. These sorts of reactions further reinforce the low levels of self-esteem of those suffering from acne.

Did You Know?

Ask for Help

You may need to speak to someone that you feel comfortable with in order to honestly discuss the sources of your anger. A professional can guide you to find new strategies to manage your anger responses or help you work through the origins of these feelings so they are not overtaking your life. Alternatively, you may need to find a way to either remove yourself from stressful situations or avoid the chronic exposure to toxic stimuli altogether.

Did You Know?

Self-Esteem Tied to Appearance

Research tells us that acne and self-esteem go hand in hand to some degree; as your skin worsens or improves, so, too, does your self-esteem. This might also imply that when you have acne, you may develop an exaggerated emphasis on image, which greatly determines your feeling of self-esteem. In other words, your perceived impression of yourself is tied to appearance. Therefore, the reported levels of self-esteem may not truly reflect an improved feeling of self-worth, but rather a transient sensation of "feeling good."

Decreased self-esteem has been shown to elevate the diurnal pattern (daily cycling) of cortisol levels. In other words, the stress response is heightened when someone has a weak self-image. In a study on students preparing for a test, it was found that their self-perceived academic abilities correlated negatively with their cortisol response — the

Self-Esteem versus Self-Worth

Self-esteem is a transient feeling that can be swayed by daily events. For example, you look in the mirror and see a new zit forming. Your self-esteem plunges and you feed into it by telling yourself some critical words. Then, later on, someone pays you a nice compliment and your self-esteem shoots up. Then you do poorly on a test at school or a performance review at work and you feel awful about yourself again. Therefore, "self-esteem" describes your short-term assessment of yourself, and it is easily shaped by external triggers.

Self-worth is a more important and stable measure of how you perceive yourself and your own value. It does not constantly fluctuate and is not as easily influenced by people's criticisms or compliments. Your feeling of self-worth develops over a longer period of time and is affected by an accumulation of events in your life. It can be shaped by the totality of positive and negative experiences throughout your development, beginning in early childhood. Self-worth enables you to feel that you are worthy of achieving certain goals, such as having a good career, a loving relationship and a supportive social circle.

worse their perception was of their ability (low self-esteem), the higher their cortisol secretion during the test. Since cortisol is a potential trigger for the development of acne, low self-esteem may also contribute to acne.

The good news is that research shows that as self-esteem increases, cortisol secretion becomes more regulated. Essentially, improved self-esteem provides us with a buffer to stress and increases our threshold tolerance.

Measuring Self-Criticism

With respect to acne, self-criticism is an important theme. Acne lesions, which most commonly appear on the face, can't be hidden from sight. They may be partially concealed with makeup, but they are nevertheless visible. Their presentation directly affects our self-perception of our image and makes us concerned about how others may perceive us. It impacts our body image and depletes our self-esteem; this is absolutely understandable.

However, the challenge is that acne can also reinforce an internal dialogue whereby we criticize ourselves. This initially impacts our self-esteem, but over an extended period of time, it can also change our sense of self-worth. When it impacts our self-worth, it greatly affects our long-term outlook on life. Not surprisingly, depression and anxiety go hand in hand with acne.

If we think of someone who criticizes himself or herself, it is easy to see that they make a much bigger deal out of small setbacks. For example, someone is doing a small presentation at work and stumbles on a couple of words. To their audience of coworkers, this tiny wrinkle in their public speaking is hardly even noticeable. If the presenter is someone who self-criticizes, this minor slipup can blow up as a complete and absolute disaster in their mind. They may feel that they have let down everyone at work, they have let themselves down and no one was able to understand the importance of their talk. They can't sleep at night, they can't make eye contact with their colleagues and they feel anxious and depressed.

Objectively, it is easy to see that things are getting blown out of proportion, especially when the presentation as a whole was received very well and understood. In the grand scheme of things, this was just a small ripple that self-criticism turned into a tsunami of emotions and negative self-reflections.

Did You Know?

Disease of Self-Criticism

Acne is a dermatological complaint that is not life threatening or typically severe, yet it dramatically influences how we and others see ourselves. It is minor in the grand scheme of disease; however, it is major in how it affects our image. It is the ultimate manifestation of self-criticism.

Acne plays out similarly, particularly in cases where it is mild to moderate. Acne causes a ripple in our state of health but does not actually affect our physical well-being; however, its presence can completely overtake and overwhelm our lives and our ability to function properly. It impacts work, relationships, socializing, self-esteem and eventually our self-worth. Acne is a physical manifestation of self-criticism.

Having acne also creates and worsens internal self-critical conversations. This, in itself, aggravates acne via the stress response. Having an acne flare-up then — again — heightens and feeds into your pattern of disrupted body image and self-sabotage. And the vicious cycle keeps going. This downward spiral continues, but only for as long as we allow it.

If we take the reins in our hand and take control of the situation, we can unravel the damage that we ourselves are creating. Consider recruiting a professional therapist or psychologist to assist you in changing your behavior and understanding where your self-criticism originates. Start to take control with the exercise below — it may help you unwind and unravel some of your ingrained patterns and turn them into positive, constructive emotions.

> Acne causes a ripple in our state of health but does not actually affect our physical well-being; however, its presence can completely overtake and overwhelm our lives and our ability to function properly.

Self-Criticism Awareness Log

Chart your self-criticisms for 1 week. Use the following steps to guide you:

1. Keep a small journal with you (or track your responses on your smartphone).
2. Be acutely aware of your dialogue with yourself throughout the day.
3. Make notes anytime you experience even a twinge of dissatisfaction with yourself.
4. Record the time you felt this way.
5. Rate your degree of self-criticism on a scale of 0 to 5 (0 = you feel minimal displeasure with yourself; 5 = you wish you weren't alive).
6. Explain the trigger that made you feel that way (it may be something concrete in the moment or it could be a memory of a traumatic event).
7. Describe the negative thoughts you had about yourself (for example, "I hate the way I look"; "I said something that sounded so stupid").

8. Give a rough estimate of how long you felt upset or angry with yourself.

At the end of the week, look back and assess your instances of self-criticism.

Making Changes

This next exercise should not be done while you are in a pattern of self-criticism. Wait until you are in a healthier emotional headspace and are feeling levelheaded about yourself and your self-esteem. You may also recruit the help of a loved one, close friend or family member whom you inherently trust to give you a more objective, positive opinion, particularly if you find that this is too hard to do by yourself.

1. Beside each instance of self-criticism, objectively evaluate your comment (for example, "I am definitely not ugly; the comment I made sounds pretty silly" or "I am sure that no one even noticed that I jumbled my words; the comment I made clearly bothered only me").
2. On a separate piece of paper, note the patterns and themes of your self-criticism, and categorize them (for example, "facial appearance" or "the way I talk").
3. Beside each of these categories, write only positive attributes about these themes that apply to you (for example, "I have incredible eyes" or "I speak to people with empathy").

For the following week, anytime you have a moment of self-criticism, recall which theme it applies to and override the negative comment with a positive-attribute rebuttal. Do this for each and every instance of self-deprecation. This is positive behavioral change and helps to rewire neural patterns that have become automatic and toxic to your existence.

For example, let's say you are walking down the sidewalk and you trip. You instantly think, "I am such a clumsy moron; everyone can see that and they have a good reason to laugh at me." Realize that this is just your negative autopilot speaking to you. Tell yourself that this fits into your theme of being "physically clumsy." Remind yourself of your positive attributes: "I am amazing at using my hands for painting, writing and sculpting; I am physically gifted and coordinated."

> Anytime you have a moment of self-criticism, recall which theme it applies to and override the negative comment with a positive-attribute rebuttal.

Recognize that your self-criticism is a part of your mind that needs to be shut down. See it for what it is, a negative voice in your head. It is not your authentic self and it prevents you from growing and flourishing. Eventually, your positive attributes will be reinforced and you can drown out the negative self-talk. Always remind yourself of your own self-worth, and let it be the strength that maintains your self-esteem from moment to moment.

Doc Talk

Be strong throughout this journey and always keep an eye on the big picture. Remember that acne is a mere ripple in the path of your life. Use what you learn constructively and turn it into something positive.

As your acne clears, your emotional and physical health will also follow. Your acne is an obstacle, but it is also the path to improving yourself.

PART 3
The Vibrant Skin Diet Plan

CHAPTER 10
Getting Started

CASE STUDY

Incorporating the Diet Plan

Elsa was a friendly, outgoing 35-year-old woman who was fed up with her facial acne, which had waxed and waned over the years and still persisted well into her 30s. She had a mix of small whiteheads and a handful of cystic pimples, primarily on her cheeks and chin. In years past, she had seen a few different dermatologists. She had been on one round of Accutane in her teens and birth control pills throughout her 20s, along with a few trials of oral antibiotics and years of continuous topical prescription formulas.

She felt that she had exhausted every conventional option and had noted only temporary improvements. She was fully on board with starting a natural approach that included a diet plan to clear her skin once and for all.

I asked her to track her diet and monitor her skin for 2 weeks, and we assessed it together. Elsa has had an "insatiable sweet tooth" since she was little, but kept her intake under control. She allowed herself a small treat of a few squares of dark chocolate twice a week. Although she did try to keep her carbohydrate intake minimal with respect to pastas and pastries, she did have toast for breakfast and a sandwich every weekday in her packed lunch.

She was ready to get started on the Vibrant Skin Diet Plan immediately. She realized that her biggest challenge would be cutting out breads during the program, but I explained to her that her cravings would substantially decrease over the first week or two.

Elsa had also suffered from digestive problems since childhood and had recently been diagnosed with irritable bowel syndrome. Her bowel movements presented with alternating symptoms of diarrhea and hard stools, and straining. Because digestion plays a role in skin health, I also started her on some gut-supportive natural supplements, including probiotics, fish oils, vitamin D, zinc and L-glutamine.

After 2 weeks, Elsa emailed me because she was quite concerned about a new cluster of cystic pimples that had developed on her jawline and neck, both areas that had been typically acne-free. I reassured her that this was not an uncommon response as her body adjusted to the major dietary modifications. She was thankful for the explanation and continued with the program.

I met with Elsa 6 weeks after she implemented the diet, supplements and other lifestyle recommendations. Her first comment was that her stools had vastly and consistently improved for the first time in decades. She was elated to finally have "perfect poops" and feel like a "normal person with normal digestion." Of course, her skin was her main reason for visiting me, and we noted that her cheeks and chin had improved by approximately 50% by this point. The new breakouts on her neck and jaw had completely subsided.

After 3 months, Elsa's skin had improved by approximately 80% since Day 1. Her digestion had remained stable, but she was starting to miss having sweets. I gave her the option of moving to the reintroduction phase, but suggested she start slowly, with careful monitoring so we would not jeopardize her progress so far.

By 6 months, Elsa's skin had cleared completely, and she was able to once again enjoy occasional sweets without flaring up. During the reintroduction phase of the program, she took note that breads tipped her skin over the edge after 3 consecutive days of consumption. This would make her skin lose luster and develop small bumps, and, if continued for longer, she would develop pimples. She said it was an "easy trade-off" to avoid breads and keep her intermittent treats. Elsa was relieved that her skin had finally grown out of its pubescent appearance 20 years after it had started.

Diet Design

The true challenge in designing a diet plan is that it must be the best possible option that suits the vast majority of the population it is trying to help. It has to take into account many individual differences, such as the following:

- Knowledge of nutrition
- Palate
- Physiological responsiveness
- Accessibility of food items
- Lifestyle
- Manageability

Most importantly, the plan has to provide you with complete nutrition, without any nutrient deficiencies. Therefore, it must provide many options within parameters that assist with the end goal — that is, to improve your acne.

In designing the Vibrant Skin Diet Plan, I took into account the most common dietary aggravators from evidence-based research and clinical experience with my acne patients. The diet plan integrates recommendations on the most effective regimen for treating acne while making it manageable and achievable for the long term.

Once you understand the rationale for controlling blood sugar and how to go about doing it, the process of sticking to a diet becomes much easier. When we realize how absurdly elevated our intake of sugar food sources has become, compared to our physiological and evolutionary needs, it helps us to comply with a healthier diet.

Once you understand the rationale for controlling blood sugar and how to go about doing it, the process of sticking to a diet becomes much easier.

Measuring Blood Sugar and Insulin Response

Controlling dietary blood sugar through the diet is a critical part of improving your acne. In order to rule in or rule out foods for the Vibrant Skin Diet Plan, I considered the glycemic index, glycemic load and insulin index, along with clinical experiences.

What Does the Glycemic Index of a Food Measure?

The glycemic index (GI) was created in 1981 by two University of Toronto researchers, Dr. Thomas Wolever and Dr. David Jenkins. It is a measure of how quickly carbohydrates in a particular food item are assimilated into the bloodstream; in other words, it assesses the extent to which that food influences blood-sugar levels.

A food that has a high GI will cause a quick and sustained elevation in blood sugar. A food with a low GI will cause a much smaller, gradual increase in blood sugar. A food that is above 70 on the GI scale is considered high. A moderate GI rating falls between 55 and 70, while a GI number below 55 is considered to be low.

Post-Consumption Blood Glucose Response to High-Glycemic Food and Low-Glycemic Food

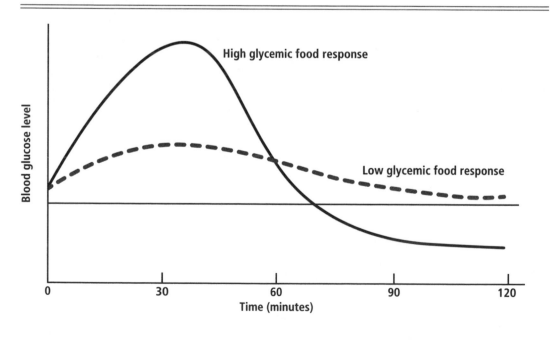

How Is the Glycemic Index Determined?

The GI is based on a standard amount of carbohydrates (50 g) for each food tested, and each food is evaluated on how it affects blood glucose relative to other foods. The upper limit on the glycemic scale is established at 100 and is set by pure glucose, which is the benchmark against which all other types of carbohydrates in foods are measured. Glucose is the form of carbohydrate that directly and most efficiently influences our blood-sugar levels.

For example, 50 g of the carbohydrates in cooked carrots has a glycemic index of about 40, whereas 50 g of carbohydrates from glucose has a glycemic index of 100.

Are There Drawbacks to the GI?

One problem with the GI is that there can be different results quoted for one particular food. The variations depend on whether the food is cooked or raw and how it is processed. Tomatoes may range anywhere from 30 to 50, based on how they are prepared (cooked versus raw versus juiced). The GI rating may also vary because some of the labs that determine GI may set white bread, which normally has a GI of about 70, to the reference point of 100 (rather than pure glucose). Together, these criteria can lead to highly variable GI ratings.

Another issue with the GI is that it does not properly take into account normal portion sizes. It is designed to measure food based on 50 g of carbohydrates, but if the tested food is actually low in carbohydrates, then a much larger portion of food would need to be used.

For example, although carrots have a high GI, the serving size required to achieve 50 g of carbohydrates is unrealistic. You would need to eat approximately 9 medium-size carrots in order to consume the 50 g of carbohydrates that is used to calculate the GI. Unless your name is Bugs Bunny, you likely would not eat that many carrots at one sitting.

This also skews how the GI rating could be used to make choices. Carrots have a relatively high GI rating (ranked anywhere from 40 to 63, based on how the carrots are processed and if they are raw or cooked), making them appear to be an "unhealthy" option. However, there are so few carbohydrates in a normal serving of carrots that the way the sugar is absorbed is irrelevant.

Is there a way to resolve this deficiency with the GI? Thankfully, there is — it is a more applicable measurement called the glycemic load.

> Glucose is the form of carbohydrate that directly and most efficiently influences our blood-sugar levels.

What Is the Glycemic Load?

The glycemic load (GL) is a concept developed in 1997 at Harvard University that adjusts the GI to account for the concentration of carbohydrates in particular foods. It is a more useful measure of how a typical serving size of a food affects our blood sugar. In essence, the GL is a GI that is weighted based on the amount of carbohydrates in a food.

GL is determined by using the number of grams of carbohydrates in a 100-gram portion of food and multiplying it by its GI. For example, let's take the highest GI rating for carrots: 63. Because a 100-gram serving of carrots contains only 10 g of carbohydrates, the conversion to GL would be:

$$63 \times 10 \text{ g}/100 \text{ g} = 6.3$$

Therefore, the moderately high GI of 63 for carrots drops to a low GL of 6.3 when weighted. This makes sense because of the low concentration of carbohydrates in carrots, and adjusts the seemingly high GI to a more realistic low GL.

Are There Drawbacks to the GL?

The GL is a reliable estimator of how a food will affect blood sugar. That being said, it is limited in that it does not specifically explain how that food will affect insulin response in the body.

To take it that step further, a scale called the insulin index measures the body's insulin secretion based on foods consumed, and it takes into account that there are more complex factors besides the carbohydrate content of a food that can determine how the body compensates with insulin release.

The insulin index was also taken into consideration when cross-referencing some "gray area" food items in the Vibrant

Research Spotlight
Low Glycemic Load and Acne

A 2012 Korean study tested the effects of implementing a low-glycemic-load diet on 32 subjects with acne. They divided the subjects into a control group and a low-glycemic-load test group. After 10 weeks, the subjects consuming a low-glycemic-load diet showed a significant clinical reduction in the number of inflammatory and noninflammatory acne skin lesions. When designing a diet to treat acne, considering the glycemic load of foods is important.

Skin Diet Plan. These needed more quantifiers to help me determine if I was going to include or exclude them. Because the insulin index rating does not include every food item, it was difficult to rely on it, so I used it as added support.

In designing the Vibrant Skin Diet Plan, I took into consideration both the GI and GL of the foods allowed. I worked within the framework of maintaining a whole-foods diet, eliminating the most likely food aggravators of acne and focusing on foods that support the health of the skin.

Preparing for the Vibrant Skin Diet Plan

The first step in adopting the Vibrant Skin Diet Plan is to ensure you have the right foods at home and to discard the foods that can aggravate inflammation and acne.

You will need to be disciplined and compliant as you follow the diet plan. This understandably takes effort and requires planning, but the diet provides your body with the right foods to support the health of your skin and reduce inflammation.

The Vibrant Skin Diet Plan is designed to provide you with proper nutrition when it comes to eating carbohydrates, proteins and fats, while also emphasizing quality foods and whole-food ingredients. Most modern-day diets don't sufficiently balance carbs, proteins and fats (the macronutrients), and many lack the proper vitamins, minerals and plant compounds (the micronutrients) that optimize our health and prevent disease. The problem is compounded by our exposure to processed, altered foods, artificial ingredients and thousands of synthetic chemicals.

Goal of the Vibrant Skin Diet Plan

The goal of this diet plan is to target acne with simple and healthy whole foods. The diet parameters are based on a combination of two main sources of information:

1. Clinical studies proven to minimize acne.
2. Additional nutritional guidelines that I have refined in my clinical practice and that have resulted in successful, achievable outcomes for my patients with acne.

Have Fun

Although implementing restrictions to your diet may seem arduous and painful at first, it can also be enjoyable. There are many healthy and, most importantly, tasty meals that can be made when following the Vibrant Skin Diet Plan. Remember that healthy eating is simple eating. This means that preparation does not have to be complicated. You do not have to have the culinary skills of Julia Child to follow this plan (likely, many of her rich, dairy-heavy dishes wouldn't make the cut anyhow). You can layer the diet with more labor-intensive skills and complex meal preparations, but only if you want to. Most people who lead time-scarce lifestyles want quick and easy.

Many of us get caught up in the ease and convenience of meal options that are available near school or work — a quick pastry and coffee in the morning, food courts for lunch and takeout on the way home. We all know that these are the options that cause the most problems to our health because of the shortcuts that restaurants take, such as the additives we don't know about, the less-than-healthy cooking methods that are quick and convenient and the poor quality of ingredients used. We use the excuses that we "don't have time," we are "starving after work," and we "can't cook" or "hate to cook." The real reason is that we have not figured out how to do these things efficiently and enjoyably without compromising great taste.

Recruit friends and family members to provide you with support and encouragement. You absolutely know more than a few people who enjoy cooking and would be happy to share their knowledge and experience with you. Make this a fun and social learning activity.

Integrating with Family

If you have a partner, be open about your health goals and your diet program and timeline. It is important to get them involved in your journey to good health. Keep in mind that the diet changes that support clear skin also support overall improved metabolism and health. You will both benefit.

Just the same, your partner may not be fully on board with all of the food restrictions; this is completely acceptable and understandable. However, it may not be realistic or fun to prepare and eat two completely separate meals. An easy compromise is to use the meals in this plan as a base, and build on them by preparing a side dish that includes a restricted food if your partner wants something else. They might choose to add toppings to the base meals to suit their own taste buds and dietary goals, such as a sprinkle of shaved cheese, bread crumbs or creamy dressing, or add on a side of bread, potato or pasta. The options are limitless, and integrating can be easy if you discuss expectations ahead of time.

FAQ

Q **I'm worried about incorporating this diet plan because of my children's picky palates. Any suggestions?**

A Try to use this as a learning tool to teach them that eating healthy can still be delicious. Children can be quite sensitive to blood-sugar fluctuations, and they are highly influenced by the sugar-focused tendencies of food marketing agencies and the unhealthy choices of their peers — not a good combination. Their developing bodies can easily become accustomed to sugar loading, and they can develop strong psycho-emotional attachments to sugar that can persist well into the adult years.

No matter how you look at it, it is very helpful to control the sugar intake of the children in your life; however, you may want to exert a lot of flexibility with them in keeping their diets varied while you embark on this plan. For example, do not feel that you need to restrict their intake of higher-sugar fruits, starchy vegetables, gluten-free whole grains or gluten-free flours. Remember that kids burn a lot of fuel with their constant activity, so they require regular doses of healthy carbohydrates.

Snacks

Your body may need time to adjust to the more stabilizing slow-release sugars found in the foods of the Vibrant Skin Diet Plan. As a result, you may initially feel hungry after meals; your body is still accustomed to expecting a sugar crash both physiologically and psychologically.

It is a good rule, particularly during the first 2 weeks, to ensure that you are enjoying healthy snacks between meals, and that you *always* eat at least every 3 hours. If you normally eat your lunch at work around noon and then eat dinner after commuting home, there may be a gap of 7 or 8 hours, when you account for meal preparation time. This is when you can expect to be hypoglycemic (low blood sugar): cranky, light-headed and with a ravenous appetite. This is also the time when people will not be able to think rationally and tend to grab some sugary or high-carb snacks or reach for a glass of wine or beer.

If you eat a mid-afternoon snack that is high in protein, good fats and healthy carbs, your body and mind (and skin!) will thank you. Make snacking a regular part of your routine in order to prevent sabotaging your efforts on the diet plan.

If there is absolutely no way to eat solid foods as snacks, sometimes drinks can be an option (say, in the case of endless back-to-back meetings). You can drink vegan protein smoothies inconspicuously from an opaque cup or covered coffee mug. It can be as easy as mixing vegan protein powder with some water or almond milk and sipping it throughout the course of a meeting.

Whatever the case may be, find creative ways to incorporate fast, easy, blood-sugar-normalizing snacks. This is a priority in the first weeks of the diet plan, but also a good general rule to incorporate into your long-term eating schedule.

Healthy Snacks

There are countless quick and easy snack options available, but here are some very simple ideas:

- A handful of nuts with a few carrot sticks
- A handful of seeds and a lower-glycemic-load fruit, such as a pear or some strawberries
- Cucumber slices dipped in homemade hummus
- Red pepper slices and up to 3 tbsp (45 mL) guacamole
- Celery sticks filled with almond butter

Taking Time to Eat

Improving digestive health is necessary to see improvements in acne. If you are eating hastily, your gastrointestinal tract will not function at its peak, and this will compromise your digestive function.

Your digestive system — its wavelike movements (called peristalsis), its carefully choreographed secretion of digestive fluids and enzymes — relies on what is called the parasympathetic nervous system. This is a component of our nervous system and it functions in diametric opposition to our sympathetic nervous system. The sympathetic nervous system is involved in our fight-or-flight response, when we are under stress and our muscles need to be activated. We are in the sympathetic state if we are running away from a bear or saber-toothed tiger (in the case of our cave-dwelling ancestors). In modern times, we are in this state when in a chronically stressed environment, such as dealing with the deadlines and pressures of work. Therefore, when we are stressed, the portion of our nervous system that regulates digestive function becomes compromised.

   This underlines the importance of taking time to eat your lunch. Make sure to take a minimum of 10 to 15 minutes away from your desk to actually focus on the act of eating. Chew thoroughly and without rushing, make sure to take deep, slow breaths in and out, and truly taste and enjoy your food. All of these steps will help activate the parasympathetic nervous system, which manages all of the necessary components of your digestive tract.

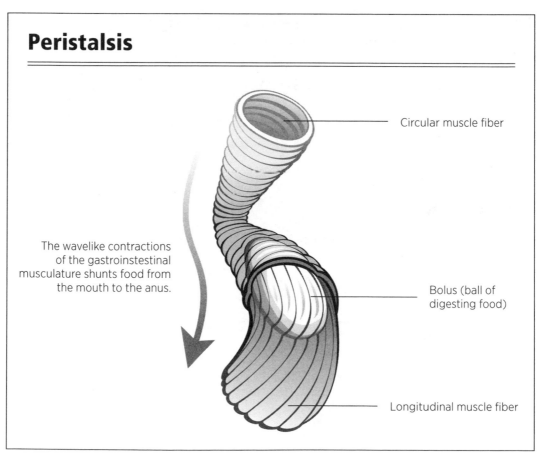

Peristalsis

Circular muscle fiber

The wavelike contractions of the gastroinstestinal musculature shunts food from the mouth to the anus.

Bolus (ball of digesting food)

Longitudinal muscle fiber

Timeline

Did You Know?

What Affects Recovery?

Factors like compliance, individual sensitivities, severity of acne, intensity of treatment plan, health status, current diet and lifestyle, past or current prescriptions, skin-care regimen, genetics and environment all play a role in determining a prognosis for acne.

Everyone wants to know when their skin will be better, and usually they want it better yesterday. However, the honest answer is: it depends.

Even conventional treatments that involve prescription medication, such as Accutane, birth control pills or antibiotics, have a timeline, typically 3 months at a minimum and up to 6 months on average, or longer.

When it comes to a dietary and natural approach to acne, there are many variables to consider when approximating a timeline.

However, a realistic expectation should not be to see acne clear in a week or two (although it is possible in certain cases). From clinical experience, I tell my patients they can typically expect a significant degree of improvement in acne intensity after 6 months. Generally speaking, the majority of cases will start to see improvements well before this point.

Approximate Expected Timeline of Acne Changes

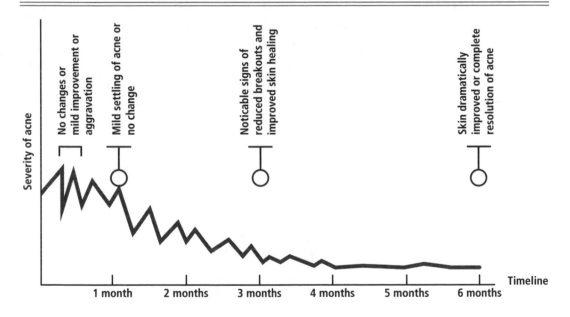

FAQ

Q What sort of adjustments should I expect when I embark on treatment and the Vibrant Skin Diet Plan?

A Be aware of the changes you are making from your current diet to the suggested Vibrant Skin Diet Plan. If just mild tweaking is involved, you are supporting your skin health by being more disciplined and giving your body extra support to normalize hormones and inflammatory processes. Alternatively, if your current diet is laden with flours, sugars and processed foods, the change may feel quite drastic. When the change in fuel for your body is dramatic, you may experience an initial period of adjustment. Our bodies are highly adaptable, which means your body has achieved a homeostasis (internal balance) that compensates for your current diet, even if unhealthy. When we give it pure, balanced nutrition, as in the Vibrant Skin Diet Plan, it has to shift from the previous homeostasis to a new homeostasis. This can result in a period of skin aggravation in certain cases.

Do not be alarmed: this is not a signal to panic and simply give up! The symptoms will gradually calm down as flare-ups settle and your body adjusts. You will eventually reach a happier, healthier, balanced state in which your skin is optimally nourished and clears.

An analogy of this scenario is the pack-a-day smoker who experiences no noticeable symptoms. Over the years, their body has acclimatized to the inhalation of cigarette smoke and inflammation in the lungs, and has adjusted its balance to tolerate the concoction of toxins and tar released by the combustion of tobacco. When this person quits smoking, it is not uncommon for their body to experience an adjustment whereby they develop a constant cough and produce mucus and congestion. Some smokers return to their comforting cigarette habit on the knowingly false premise that they were "healthier and symptom-free" when they were smoking regularly. The body had adjusted its homeostasis, and with the aggravating stimulus removed, it was finally able to harness its resources to clear out the inflammation.

In the same way, your skin may adjust and "release" by flaring up, but in the long run, it settles and becomes clearer than it was before.

Patients will typically begin to see some signs of improvement after approximately 1 month of implementing the treatment plan. This may be after an initial period of aggravation, which can occur with some patients.

I regularly encounter setbacks with some patients. I often need to talk them through the process, manage their expectations, calm their emotions and assure them that they are on the right path. The good news is that in the vast majority of cases, if these patients stick with the plan, their skin will improve.

Here are the expected timeline results after full implementation of the treatment plan:

- **Weeks 2–3:** Very gradual improvement, no changes noted or a distinct aggravation
- **At 1 month:** Symptoms settle; some improvements typically noted; in cases of aggravation, flare-up mellows
- **At 3 months:** Notable and obvious signs of skin healing; patients experience improved motivation to continue with the plan, based on results
- **At 6 months:** Skin is dramatically improved, many times with complete resolution of acne

Foods to Avoid

Part 1: The Ditch-the-Sweets Rules

These rules outline the foods that are most likely to aggravate sugar fluctuations in the blood. It is important to avoid both obvious and more inconspicuous forms of sugar in order to heal acne.

Sweet Foods to Avoid

- Refined sugar
- Natural sugar alternatives
- Sugar-free natural sweeteners
- Artificial sweeteners
- Soft drinks
- Juices
- Dried fruits
- High-sugar fruits
- Foods containing flour
- Starchy vegetables

No Refined Sugar

Refined sugar is the most obvious perpetrator of blood-sugar spikes. We find huge amounts of sugar in packaged foods in one form or another. Refined sugars are categorized as those that are highly processed or isolated in their basic sugar form. These forms of sugar have become more ubiquitous in our food supply since the 1950s.

Refined sugars appear on labels as:

- Dextrose
- Fructose
- Galactose
- Glucose
- Glucose solids
- Glucose-fructose
- Granulated sugar
- High-fructose corn syrup
- Invert sugar
- Isoglucose
- Lactose
- Levulose
- Maltodextrin
- Maltose
- Sugar
- Table sugar
- White sugar

Natural sugar alternatives are deceptive because they can be touted as a healthier alternative to refined sugar and described as "natural sweeteners." They may even be promoted as having additional health benefits based on the compounds that are part of their makeup. Unfortunately, sugar is sugar.

No Natural Sugar Alternatives

Natural sugar alternatives are deceptive because they can be touted as a healthier alternative to refined sugar and described as "natural sweeteners." They may even be promoted as having additional health benefits based on the compounds that are part of their makeup. Unfortunately, sugar is sugar, and these are just raw variants of sugar with different names — they will still raise your blood sugar and lead to worsened skin health.

These are some examples of the natural sweeteners derived from either cane sugar or other sources:

Sugarcane Derivatives

- Brown sugar
- Cane juice
- Demerara sugar
- Evaporated cane juice
- Golden syrup
- Jaggery
- Molasses
- Muscovado sugar
- Panela
- Rapadura
- Raw cane sugar
- Sucanat
- Treacle
- Turbinado sugar

Natural Sugars Derived from Other Sources

- Agave syrup
- Amazake (amasake)
- Arenga sugar
- Barley malt
- Beet sugar
- Brown rice syrup

- Caramel
- Coconut sugar
- Corn syrup
- Corn syrup solids
- Date sugar
- Fruit juice
- Honey
- Malt syrup
- Maple syrup
- Palm sugar
- Sorghum syrup

No Sugar-Free Natural Sweeteners

There are sugar-free low- to no-calorie natural sweeteners available as well, and these theoretically sound like a great alternative to sweeten your foods, since they do not affect your blood sugar and therefore would not aggravate your acne. Although this may be true, the issue with sugar-free natural sweeteners is that they do not serve to dampen your cravings for sweets.

One of the purposes of the Vibrant Skin Diet Plan is to ensure that you reduce your sugar intake in the long term, not just until your skin clears up. The most effective way to do this is to limit your taste for sweet things. For this reason, avoid any type of sweetener, even if it is natural and sugar-free, while on the Vibrant Skin Diet Plan. Remember that we are putting your taste buds through a reprogramming regimen!

Here are some examples of sugar-free natural sweeteners:

- Arabitol
- Erythritol
- Galactitol
- Glycerol
- Glycyrrhizin
- Isomalt
- Maltitol
- Mannitol
- Monk fruit (*luo han guo*)
- Ribitol
- Sorbitol
- Stevia
- Stevioside
- Whole-leaf stevia
- Xylitol

No Artificial Sweeteners

Artificial sweeteners may be considered GRAS (generally regarded as safe), but this does not equate with being safe for regular use and for every person. There is inadequate information about the long-term health effects of artificial sweeteners on various systems in our body.

They are completely unnecessary from a health perspective and will sabotage your progress in retraining your body to reduce its taste for sweeteners.

Here are some examples of artificial sweeteners:

Did You Know?

Sweet Tooth

The prevalence of sugar in our food supply is due, in big part, to the fact that we are all now accustomed to tasting and needing sweetness in order to feel satisfied. By retraining your psychological dependence on sweetened foods, you will be less likely to succumb to a regular intake of sweetened foods in the long term.

- Acesulfame K (contained in Sunett and Sweet One)
- Aspartame (contained in Equal and NutraSweet)
- Cyclamate
- Neohesperidin dihydrochalcone
- Neotame
- Saccharin (contained in Sweet'N Low and Hermesetas)
- Sucralose (contained in Splenda)

No Soft Drinks

Soft drinks seem pretty obvious to avoid; however, it is important to single them out for a few reasons.

Some people may still consider high-fructose corn syrup to be a safer form of sugar. Do not be deceived: high-fructose corn syrup has been proven to be one of the most dangerous food ingredients, based on its omnipresence in foods and its continuous consumption by the majority of the population. It has been linked to diabetes, high cholesterol, heart disease and obesity, all of which have become increasingly common since the inception and common use of high-fructose corn syrup.

A regular 12-ounce (355 mL) can of cola contains high-fructose corn syrup in an amount equivalent to more than 9 teaspoons (45 mL) of sugar. There is no question that soft drinks are a terrible option for inflammation in the body and, therefore, acne.

What's more, the other ingredients in soft drinks are artificial and have no discernable health benefits in the body. Many people argue that diet soft drinks are a suitable alternative because of their lack of sugar. In diet soft drinks, however, sugar is just traded out for a chemical sweetener replacement that again is not useful in any way for our health. Essentially, they are a witch's brew of chemicals that aggravate inflammation.

Doc Talk

In my practice, I consider the daily consumption of diet soft drinks to be as serious as a cigarette addiction. I commonly see patients consume diet soft drinks on a daily basis; a handful of patients reported drinking in excess of 68 to 100 ounces (2 to 3 L) a day. Overcoming an addiction to diet soft drinks takes a lot of willpower and motivation, and may require working together with a health-care professional. No soft drinks or variations thereof are permitted on the Vibrant Skin Diet Plan.

No Juices

Juices are fiber-free forms of fruit in a concentrated liquid medium. Essentially, this adds up to a highly accessible and absorbable fructose vehicle; these are quick blasts of sugar.

Juice has long been considered a health food because it is an easy way to increase your fruit intake. The tide is finally turning, and more people are beginning to acknowledge juice for what it is. But there is still a lot of confusion.

Processed packaged juices with added sugars are more obvious sugar perpetrators. The confusion lies in the more deceptive "natural" blends of juices.

The other trouble lies in the growing popularity of home-pressed, centrifuged juices. The fruits and vegetables in these are consumed in quantities that would not normally be eaten in one sitting if in their natural form.

A tall glass of juice may contain the sugars from 3 beets, 2 apples and 3 pears. This glass of juice may be consumed in less than 2 minutes. In this case, our satiety receptors are not activated as they would be if we were eating these in their whole forms. In fact, we simply would not consume this much produce all at once.

As a result, along with the intake of numerous beneficial plant compounds and antioxidants, we also take in a large amount of naturally occurring plant sugars.

In essence, no matter the form, juices are a no-go on the path to clear skin.

No Dried Fruit

Dried fruit is problematic to acne for a couple of reasons.

First, dried fruit contains more concentrated fruit sugars compared to the same volume of fresh fruit. This is attributed to the removal of water in the dehydrating process. This means that you will consume much more sugar in a dried fruit than you would in a fresh fruit, particularly when you take into account the high water content of fruit. This also means that you would likely consume more of the same fruit than you would of its fresh counterpart.

One cup (250 mL) of raisins contains almost 100 g of sugar, whereas 1 cup (250 mL) of grapes contains less than 25 g. In this example, eating the same volume of dried fruit as fresh fruit provides quadruple the intake of sugar.

Another reason why dried fruit is problematic is because it often contains added sugar. This is usually the case with fruits that are tarter in taste, such as dried cranberries, which almost always contain added sugar.

> Fruits that are tarter in taste, such as dried cranberries, almost always contain added sugar.

No High-Sugar Fruits

Tropical fruits, as a general rule, contain higher concentrations of sugars. The warmer climates concentrate the sugars. Avoid all types of tropical fruits — mangos, bananas, pineapples — as well as grapes and melons.

Fruit is not altogether banned on the Vibrant Skin Diet Plan, since that would be an overly extreme and unnecessary measure, particularly when there are many powerful anti-inflammatory antioxidants in fruit that may be beneficial in healing skin. The emphasis is on understanding the differences in sugar content, glycemic index and glycemic load between different types of fruits, and choosing fruits that help keep blood sugar stabilized.

Tropical versus Temperate Fruits

The following lists outline the sugar content per cup (250 mL) of tropical fruits compared to fruits from a temperate climate:

Tropical Fruits
Mango: 23.0 g
Banana : 18.3 g
Pineapple: 16.5 g

Temperate Fruits
Peach: 13.0 g
Green apple: 12.0 g
Cherries: 9.0 g
Strawberries: 6.5 g
Raspberries: 5.5 g

Exception to the temperate-climate rule: Melons and grapes have a glycemic index and/or glycemic load that makes them unacceptable on this diet plan.

No Foods Containing Flour

Flour does not taste sweet, and for this reason it is not generally regarded as a problem for keeping blood sugar controlled. But remember this statement: flour equals sugar. It makes it much easier to implement and understand the concept of hidden sugars this way.

Flour is a starch, and starches are essentially chains of sugar molecules strung together. Flours are grains that have been mechanically macerated to a powder, a highly processed food ingredient.

With the commonly used refined flour, the bran and germ have been removed during production. The bran is the fibrous covering of the whole grain, while the germ is the inner region (the embryo of the plant) that contains the nutrients and building blocks to germinate a grain. The removal of these naturally occurring components of the grain accelerates the absorption of glucose into the bloodstream.

When you think of any food made with flour, whether gluten-free or not, regard it as a sugar. This means that you will have to exclude all flour-based foods, including breads, pastas, wraps, noodles and baked goods.

No Starchy Vegetables

Starchy vegetables by definition are much higher in carbohydrates, meaning they have a high concentration of starches. Starch, as discussed earlier, readily converts to sugar in the body.

If these vegetables are cooked, the heating process predigests the starch and actually further increases our body's access to its sugar content. Essentially, cooked starchy vegetables are even more likely to act as a sugar source than their raw counterparts.

The vegetables with the highest glycemic index and glycemic load are primarily root vegetables, plus a few others that grow above the soil.

Starchy Root Vegetables

- Beet
- Edo
- Parsnip
- Potato
- Rutabaga
- Sweet potato
- Taro
- Turnip
- Yam

Starchy Vegetables That Grow Above the Soil

- Corn
- Peas
- Plantain
- Pumpkin
- Squash

FAQ

Q Are there any exceptions to eating starchy vegetables while on the Vibrant Skin Diet Plan?

A All forms of starchy vegetables should be avoided on the plan, with one exception to this rule: starchy vegetables can be enjoyed within 2 hours before or after a moderate-to-intense workout to provide energy. In other words, they do not have to be completely excluded if you are on a fairly intense goal-specific exercise regimen, or training program. In these cases, your body will need the additional complex carbohydrates to provide energy and replenish glycogen (your body's storage form of carbohydrates in the liver and muscle tissues). If you are too limited in your carbohydrate intake and are following an intense exercise regimen, your body may resort to breaking down muscle proteins in order to access energy (a process called gluconeogenesis).

Part 2: The Heal-Your-Inflammation Rules

The crux of the acne issue is to control foods that instigate blood-sugar spikes. However, there are other foods that also create inflammation or perpetuate inflammatory cycles in the body. While healing acne, we want to enjoy a diet that reduces inflammation. Incorporating these guidelines in combination with the Ditch-the-Sweets Rules (page 146) is paramount to properly addressing acne.

The rules outlined in this section advocate eliminating the major food sensitivities that may be linked to acne and focus on a clean, whole-foods diet that reduces your exposure to synthetic ingredients and chemicals that your body is not accustomed to processing. When your body is not physiologically designed to handle certain chemicals or food derivatives in unnatural concentrations, your body's metabolic processes may be disrupted, setting the stage for inflammation to continue.

> When your body is not physiologically designed to handle certain chemicals or food derivatives in unnatural concentrations, your body's metabolic processes may be disrupted, setting the stage for inflammation to continue.

Inflammation-Inducing Foods to Avoid

- Dairy products
- Gluten
- Eggs
- Processed foods
- Artificial ingredients
- Alcohol
- Caffeine

No Dairy Products

Dairy products cause one of the most common food sensitivities that aggravate acne. During the Vibrant Skin Diet Plan, all forms of dairy must be strictly avoided.

Keep in mind that although this is a large and challenging category of foods to eliminate, you may be able to reintroduce certain forms of dairy with lower allergenic properties (for example, hard aged cow's milk cheese, goat's milk cheese,

Cow's Milk versus Other Mammal Milks

The added problem with cow's milk is the potential health concerns regarding the mutation of A2 beta-casein to A1 beta-casein. This milk mutation has occurred over a few thousand years of bovine domestication. The A1 protein is prevalent in the majority of the Western world's milk supply.

Regular consumption of the mutated A1 beta-casein in dairy products has been connected to heart disease and type 1 diabetes.

Some emerging dairy companies are now producing and testing cattle to produce only A2 milk and A2 dairy products in response to these concerns.

It has not been investigated if this mutation is the potential cause of dairy products' negatively impacting acne. Regardless of the causative factor, dairy is to be avoided on the Vibrant Skin Diet Plan because of its correlation to acne.

Milk and dairy products from other mammals, such as goats, sheep, camels and buffalo, may be safer to consume in the long term for the following reasons:

- Their unique proteins differ from those in cow dairy. We are overexposed to cow's milk, cow dairy products and cow dairy derivatives in our food supply, but we are exposed only minimally to dairy from other mammals. Not surprisingly, dairy products from non-cow mammals have less potential to be allergenic.
- These other milks do not contain mutated casein proteins.

For the purposes of the Vibrant Skin Diet Plan, it is recommended to avoid all forms of dairy, from cows and other mammals. When you reintroduce foods into your diet, start with non-cow dairy sources before reintroducing cow dairy products (see Protocol for Reintroducing Foods, page 193, for more information).

sheep's milk cheese or fermented dairy, such as yogurt or kefir) into your diet after your skin and inflammation have settled (see Vibrant Skin Maintenance Diet Plan, page 191, for more information). The main goal is to eliminate dairy for the duration of the diet plan and thereby allow the body to clear inflammation, which may present as other symptoms besides just acne. Eventually, with the restricted exposure to dairy, other systemic symptoms may subside along with acne as the body resets to a healthier homeostasis.

Dairy Products

- Butter
- Buttermilk
- Cheeses (all)
- Cream cheese
- Gelato
- Ice cream
- Kefir
- Milk (including lactose-free)
- Milk chocolate
- Milk powders
- Sour cream
- Whey protein powder
- Yogurt

Derivatives of Dairy

- Casein
- Lactalbumin
- Lactoglobulin
- Modified milk ingredients
- Sodium or potassium caseinate
- Whey

FAQ

Q Can I have lactose-free dairy options on the diet plan?

A It is important to distinguish a dairy sensitivity from a lactose intolerance.

When you have a lactose intolerance, your body lacks the lactase enzyme, which catalyzes the breakdown of the milk sugar called lactose. This leads to bloating, abdominal discomfort and diarrhea after consuming milk and most other dairy products.

A dairy sensitivity is a delayed reaction to the hundreds of types of proteins found in milk, not the lactose sugar. The main protein classes are casein and whey proteins.

Lactose-free milk may not contain lactose; however, it still contains the many other milk proteins to which you are likely sensitive. Therefore, lactose-free milk is not an option.

No Gluten

Gluten has been one of the most talked-about causes of food allergies and sensitivities in recent years, with a lot of attention coming from various media sources either extolling the virtues of going gluten-free or, conversely, questioning whether this is just a fad. Various medical conditions have been associated with gluten consumption, and these fall along a spectrum of severity. The most serious presentation of a gluten condition is celiac disease.

In addition to celiac disease, the conventional medical community has also finally acknowledged non-celiac gluten sensitivities. Symptoms can be mild to moderate, but in this case, continuing to eat gluten-containing foods may contribute to increased inflammation in the body. This may disrupt normal levels of hormones, leading to increased breakouts. This can occur with premenstrual estrogen spikes or with the sebaceous glands being exposed to stronger androgens, both of which trigger acne.

Gluten-containing products by their nature are also foods that are easily digested into sugar. Breads, pastas, breaded foods, baked goods and anything that is made of regular white flour or whole wheat flour (or any derivative of these) will both contain gluten and aggravate sugar fluctuations in our blood. Gluten-containing foods may be a double whammy in terms of how they can influence your acne, as a food sensitivity and from a blood-sugar-control perspective.

Even if a bread or pasta product is made from gluten-free grains, it will need to be eliminated from the diet because it still contributes to sugar spikes. Remember that flour has a similar effect to sugar in your body, even if it is gluten-free.

Because one of the main rules from the Vibrant Skin Diet Plan states that you should avoid any flour-based foods, you will also be avoiding the main sources of gluten-containing foods.

There is extensive overlap between flours and gluten. Essentially, in the Vibrant Skin Diet Plan, you will be avoiding all of the foods below.

> Gluten-containing foods may be a double whammy in terms of how they can influence your acne, as a food sensitivity and from a blood-sugar-control perspective.

Gluten-Containing Flours

- All-purpose (white) flour
- Barley
- Bulgur
- Dinkel
- Durum
- Einkorn
- Farina
- Faro
- Freekeh
- Fu

- Graham
- Kamut
- Khorasan
- Matzoh
- Mir
- Oats
- Rye
- Seitan
- Semolina
- Spelt
- Triticale
- Wheat berries
- Whole wheat

Gluten-Free Flours

- Amaranth
- Buckwheat
- Corn
- Cornmeal
- Maize
- Millet
- Potato
- Potato starch
- Quinoa
- Rice
- Sorghum
- Tapioca
- Teff

Gluten-Containing Grains

- Barley
- Barley grass
- Couscous (actually not a grain, but included here because it is commonly mistaken for a gluten-free grain)
- Durum semolina
- Kamut
- Oats
- Spelt
- Sprouted wheat
- Wheat
- Wheat berries

No Eggs

Eggs are another very common food sensitivity cause. Eggs do not adversely affect our blood sugar, and they are low in carbohydrates and high in protein. However, as a food sensitivity cause, they have the potential to increase inflammation and should be avoided.

Egg-Containing Foods

- Almost all baked goods
- Dressings
- Mayonnaise
- Pastries
- Sauces

Egg Ingredients

- Albumin
- Binder
- Coagulant
- Emulsifier
- Lecithin
- Ovalbumin (and most ingredients that start with the prefix *ova-* or *ovo-*)

Did You Know?

Egg Exception

If your IgG food sensitivity testing shows that eggs are not problematic for you, you can continue eating them on the Vibrant Skin Diet Plan. The results show that they will not aggravate inflammation and are nutritionally suitable to prevent blood-sugar spikes. However, this has to be confirmed before eggs are included.

No Processed Foods

What exactly is a processed food? It is a hard question to answer concretely. Essentially, it is a food item that is altered, packaged or manipulated from its natural state to such a degree that it is cheaper to manufacture, suitable for a longer shelf life and made to sell more efficiently.

The best question to ask yourself when assessing a food item is "Has this been made primarily to be healthy or to be sellable?"

The category of processed foods includes all fast foods as well as most boxed, bagged or canned foods. Also avoid food products with multiple ingredients, particularly ingredients you would never use when you cook at home, which usually means that they are not real food ingredients. For example, a healthy ingredient would be basil, but pass on a food containing disodium guanylate.

Also included in processed foods would be most foods with labels such as "low-fat," "low-sugar," "sugar-free," "imitation," "flavored" and "refined."

Genetically modified (GM) foods are also considered processed. Genetic material has been spliced into their DNA to improve their ability to grow in various conditions. We still do not know the long-term implications of eating GM foods. Let's go back to the test question to assess a food's quality and level of processing — "Has this been made primarily to be healthy or to be sellable?" With respect to GM foods, it is clear that these foods have not been genetically manipulated to be healthier. They are altered to produce higher yields and, therefore, to be more sellable.

When possible, choose certified organic whole foods to ensure they are not only devoid of pesticides, fungicides and herbicides but are also not manipulated genetically.

No Artificial Ingredients

Artificial ingredients are synthetic and created in a laboratory rather than grown from a natural source. You could consider them a subcategory of processed foods. They generally include the following categories: artificial sweeteners, preservatives, artificial colors, artificial flavors and artificial additives.

Additives are a category that includes miscellaneous other chemicals that may be added to foods for texture or emulsification, or to regulate pH, to prevent bulking or caking, or to stabilize. They may also be used for glazing or to buffer the effect of humidity.

With literally thousands of these chemicals used as artificial ingredients, we just do not know what they may do individually or in combination to our body. Normal physiology may be disrupted if there is chronic exposure to these ingredients. As a result, these ingredients may potentially disrupt hormones or initiate inflammatory processes in the body, which may aggravate acne.

It is recommended to avoid these man-made compounds, which are not designed to benefit your health but rather to improve a food's shelf life, flavor, color and texture.

No Alcohol

Alcohol should to be avoided for several reasons.

- In traditional Chinese medicine, alcohol is considered a yang type of food (meaning it aggravates "heat" in the body). Heat in the body appears in conditions where there is warmth, redness, irritation, dryness and growth. Acne typically fits all of these descriptors. This means that acne is typically a yang condition, and consuming a yang food such as alcohol will aggravate it.
- Fermented alcoholic beverages, such as wine, beer, cider, mead, sake and soju, contain yeast. Because yeast is a fairly common food sensitivity cause, fermented alcohol should be avoided, since it may perpetuate the cycle of inflammation in someone with acne.
- Alcohol often disrupts fluid balance in the body, aggravating dehydration and causing constipation or overstimulating the digestive tract, which can lead to diarrhea and later dehydration. Because acne is typically a condition of suboptimally hydrated skin — whether it appears as oily skin or dry skin — alcohol will aggravate the underlying problem.

No Caffeine

Caffeine is most commonly consumed in the naturally occurring form of coffee. It is also found in black tea, green tea and white tea — in lesser concentrations compared to coffee. Energy drinks, energy pills and sodas also contain caffeine.

From a traditional Chinese medicine perspective, caffeine is similar to alcohol in that it is a yang food that can aggravate yang conditions like acne.

The other issue with caffeinated drinks is that they are a common vehicle for sweeteners and/or dairy products, the two big no-nos for people with acne. It is usually easier to just eliminate the caffeinated drinks altogether, since caffeine, dairy and sweeteners are all consumed together in an acne-supporting concoction.

For these reasons, keep caffeine out of your diet when treating acne. Caffeine may be reintroduced cautiously when acne has cleared and aggravation can be monitored. As a general rule, keep caffeine to 1 medium coffee or 2 medium caffeinated teas a day in the long term.

Foods to Incorporate

These whole foods can be incorporated into the Vibrant Skin Diet Plan:

- Naturally raised meat, wild-caught fish, vegetarian proteins and pulses
- Healthy oils
- Non-starchy vegetables
- Low-sugar fruits
- Nuts and seeds
- Whole grains (gluten-free), within specific parameters
- Water and herbal tea

Naturally Raised Meat, Wild-Caught Fish, Vegetarian Proteins and Pulses

Protein is important to support collagen production in the skin and should be consumed regularly throughout the day. For your main three meals, be sure to incorporate approximately 20 to 30 g of protein.

Sources of Animal and Fish Protein

- Grass-fed beef, lamb or wild game
- Free-range chicken or turkey
- Wild-caught fish

Sources of Vegetarian Protein

- Tofu, tempeh and natto
- Lentils, chickpeas, black beans, navy beans, lima beans, adzuki beans, broad beans, black-eyed peas, pinto beans and other types of pulses

Meat

The problem with the majority of modern-day commercially available meat is that it is mass-produced and, as such, the animals have been fed unnatural sources of food and have lived in unnatural environments. Both of these factors affect the health of the animals and, hence, the nutritional quality of their meat.

If you choose to consume meat, ensure that it is certified organic and ethically raised, and that the animals were fed the right food. Cows, for example, are most commonly fed corn or grain. This is an easy way to increase their fat content, which thereby increases the desired marbling (tenderness) of the meat. From a nutritional standpoint, however, this also increases the inflammatory nature of the meat. Even organic meats may have come from animals that were fed organic grain and corn. Therefore, they may suit all the criteria for being organic, but they are still not ideal. Consuming a corn or grain diet increases an animal's levels of omega-6 fatty acids, which aggravate inflammation upon consumption.

Ruminants that consume a diet of grass, however, synthesize a nutrient called vitamin K_2, which we humans can't produce in our own bodies. This is important because vitamin K_2 shunts calcium out of our blood vessels and into our bones. Therefore, grass-fed meats improve our cardiovascular health by keeping our blood vessels supple while simultaneously increasing our bone density.

Vitamin K_2 is a fat-soluble vitamin, meaning that it is stored in the fat of grass-fed animals. Therefore, don't be shy about consuming the fat components of grass-finished organic meats. However, if you are consuming conventional (non-organic) grain-fed meats, remove the fat and choose leaner cuts. The fats in conventional meat will not only be devoid of vitamin K_2 and contain pro-inflammatory fats, but they also harbor residues of any antibiotics and hormones that the animal may have been given.

Note that some smaller farms may produce meat that meets all the criteria of being organic, ethically raised and grass-finished, but they are not *certified* organic. This is because the certification process is expensive, and small farms may not be able to afford the fees. If you know and trust a farm or a distributor of small farm products that meet the parameters of being "naturally raised," this works, too.

Poultry

Your poultry cuts should also be organic and naturally raised. Ideally, find poultry that is not only free-range (which is a loose term meaning that the fowls were not constantly kept in restrictive cages) but is also preferably pastured. *Pastured* means that the animals had access to outside pastures, and that they also consumed a more varied diet that included insects. The animals will have been supplemented with a grain diet, but fowls that have consumed a balanced diet (including foraged insects) will have better-quality meat and fat.

"Grass-fed poultry" is a bit of a misnomer, since the birds do not actually digest grass (as do ruminants). They may consume grass, but they do not digest and extract its constituents the way cows, lambs and wild game do.

Fish

Fish can be more complicated to source. The label "organic" is not reliable when it comes to fish. Organic farming can be managed only in controlled situations, meaning that the only way fish can be considered truly organic is if they are raised on fish farms. Fish farms provide an overcrowded and unnatural environment for fish, and many people question whether the organic label for fish is even relevant.

Ideally, choose fish that are wild-caught. Wild-caught fish lived in their natural habitat and consumed a balanced natural diet from their ecosystem. In addition, choose fish that are not high up on the food chain (large fish) since these are more prone to bioaccumulate pollutants from their environment. Mercury and other heavy metals, volatile organic compounds, polychlorinated biphenyls (PCBs) and other impurities are examples of these pollutants.

Vegetarian Proteins

Non–genetically modified organic tofu and tempeh are suitable vegetarian protein sources with high concentrations of minerals, such as calcium and iron, and are exceptionally well suited for the Vibrant Skin Diet Plan. Tofu and tempeh are high in protein and low in carbohydrates. This is a preferable option for vegetarians compared to the possible overconsumption of carb-heavy pulses.

Avoid processed soy products such as vegetarian meats, products supplemented with soy protein, soy flours and soy oils, all of which contribute to inflammation in the body.

Research Spotlight: Soy and Breast Cancer

There's been much debate about the connection between soy products and an increased incidence of breast cancer due to its estrogen action in the body. However, there is also evidence that a compound in soy called soy isoflavones may offer some protection against breast cancer.

A large American study in 2014 investigated the relationship between the intake of soy and incidence of breast cancer risk across a multiethnic group of 84,450 women. The study population included Japanese Americans, Latinas, Caucasians, Native Hawaiians and African Americans. This study showed that there was no correlation between low levels of soy intake and increased risk of breast cancer, nor any protective effect. However, at higher levels of soy intake, the study suggested that there was a decreased incidence of cancer.

A study from China in 2014 used a meta-analysis (a statistical analysis of the results of a group of prior studies) to examine the link between soy isoflavone intake and breast cancer. The researchers looked at 35 studies and divided the subjects into premenopausal or postmenopausal categories. In Western women, soy intake was not shown to have any statistically significant correlation to breast cancer risk. On the other hand, soy intake showed a protective effect in both premenopausal and postmenopausal women in Asian countries.

It is difficult to discern why the protective effects of soy are not evident in Western countries as they are in Asia. This may be related to ethnic genetic differences, but is more likely related to the types and quality of soy products consumed.

The whole-food forms of soy — such as tofu and tempeh, which are used regularly in Asia — are preferable to support a healthy balance of hormones and reduce inflammation.

Pulses

Pulses is the category of food that includes all types of what we commonly (and mistakenly) refer to as beans. *Legumes* is the broad categorization of any plant whose fruit is contained in a pod, and also includes soybeans, peanuts, peas, string beans and green beans. *Pulse* refers only to the dried seed component of the legume family of plants, and includes dried beans as well as lentils and chickpeas.

If you are consuming pulses as your main protein source, eat them with low-carbohydrate vegetables and do not combine them with grains, since pulses are also high in carbohydrates. Consider pulses protein-carbohydrates — if you eat them with grains, which are primarily a carbohydrate, then you are essentially doubling up on carbohydrates for that meal. This is often why vegetarian diets can be high in carbohydrates, which increases blood-sugar fluctuations and aggravates acne.

Doc Talk

Soy contains plant-based estrogen, or "phytoestrogen." There is much confusion about how this affects our body's hormone levels. Women are concerned that the estrogen may increase their risk of breast cancer (despite the fact that numerous studies demonstrate the opposite).

Men, on the other hand, seem to avoid soy like the plague out of fear that it will increase their estrogen, depress their testosterone and cause them to grow breasts. I tell my male patients who have these fears that beer is also estrogenic (because of its hops content, which is also a phytoestrogen). This usually puts the issue into perspective pretty quickly.

Here is the explanation I give to my patients to ensure they better understand what is happening in their body with respect to soy's estrogenic effects:

1. The main problem related to estrogen overload is our exposure to xenoestrogens — artificial foreign estrogens that are pervasive in plastics, pesticides and other common industrial chemicals. These estrogens have a much stronger effect in our body than do our own natural estrogens. The overexposure to estrogens in general is already making an impact globally on humans, such as the earlier onset of puberty. It has declined from about 17 years to 13 years of age over the past couple of centuries.

2. Phytoestrogens, such as soy, also act on the estrogenic pathways of our body, but they do so at a weaker level than both xenoestrogens and our own naturally produced estrogens. The increased intake of soy isoflavone (one of the compounds in soy that is theorized to be protective against breast cancer) in Western countries does not indicate a lessened risk of breast cancer, whereas increased consumption in Asian populations does correlate to a significantly reduced risk.

3. All estrogens in the body compete for access to the same estrogen receptors on our cells, because they are similar in their chemical structure.

4. In cases of estrogen excess, phytoestrogens reduce our total estrogen load by displacing the much stronger xenoestrogens.

5. If your estrogen levels are too low (a common occurrence after menopause), adding phytoestrogens can help return your estrogen levels to normal.

6. Because phytoestrogens can normalize low or high estrogen levels, they are described as having a normalizing effect on your body's estrogen levels. When assessing how different estrogens play a role in your body, think of a tug-of-war with you and several friends against an opposing team (your natural estrogens) — and you are in an even deadlock. If the opposing team substitutes in several bodybuilders (powerful xenoestrogens), you will be yanked down pretty quickly. But if a few kids (weaker phytoestrogens) replace some of the bodybuilders, the net effect balances out, and the tug-of-war evens out again.

   The confounding factor in this conundrum is likely what type of soy we consume. Asian populations consume soy in whole-food forms, whereas Western populations typically consume soy in heavily processed forms, such as soy protein, soy oils and soy flours. For this reason, I recommend sticking to organic tofu and tempeh (as well as natto, tamari and miso) while avoiding other forms of soy.

I also recommend soaking pulses overnight and cooking beans and chickpeas for at least 2 hours (lentils can be cooked for less than an hour since they are smaller). This ensures that the pulses' lectins and saponins, which are potential inflammatory compounds, are broken down. Also, eat legumes in moderation.

Healthy Oils

Oils are important for the skin because they reduce inflammation. If your skin is overproducing oil because it is dehydrated, the best way to compensate for this is to consume more healthy oils.

Eating more omega-3 fatty acids (found in fish, nuts, seeds and grass-fed meats) along with healthy oils helps to shift the body's balance from a state that promotes inflammation to one that reduces it. Acne and its accompanying redness are both types of skin inflammation; adding healthy oils regularly to your diet is critical in settling acne in the long term.

Overconsumption of omega-6 fatty acids, on the other hand, can promote inflammatory cycles in the body. Omega-6 oils are plentiful in grain-fed meats, peanuts, vegetable oils (safflower, canola, soybean, corn), wheat products and whole-grain bread. If you consume more omega-6 oils than omega-3s, you shift the balance to a pro-inflammatory state, which sets the stage for acne.

The body's cell membranes — the sacs that enclose each cell — are made up of omega-3 fats. To support the cell membranes of the epidermis most effectively, a good intake of omega-3s in our diet is required. Patients with acne are usually diligent about drinking an adequate amount of water to support hydration of their epidermis. To keep the skin hydrated, you also have to target the integrity of the cell membranes, and the best way to do that is to increase omega-3 fat consumption through diet and supplementation.

Non-starchy Vegetables

Vegetables are perfectly suited for the Vibrant Skin Diet Plan; they are dense in nutrients, high in fiber and water content, and anti-inflammatory. The exception is starchy vegetables, which we want to avoid to prevent acne flare-ups. That is because starchy vegetables have a moderate to high glycemic index and glycemic load, which creates sugar spikes (see Measuring Blood Sugar and Insulin Response, page 136, for more information).

Did You Know?

Ideal Ratio

To optimize health outcomes and mitigate inflammation, the body's ideal ratio of omega-3 to omega-6 fatty acids ranges from 1:1 to 4:1. The typical Western diet is heavily weighted to omega-6 consumption, averaging a 1:15 to 1:17 ratio.

There are countless non-starchy vegetables that support skin health. It is recommended that you consume large amounts of these on the diet plan. The non-starchy vegetable list is quite extensive, but here is a partial list to give you an indication of the many options available:

- Artichoke hearts
- Arugula
- Asparagus
- Bamboo shoots
- Bell peppers
- Beet greens
- Bok choy
- Broccoli
- Brussels sprouts
- Cabbage
- Carrots
- Cauliflower
- Celery
- Chile peppers
- Chives
- Collard greens
- Cucumbers
- Daikon
- Dandelion leaves
- Eggplants
- Endives
- Garlic
- Iceberg lettuce
- Kale
- Kohlrabi
- Leeks
- Mushrooms
- Mustard greens
- Okra
- Onions
- Parsley
- Radicchio
- Radishes
- Romaine lettuce
- Shallots
- Spinach
- String beans
- Swiss chard
- Tomatoes (although properly classified as a fruit, tomatoes are normally considered a vegetable)
- Water chestnuts
- Watercress
- Zucchini

Did You Know?

Carrots and Tomatoes

Carrots and tomatoes are sometimes considered starchy because of their high glycemic index; however, their glycemic load — which gives an indication of sugar concentration based on a realistic serving size — is actually low.

Non-starchy vegetables can be juiced, made into smoothies, eaten as salads, baked, grilled, stir-fried or steamed. All of these vegetables are supportive of clearing your skin and should be the largest portion on your plate during main meals.

Low-Sugar Fruits

Fruits contain ample phytonutrients to support the healing of the skin and to dampen the inflammatory processes that can lead to acne. They contain fiber, vitamins, minerals and antioxidants. However, they also contain the fruit sugar fructose, which can impact blood sugar. Certain fruits contain higher concentrations of fructose than others, and

Low-Sugar Fruits

- **Stone fruits:** apricots, cherries, nectarines, peaches, plums
- **Berries:** blackberries, blueberries, boysenberries, cranberries, currants, elderberries, golden raspberries, gooseberries, loganberries, red raspberries, Saskatoon berries, strawberries
- **Pears and apples:** cooler-climate fruits with a relatively low glycemic index and/or glycemic load; within each of these types of fruit are several different varieties
- **Exceptions to tropical fruits:** clementines, figs, grapefruit, kiwis, lemons and oranges; these are relatively low in their glycemic index and/or glycemic load
- **Coconut and tomatoes:** also acceptable (both classified botanically as fruit)

this determines their inclusion or exclusion on the Vibrant Skin Diet Plan.

As a general rule, tropical fruits are higher in their concentration of sugars, with a few exceptions (see box, above). That being said, the cooler-climate options are your best bet to keep sugar controlled while reaping their health benefits. Stone fruits (fruits with pits) and berries are two broad categories that fit into this cooler-climate category, along with apples and pears. The exceptions to this general rule are melons and grapes, which have a high concentration of fruit sugars, making them unsuitable for consuming while actively treating acne. Making fruits a regular part of your diet will enable you to meet nutritional requirements without sabotaging your goals for clearer skin.

> Making fruits a regular part of your diet will enable you to meet nutritional requirements without sabotaging your goals for clearer skin.

Nuts and Seeds

Nuts and seeds work well as a snack, since their healthy fat content makes us feel full. They are low in carbohydrates and high in both protein and omega-3 oils, making them well suited for supporting clear skin. Nuts and seeds both contain good amounts of various minerals (such as potassium, calcium, zinc and selenium) and vitamins (vitamin E and most of the B vitamins).

These seeds offer the most anti-inflammatory nutrition:

- Chia
- Flax
- Hemp
- Pumpkin
- Sesame
- Sunflower

These nuts are also beneficial:

- Almonds
- Brazil nuts
- Cashews
- Macadamia nuts
- Pecans
- Pine nuts
- Pistachios
- Walnuts

Gluten-Free Whole Grains

Yes, whole grains are carbohydrates, and, as such, are converted into sugars in your body. That said, when they are consumed in their actual whole-grain form (as opposed to whole-grain flour), the breakdown of their sugar is slowed.

Any whole grains you consume must be gluten-free to account for potential gluten sensitivities. To slow their absorption further, ensure that you consume these grains with proteins by either accompanying them as a side dish or mixing them together with healthy meat, fish, tempeh or tofu options. Avoid eating whole grains with pulses, since the combination adds to the carbohydrate count and creates an environment that is less conducive to healing acne.

Limit whole grains at mealtime: just $1/4$ cup (60 mL) in total over 2 meals a day (for example, lunch and/or dinner). Although this is a relatively small quantity, it will make adjusting to and maintaining the Vibrant Skin Diet Plan more manageable for a longer period of time. Moderation and balance are key to achieving and maintaining your goals for skin health.

> Any whole grains you consume must be gluten-free to account for potential gluten sensitivities. To slow their absorption further, ensure that you consume these grains with proteins.

Allowable Gluten-Free Whole Grains

(Note: Some of these so-called grains are actually seeds by definition.)

- Amaranth
- Brown rice
- Buckwheat
- Millet
- Quinoa
- Red rice
- Sorghum
- Steel-cut oats
- Teff
- Wild rice

Increasing Grains with Exercise

If you exercise regularly at moderate to intense levels, you may need additional carbohydrates pre- or post-workout. Higher levels of intensity may require the added sugar conversion for energy during your exercise program, and the exercise will efficiently metabolize the carbohydrates so it does not exacerbate your acne. In these cases, you can eat whole grains within 1 hour before or after a workout.

For specific quantities of carbohydrates that will serve your exercise needs but won't aggravate your acne, discuss options with a naturopathic doctor or registered dietitian who is knowledgeable about sports nutrition.

Checklist for Consuming Whole Grains

☐ Limit consumption to a maximum of $\frac{1}{4}$ cup (60 mL) in total for lunch and/or dinner each day.

☐ Add only to main meals that contain protein, to slow sugar absorption.

☐ Do not combine with pulses, since this will essentially double your carbohydrate count.

☐ Consume in higher quantities to reflect your moderate to intense physical exercise, which may require additional blood glucose.

Why Pulses and Whole Grains Are Included in the Vibrant Skin Diet Plan

As discussed earlier in the book, a healthy digestive tract and proper bowel regularity are critical before acne can be properly addressed. Therefore, the benefits from moderate quantities of pulses and grains in terms of regulating the stool and bowel function are more important than their minor impact on blood sugar at the quantities recommended. Also, their effect on blood sugar is not significant when consumed in combination with proteins, vegetables and fats, and when eaten in their natural whole-grain form.

Soaking, Sprouting, Fermenting and Long-Cooking Grains and/or Pulses

Soaking, sprouting, fermenting and cooking legumes and grains at high heat for at least $1\frac{1}{2}$ to 2 hours will significantly reduce lectin levels. Some of these methods are more involved than others, but do get into the habit of soaking your dried pulses and grains for several hours (or even overnight) before cooking with them.

To cook them, combine legumes with two to three times the volume of water and bring to a boil for at least 10 minutes. Simmer for $1\frac{1}{2}$ to 2 hours to maximize the

Did You Know?

Cooking Pulses
Cooking legumes at 158°F (70°C) — below a boil or a simmer, such as in a slow cooker — for several hours was shown to have only minimal effects on the digestion of various plant lectins. However, presoaking kidney beans overnight resulted in neutralization all the negative effects of lectin after just 10 minutes of cooking at a boil (212°F/100°C).

FAQ

Q There are claims that grains and pulses are anti-nutrients and have gut-irritating effects. Should I be worried about eating them?

A Some groups (for example, advocates of the paleo diet) advocate avoiding grains and pulses because of their lectin content; however, it is safe to eat them and they will not cause adverse effects on your acne to a certain degree. Lectin is a naturally occurring protein found in plants that deters pests from consuming them; it acts as a weak toxin. Studies show that overconsuming lectins irritates the digestive tract, leading to functional and structural changes in the colon, and prevents the assimilation of nutrients into our body. This would then weaken the immune system and energy in the body. Lectin is often viewed as a type of anti-nutrient, and it is speculated that it may exacerbate leaky gut syndrome.

However, when grains and legumes are consumed in small to moderate amounts and are properly prepared (soaking, sprouting, fermenting, long cooking) in a balanced, varied diet, this effect is negligible.

Doc Talk

From my clinical experience, eating grains and legumes will not hamper your progress to good health as long as they are prepared with appropriate methods to maximize their health benefits and prevent any adverse effects.

From a compliance perspective, it is more practical to recommend an attainable diet plan that works over a longer period of time rather than a stricter plan that fewer people will be able to maintain for a shorter period of time. Because achieving a healthy gut may take up to 6 months or longer, it is best to use a marathon approach rather than a short-sprint mindset.

The other issue with excluding grains and sticking to a completely grain-free diet is that it may aggravate the consistency of your stool. I have seen time and again patients with incomplete, infrequent, hard or even loose stools because they avoid consuming grains. Adding even a minimal amount of grains to their diets can help improve their stool and enhance its consistency.

Grains essentially help normalize stool. With hard, small or infrequent stools, grains serve to "fluff" them up to make them softer, easier to pass and more frequent. On the flip side, grains help provide bulk to loose, overly frequent or urgent stools, slowing their frequency and making them more formed. Improved bowel movements and stool consistency reduce irritation of the gut.

Taking this into account, grains can actually serve to improve gut function. While the issue is contentious, it boils down to this: keep a moderate, varied approach to your diet and implement proper, simple methods to improve the health benefits of grains and pulses.

breakdown of lectins, some of which may be resistant to lower-heat cooking.

The process of sprouting grains releases enzymes from the seeds, readily breaking down the lectins and other anti-nutrients, such as trypsin inhibitors, amylase inhibitors and tannins, found in legumes and grains. There are many methods of do-it-yourself grain or legume sprouting available (a brief search online will give you many options), or alternatively, you can purchase various sprouting kits from health food stores.

A combination of more than one of these methods is even more effective in inactivating the anti-nutrient effects of grains and pulses.

Water and Herbal Tea

For beverages on the Vibrant Skin Diet Plan, water and tea will be your staples. Beverage options become fairly limited when you avoid sugars, milk products, soft drinks, caffeine, juices and alcohol to target clearer skin. However, consuming an adequate amount of fluid (6 glasses a day is sufficient) provides the proper level of hydration for your skin, thereby preventing the sebaceous glands from overproducing oils (see FAQ, page 172).

If you drink a liquid that contains sugar, the sugar is easily absorbed across the gut wall and enters your bloodstream. Since a majority of commercial drinks include sugar, artificial sweeteners and other harmful ingredients, your best option is to stick to water.

If you dislike the taste of water on its own or find it boring, consider whether your aversion is a result of cravings or addictions to unhealthy/sugary drinks (even juices) that may have become ingrained at an earlier age. Train yourself to consume plain filtered water regularly so that you become accustomed to its taste and get a feel for how your body reacts. Avoid all water-flavoring products, too; these are chemical concoctions that artificially flavor, color and sweeten water.

Teas are a great way to add variety to your fluid intake. As well as drinking hot teas, consider adding herbal teabags or lemon/lime slices to your regular water bottle for the day. These will steep slowly over a few hours at room temperature or in the fridge.

Did You Know?

Tea Variety

If you need some variety in your fluids, try non-caffeinated herbal teas, such as chamomile, peppermint, lemon, ginger, fennel, cinnamon, rooibos, raspberry leaf and nettle. These help modify the taste of water into a more palatable drink while supporting the health of the skin.

FAQ

Q How much water do we need?

A We often hear that the standard recommendation for optimal hydration is 8 to 10 glasses (8 to 10 cups/2 to 2.5 L) of water a day. We require this range of water to replenish fluids lost through respiration and perspiration over the course of 24 hours. The truth is, most of the foods we consume contain a large proportion of water, so the 8-to-10-glasses figure should include the fluid that is contained in the food we consume throughout the day.

Consider an eye of round roast, for example. Keep in mind that muscle tissue is approximately 75% water. Surprising to most people, a roast is approximately 73% water by weight before cooking; after roasting, it is still approximately 65% water. Fruits and vegetables have a much higher water content, somewhere in the 80% to 90% range. Cooked grains, by comparison, fall into the 50% to 70% range for water content. All in all, the foods we eat throughout the day provide a substantial amount of water — approximately 2 to 4 cups (500 mL to 1 L) of water — which we can subtract from the 8 to 10 glasses recommended.

From an evolutionary perspective, people in North America have never had such easy access to drinkable water in our entire existence on the planet. Naturally, our bodies, which are highly adaptable, do not absolutely require the large amount of fluids expected for us to survive. However, it can be counterargued that we may potentially function better with an increased water intake to help flush out the overabundance of modern environmental chemicals.

The truth likely lies somewhere in the middle ground, and no matter what, water should be consumed regularly throughout the day. If you feel better drinking 8 to 10 glasses of water a day, there is no harm in doing so (besides extra trips to the bathroom), but it is likely an overestimated volume.

In practicality, 6 glasses of water (approximately 6 cups/1.5 L) should be adequate to provide your blood, tissues and skin with sufficient hydration. Many of us do not achieve this volume in a given day, but it is much more realistic to attain compared to the inflated, but unnecessary, 8 to 10 glasses we always hear about. The 6 glasses can be consumed in either water or herbal tea form.

Keep in mind that for every 1 hour of moderate to intense exercise, 4 cups (1 L) of fluids are required to replenish fluid lost though perspiration.

Importance of Fats and Protein

Fatty Acids

Essential fatty acids support the structure and integrity of cell membranes. Regular intake of essential fatty acids through diet and/or supplementation will ensure that the water barrier of the stratum corneum (the upper layer of the epidermis) will stay hydrated. The stratum corneum is composed of a protective layer of lipids (fats) that prevents water evaporation from the layers of skin below. The lipids are made up of the following fatty compounds: ceramides, cholesterol, cholesteryl sulfate and free fatty acids. Therefore, increasing your intake of fatty acids will provide additional building blocks for the protective upper layer of your skin.

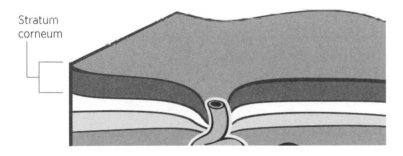

Stratum corneum

Protein

Protein is also crucial in supporting the strength of your skin; it also helps you feel full and stabilizes your blood sugar.

Protein is what makes up much of the structure in our bodies. Collagen is a high-tensile protein (think of it as rope) that provides strength to our blood vessels, bones, tendons, ligaments and skin. It actually constitutes 25% to 35% of our body's protein content. A proper supply of dietary protein ensures that our skin's collagen is rebuilt efficiently. Aim to incorporate a palm-size portion of protein — the equivalent of approximately 25 to 30 g of protein — with each meal.

Adding protein to your meals and snacks (via seeds or nuts) helps regulate the uptake of sugars and provides you with satiety, which is very helpful in this diet because of the restriction of high-carbohydrate foods.

Did You Know?

Replenishing Sebum

Sebaceous glands are more prone to overproduce and over-excrete sebum in people with acne. Sebum consists of fats and waxes, so when this happens, the protective lipid layer of the epidermis becomes deficient in essential fatty acids and there is an overproduction of proteins in the epidermis (hyperkeratosis), which leads to acne. Maintaining a regular intake of essential fatty acids can help prevent acne.

Did You Know?

Building Blocks

Proteins and fats are converted into messengers that function in both the immune system and the endocrine (hormone) system. These messengers assist with the regulation and normalization of our immunity and hormones, which are important for the health of your skin.

CHAPTER 11

Additional Skin Support

CASE STUDY

Nutrient Support

Benson, a computer programmer, had suffered from acne for 10 years. At 26 years old, he was quite laid-back and had a good disposition and perspective regarding his skin. Initially, his approach to his acne had been "it is what it is" and he had wanted to wait it out until it settled on its own. But when he came to see me, he felt that he had given his skin plenty of time to normalize, and realized that he should take more control of the situation to clear it up.

Benson presented with moderate acne. A mix of whiteheads and blackheads presented on his temples and jawline, with milder acne on his chest and back.

Because he was not in a rush, he wanted to do only what was absolutely necessary to clear up his skin. If the first, limited treatment plan did not deliver, he would incorporate additional recommendations. Essentially, he wanted to undergo treatment in a stepwise fashion.

This was not the typical mindset of most of my acne patients, who want their skin to improve as quickly as possible and will use whatever means are necessary. Benson's approach made sense logically, because we could clearly see what effect each modification would have on his acne.

I presented him with the Vibrant Skin Diet Plan, and we strategized a way to incorporate it one step at a time to meet his goals and timeline. After 3 months, Benson's back and chest had completely cleared, but he still experienced recurrent mild facial acne.

I suggested incorporating some additional nutrients to normalize his hormones, digestion and immunity, and to support his skin. We incorporated fish oils, probiotics and zinc over 2-week intervals. The fish oils were recommended to target inflammation and support the hydration of his epidermis. The probiotics were recommended to support his gut and immune system, while the zinc was important to stabilize his androgenic hormones.

We met after another 2 months and, although the fish oils and probiotics had offered some noticeable minor improvements, it was the zinc that finally pushed his skin to clear up. He was pleased that he finally got his skin to a point where he did not have to wait around for it anymore. He had also experienced improved energy and digestion, which motivated him to continue with the bulk of the diet modifications and supplement support.

Skin-Boosting Foods

If you are incorporating the foods outlined in this section, make sure you add them regularly to maximize their benefits to your skin. These foods are widely available, are versatile to cook with and can be easily added to your weekly menus. Try to make them staples in your diet and eat them at least two to three times a week.

These foods are all suitable for the Vibrant Skin Diet Plan: they are not known to cause food sensitivities and do not lead to sugar spikes. Be creative and find many ways to add these foods to your diet.

Avocado

Remember that fats comprise the cell membranes of your epidermis. Adequate fat levels help your skin maintain and retain water. Avocado is replete with healthy fats that support the skin and its hydration.

Avocados are rich in glutathione, a compound that supports our detoxification system not only by reducing the body's toxic burden but also by normalizing liver function. The liver helps metabolize hormones, which can thereby assist with skin health.

Cucumber

Cucumbers are high in a mineral called silica, which provides strength and structure to not only your skin but also your hair and nails. They also have a high water content, which supports skin hydration. They are delicious as a snack or in salads, and they combine well when juiced with other non-starchy vegetables or added to smoothies.

Extra Virgin Olive Oil

Extra virgin olive oil supports the skin with its anti-inflammatory effects. It is high in monounsaturated fats (MUFAs), which are known for their many heart-health protective effects, and they also help stabilize blood sugar and improve insulin sensitivity. Oleic acid is the main MUFA in olive oil, and it is this compound that instigates a lot of its anti-inflammatory activity, which helps inflammatory conditions like acne.

The important caveat with olive oil is the label of "extra virgin" — because it is not carefully regulated in North America, the quality of the olive oil can be compromised.

> **Did You Know?**
>
> **Antioxidants in Olive Oil**
>
> Olive oil also includes many polyphenol compounds that protect the skin through their powerful antioxidant activity. Polyphenols mitigate free-radical damage, reduce inflammation and have antimicrobial effects.

Good-quality, properly sourced and less processed extra virgin olive oils should taste spicy or grassy. That taste profile is produced by a high concentration of polyphenols. The "smoother" extra virgin olive oils that we are accustomed to have greatly reduced amounts of polyphenols, and as a result, their major health benefits are sacrificed. Source your olive oil from a reputable supplier who knows how to distinguish a low- from a high-quality oil.

Fish

Packed with protein and healthy oils, fish is an important part of a diet that aims to regulate acne. If you are not a fan of fish, you can always take a high-potency fish oil supplement to compensate. The eicosapentaenoic acid (EPA) and docosahexaenoic acid (DHA) — omega-3 fatty acids — in the fish oil help dampen inflammatory processes and support hydration of the skin.

Opt for cold-water fish, such as mackerel, sardines, anchovies, herring and salmon. Smaller species of fish are generally lower in mercury and other contaminants, as they are lower on the food chain.

Ginger

Ginger is a diaphoretic herb, meaning that it encourages perspiration. It also stimulates circulation and is a powerful anti-inflammatory. Its potent qualities help rejuvenate and restore the tissues comprising the skin. Ginger can be regularly added to and cooked with your meals. It also blends nicely in smoothies and juices. Alternatively, you can make a ginger tea by cutting a knob-sized piece of ginger into thin slices, boiling the slices in 4 cups (1 L) of water for 20 minutes, then straining out the ginger.

Lacto-fermented Vegetables

Fermented foods support a healthy microbiome (the ecosystem of bacteria in your digestive tract). Supporting the digestive tract assists the proper metabolism of hormones, the immune system and, therefore, acne. Fermenting vegetables at home is surprisingly easy to do, and these can be consumed as a side dish with your main meals. Consuming fermented foods also assists with the secretion of acids in your stomach, which improves digestion of proteins. Include fermented vegetables as an accompaniment to your meals on a regular basis.

Use the accompanying recipe to lacto-ferment vegetables at home. The bonus of this historical method of food preservation is that fermented vegetables keep in your fridge for a much longer time than fresh vegetables.

Lacto-fermenting Vegetables

Tips

Plastic lids for canning jars can be found at food or hardware stores or ordered online.

Make sure to purchase sea salt that is unadulterated by additives, such as anticaking agents.

For the vegetables, try carrots, mini cucumbers, cabbage, peppers, green beans or cauliflower, alone or in combination.

For the herbs, try basil, dill, bay leaves, rosemary, tarragon, sage, thyme or mint, alone or in combination.

As the vegetables ferment, check carefully each day and discard if any sign of mold appears or there are any off aromas.

- **1-quart (1 L) mason jar with plastic lid (see tip, at left)**

3 tbsp	sea salt (see tip, at left)	45 mL
4 cups	boiling-hot filtered water	1 L
	Vegetables (see tip, at left), cut into strips, chunks or sticks	
	Fresh herbs (see tip, at left), torn	

1. Dissolve sea salt in filtered water to make brine. Let cool to room temperature.

2. Pack vegetables and herbs into jar, leaving 1½ inches (4 cm) headspace. Fill with brine so that vegetables and herbs are fully submerged. Insert a narrow utensil into the jar in several places to remove any air bubbles. If vegetables float above the surface of the brine, wedge a piece of cabbage leaf into the jar to hold them down. Cover the jar with the plastic lid.

3. Place the jar in a baking dish (in case of spills or leaks) and let stand at room temperature for 3 to 7 days. Starting on Day 2, burp the lid (open it to allow gases to escape) at least once a day to prevent gas buildup (otherwise, the jar could potentially burst).

4. When the vegetables smell and taste fermented, transfer the jar to the refrigerator to slow the fermentation process. Continue to open the jar periodically to release any accumulated gas. Store in the refrigerator for up to 3 months.

Lemon

Lemon is an acidic fruit and is naturally low in sugars compared to other fruits. It works as an anti-inflammatory agent by buffering the blood to become more alkaline after consumption.

Its skin contains a phytochemical called d-limonene, which is shown to induce peristalsis (wavelike) contractions, which assist with digestion. This compound has also been shown in rats to reduce inflammation in the liver as well as reduce insulin resistance.

As discussed earlier, targeting liver, digestion and sugar regulation are keys to treating and preventing acne, so lemons are a good food to include as a regular part of your diet.

Lentils

Lentils are a type of legume and they come in many varieties. They are widely used in vegetarian dishes and have a good protein and nutrient profile. One cup of lentils (250 mL) has approximately 18 g of protein, which makes it a significant vegetarian source of protein.

Nutritionally, lentils are replete with B vitamins, iron, zinc, folic acid, manganese and magnesium. Because of their excellent soluble fiber content, they help stabilize blood sugar, which is critical in regulating acne. Lentils, as a general rule, are less likely to aggravate digestion and cause a food sensitivity than other legumes.

The one caution in cases where acne is very sensitive to carbohydrate intake is to ensure that lentils are not combined with large amounts of grains. Lentils are high in protein but also carbohydrates, so when they are combined with another carbohydrate (grains), they can cause blood-sugar spikes.

Strawberries

Berries are packed with antioxidants and many beneficial phytochemicals. Antioxidants should be a regular part of your diet to protect the health of the skin by reducing free-radical damage. Their low-fructose content also makes them an ideal fruit to add to your breakfast.

Strawberries are also exceptional for their rich levels of vitamin C, which is an important cofactor in the skin's collagen production. Just 100 g of strawberries (approximately $1/2$ cup/125 mL) will provide you with almost 100% of your recommended daily amount of vitamin C, which is a better bang for your buck than the better-known orange.

Swiss Chard

Swiss chard contains compounds that inhibit alpha-glucosidase, an enzyme that helps break down starches into sugars. Eating Swiss chard helps regulate blood sugar by slowing down their availability from food. Since controlling sugars is a critical part of the Vibrant Skin Diet Plan, Swiss chard is a helpful ally on the menu. It is also replete with vitamins A, C and E, all of which are important for improving cell turnover and strengthening collagen in skin. It is relatively high in zinc, a mineral that is crucial in the fight against acne (see Additional Nutrients to Support Clear Skin, page 182). Additionally, Swiss chard contains other phytochemicals that are powerful antioxidants and have anti-inflammatory effects, both of which support skin health.

Tofu (Non-GMO)

Tofu is a quality low-carbohydrate vegetarian protein source. It has substantial amounts of calcium, iron, potassium, phosphorus, magnesium and selenium.

The soy in our food supply is heavily processed, its components separated and concentrated and added as filler to numerous packaged foods, unbeknownst to most consumers. The other issue with soy is that approximately 95% of soy crops in North America are genetically modified organisms (GMOs). We do not yet know the health implications of GMOs, and it is always advisable to choose a certified organic form of tofu or tempeh, which by definition is non-GMO.

The Japanese diet consists of a daily intake of soy products; however, these are consumed in food forms that are naturally derived from the whole soybean. Japan has strong regulations regarding the import of non-GMO soy because of the questionable nature of GMO foods from a health standpoint. GMO foods were introduced to Japan in 2013 and must undergo a rigorous safety screening protocol prior to approval. Furthermore, GMO foods require mandatory labeling.

The health benefits of soy have been touted and demonstrated for years, but many of these results do not seem to translate to the North American population, despite our somewhat high intake of soy derivatives. The main red herrings in the soy debate are the types of soy foods we eat and whether they are GMO crops. The added benefit of choosing non-GMO soy is that it is an ethically sound vegetarian source of protein.

The health benefits of soy have been touted and demonstrated for years, but many of these results do not seem to translate to the North American population, despite our somewhat high intake of soy derivatives.

Walnuts

Walnuts are high in omega-3 fatty acids, particularly alpha-linolenic acid, which decrease inflammation and improve hydration of the epidermis. Walnuts are also high in vitamin E, which is helpful in maintaining the integrity of the skin by providing UV protection and supporting normal sebum production.

Skin-Boosting Herbs

Because of the potential adverse effects that may be caused by any nutritional health products — including herbs, plant or animal extracts, vitamins and other nutrients — please consult your health-care provider before implementing the following recommendations in your health regimen. Natural health products may be perceived as being safe to use, but there is a potential for interactions between supplements, medication and health conditions that can be harmful to your health.

Herbs for Hormonal Acne

Spearmint and Fennel

Spearmint and fennel both dampen the effects of androgen hormones, such as testosterone, on the body. Because androgen hormones are a common contributing factor to acne, either or both of these herbs can help settle hormonal acne caused by an elevated androgen response.

I recommend a 1:1 ratio of these two herbs, drinking 2 to 3 cups (500 to 750 mL) a day in tea form. The tastes of spearmint and fennel complement each other well. They are also both carminative herbs, meaning that they settle

Research Spotlight
Reducing Androgens

A study in 2007 demonstrated that tea made from *Mentha spicata* (spearmint) led to a decrease in free testosterone levels in women with excess hair growth (hirsutism, caused by excess androgens). This suggests that spearmint would work as a natural antiandrogenic treatment option.

Women with hirsutism who applied fennel extracts topically showed a decrease in hair growth. This suggests that fennel, like spearmint, plays a role in reducing excess androgens.

the smooth muscles in your stomach and calm digestion. Improved digestive function also translates to healthier skin.

This concoction is particularly useful in situations where medication (Diane-35, Ortho Tri-Cyclen, Estrostep, Yaz and spironolactone) has suppressed testosterone and there is likely to be a rebound surge — with accompanying acne flare-up — after ceasing its use. Essentially, spearmint and fennel help buffer against abnormal elevations of androgens, such as testosterone.

Red Clover

Red clover has been used for centuries as a "female tonic," to support childbirth, improve premenstrual syndrome and help relieve menopausal symptoms. It has a balancing effect on progesterone and estrogen in the body. Acne that flares in a cyclical pattern related to a woman's menstrual cycle responds best to red clover.

Drink 2 cups (500 mL) of red clover tea a day, being particularly diligent during the second half of your cycle. This means consuming the tea regularly leading up to ovulation (mid-cycle) and continuing regularly until you get your period. This is usually the interval when imbalanced hormones are most likely to trigger acne.

Blood-Purifying Antioxidants
Nettle, Parsley and Turmeric

Traditionally, nettle, parsley and turmeric are used to assist with chronic inflammatory conditions, and they have a special use for diseases that appear in the skin. Being powerful antioxidants, they help reduce the compounds called free radicals in the blood, which disrupt normal metabolism and function.

Did You Know?

Balance Progesterone and Estrogen

Typically, acne that flares premenstrually is known to be caused by an excess of estrogen versus progesterone, so the progesterone-to-estrogen ratio is too low. Red clover tea can help normalize these hormones.

They have also been used historically to reduce allergic hypersensitivity reactions and to provide antimicrobial activity. The combination of their effects may help improve acne.

These can be used in teas, cooked in foods or blended into beverages.

Liver Detoxification Herbs
Milk Thistle, Dandelion and Burdock

These three herbs have been used for centuries in traditional herbal medicine, and have the effects of stimulating bile production and bile excretion (termed cholagogue and choleretic, respectively). Improving the creation and removal of bile helps to bind fat-soluble toxins and by-products in the liver, helping to keep things moving, so to speak.

Part of the goal of improving bile flow is to assist with the removal of excess hormones — as well as medications, chemicals and toxins — from the liver. Optimizing bile's role in improving the removal of hormones helps to improve your acne.

Use these herbs in a tea or tincture, or as extracts, which may come in liquid or capsule form.

Additional Nutrients to Support Clear Skin

Nutrients can make a big difference in clearing acne, depending on its possible causes. The Vibrant Skin Diet Plan is a foundation base for improving your skin by controlling food sensitivities and sugar fluctuations. However, there are usually multiple reasons for your acne.

To accelerate the healing of acne, added nutrients are often required to support metabolic processes and heal functional problems.

The nutrients I typically recommend are listed below and they are based and categorized according to their function in healing your acne.

Healing the Gut
L-Glutamine

L-glutamine is an amino acid, and it is the fuel source for enterocytes, the cells that comprise the lining of

Did You Know?

Herbal Tea Preparation

Use approximately 1 tbsp (15 mL) dried herbs per 1 cup (250 mL) of boiling water. Steep for at least 10 minutes to extract and concentrate the active constituents into the tea.

Did You Know?

Nutrient Therapy Targets

The goals of nutrient therapies that target acne may involve a combination of the following: heal the gut, correct nutrient deficiencies, decrease inflammation, increase hydration of the skin and balance hormones.

your digestive tract. L-glutamine is the chemical form of glutamine that is used by our body, but as a supplement it is typically labeled just "glutamine" for simplicity. Taking glutamine helps repair and strengthen the integrity of the intestinal wall. A healthy gut wall is highly selective in filtering out unwanted foreign material so that it doesn't reach the bloodstream. This is important for skin health because inflammatory substances that get into the blood can manifest on the skin. People with a history of recurrent antibiotic use, anti-inflammatory medication, birth control pills, multiple food sensitivities or digestive problems should consider implementing a regimen of L-glutamine for 3 to 6 months.

> Glutamine helps repair and strengthen the integrity of the intestinal wall. A healthy gut wall is highly selective in filtering out unwanted foreign material so that it doesn't reach the bloodstream.

Recommended dose: 3–5 g powder daily

Probiotics

Probiotics are an integral part of the digestive filter and help regulate the immune system. As a result, ensuring that your microbiome is optimized improves unwanted inflammatory particles from penetrating into the bloodstream and, subsequently, decreases the propensity for developing acne. Probiotic supplementation has been shown to have potential benefits in treating and preventing certain skin conditions, including acne and eczema.

Establishing a healthier digestive tract leads to improved skin health. I recommend taking a high-potency, multi-strain, enteric-coated probiotic for 3 to 6 months to adequately colonize the intestines.

Recommended dose: variable, based on probiotic makeup

Research Spotlight
Probiotics versus Antibiotics

A 2013 Canadian trial investigated the treatment of acne in three groups: subjects treated with an antibiotic (minocycline), subjects treated with probiotics and subjects treated with a combination of both. The study revealed that probiotic treatment is a useful therapeutic option to reduce inflammation in acne, as well as to reduce the adverse effects of antibiotic therapy when used together.

Choosing a Probiotic

There are so many variables among probiotic brands that they can be hard to compare. Use these parameters to determine if you are choosing a good probiotic.

- It contains a minimum of 10 different strains of bacteria (including multiple strains of lactobacilli and bifidobacteria).
- It contains a minimum of 10 billion live CFUs (colony-forming units) per capsule.
- It is an enteric-coated capsule (the capsule dissolves after it passes the stomach and is in the small intestine).
- It contains prebiotics, which are essentially food for the bacteria. These are most commonly fructooligosaccharides (FOSs), inulin and galactooligosaccharides (GOSs).

Resolving Nutrient Deficiencies

Zinc

Low zinc has become a common mineral deficiency. Part of the reason is our overexposure to copper. Copper and zinc have an antagonistic relationship in the body — the more copper our tissues store, the more zinc they release. We are chronically exposed to copper through copper piping for plumbing, cookware, wires, jewelry, soil, water and air contamination, agriculture and fertilizers. Zinc is an important cofactor that supports our hormone metabolism and immune system. It has also been demonstrated that zinc inhibits the conversion of testosterone to dihydrotestosterone, which leads to acne in the skin. In blood tests, zinc serum levels were shown to correlate to the severity and type of acne. For these reasons, zinc can help restore balance to hormones in the body and, as result, improve acne.

Recommended dose: 30–50 mg daily of zinc citrate (take on a full stomach, since zinc can cause nausea on an empty stomach)

Vitamin D$_3$

Vitamin D$_3$ deficiency is a common phenomenon, particularly in regions away from the equator, which experience decreased sun exposure. The UV from sunlight catalyzes our body to produce vitamin D$_3$. Vitamin D$_3$ helps decrease the proliferation of cell growth in the sebaceous glands, thereby mitigating the likelihood of acne formation.

It also promotes the growth of antimicrobial proteins called cathelicidins in the skin, which may also improve acne.

Recommended dose: 1,000–3,000 IU daily of vitamin D_3, depending on sun exposure

Decreasing Inflammation and Increasing Hydration
Fish Oils

Fish oils are important for their well-studied effects of decreasing inflammation in the body. The other reason fish oils help with acne is that they act as an internal moisturizer for the skin.

Choosing a Fish Oil

Fish oils are not all created equally. As a general rule, you get what you pay for. Use these parameters to better compare prices between fish oils, based on concentration and quality.

- Choose a fish oil that is molecularly distilled, a purifying process that removes the heavy metals, polychlorinated biphenyls and dioxins that are concentrated in their tissues (from the contaminated waters the fish swim in).
- Make sure the fish oil contains high-potency EPA (eicosapentaenoic acid) and DHA (docosahexaenoic acid), translating to 1,000 mg combined EPA+DHA per capsule, or per 1 teaspoon (5 mL) for liquid fish oils.
- Choose a fish oil that uses oils from smaller fish (sardines, anchovies, herring, krill), which are more sustainable and less likely to contain toxins.
- If you are vegetarian or vegan, choose an oil derived from algae, which contains DHA as well as stearidonic acid (SDA) — it converts in the body to EPA much more efficiently than other plant-based oils, such as flax.

Consuming high-potency fish oils not only works as an anti-inflammatory, but fish oils also help the epidermis maintain its hydration. I consider fish oils — or a vegetarian algae-based oil equivalent — an important component of an acne regimen.

Recommended dose: 2,000 mg daily of combined EPA+DHA fish oil

Normalizing Hormone Imbalances

Calcium D-Glucarate

The important component of calcium D-glucarate is not the calcium but the glucarate, which is converted to glucaric acid in the body. It assists with metabolizing toxins through the liver using a process called glucuronidation — essentially, it modifies toxins to become more water-soluble, readying them to be eliminated by the body (via urine, feces and sweat).

Recommended dose: 500 mg, three times daily

Indole-3-Carbinol

Indole-3-carbinol is a compound that naturally occurs in the cruciferous family of vegetables, such as broccoli, Brussels sprouts, cabbage, kale and cauliflower. The body converts it to diindolylmethane, which is a compound responsible for buffering the effects of excess estrogens. With cyclical acne that occurs premenstrually, indole-3-carbinol helps reduce the surge of estrogen that can aggravate acne.

Recommended dose: 200 mg, two times daily

Diet Guidelines

To make this diet overhaul easier to accept, focus on the foods you can consume rather than those you must avoid. In essence, you are going to be eating meals with healthy whole foods that provide you with complete nourishment.

In a nutshell, your diet will consist of:

1. Three main meals that will comprise healthy proteins (naturally raised meats, wild-caught fish and legumes), plenty of non-starchy vegetables and a limited amount of gluten-free whole grains, if you choose.

Did You Know?

Pushing Out Estrogen

Glucuronidation coaxes estrogen to be released from the body, which is helpful since excess estrogen impacts acne, particularly those flare-ups that occur during the second half of the menstrual cycle. This type of acne also typically manifests on the jawline, around the mouth and on the neck.

---

2. Snacks in between meals that will be one or a combination of nuts, seeds, non-starchy vegetables and low-sugar fruits (stone fruits, berries, pears and apples).
3. Fluids that include herbal teas, non-caffeinated teas and filtered water.

Complying with these simple guidelines ensures that you are avoiding the intake of sugars, derivatives of sugars and carbohydrates that convert quickly into sugars (think: flours). The diet plan also eliminates the major causes of food sensitivities that can trigger acne and foods that can aggravate hormone surges.

This is essentially a very simplified, condensed iteration of the Vibrant Skin Diet Plan. If the details of the plan seem overwhelming, go back to these three simple rules to make the process seem more manageable and enjoyable.

Making the Adjustment

As you adjust to the plan, you will find it gets easier and easier for these reasons:

1. You become accustomed to the allowable foods and understand what to shop for, where to eat, what to prepare in advance to prevent sabotage, and how to make tasty meals. It is about creating new habits.
2. As you get further along on the diet plan, your body will adjust and you will notice a decrease in physical cravings for sweets and other food triggers that are eliminated in the plan.
3. Psychological cravings usually take the longest to resolve, but they will eventually subside. The foods that are excluded are not essential to your survival; they are simply foods that we have become emotionally dependent on. Foods can be our crutches and our stress relief, and they can remind us of family and loved ones. We need to be aware of these emotional triggers in order to let go of them.

If You Absolutely, Positively Can't Commit

Most patients with acne are extremely compliant and will follow a diet plan to the letter, particularly if there is an indication their skin is healing. Typically, if you have acne, it affects you to the point that you are very motivated to take measures to improve it (including taking potentially toxic medication).

Did You Know?

Building Motivation
When you understand the physiological responses to eating in a way that nourishes and calms your skin, you will be motivated to maintain and stick to the diet plan. When you realize that having "just a cheat" here or there in the early stages of the diet can set back your progress quite a bit, it makes it much easier to eat healthfully.

No Excuses

"I don't like cooking" and "I don't know how to cook well" are not legitimate excuses in most cases, because eating healthy can actually be very simple. It can be complicated if you want it to be, but you can make healthy, delicious meals with just a few basic ingredients. If you know your skin is likely to improve by eating a healthier diet, and you still tell me "I don't like cooking," what I hear is "I don't really want my skin to get better."

However, I understand that in some situations it may be just too much to follow this whole program because of external circumstances. It is an important distinction to make, though, whether you are not motivated to follow the diet plan or you actually can't because of your situation.

For example, it is understandable that there may be variables beyond your control that make it difficult to fully comply with the plan (for example, regular work-related events where there are no options except catered food). If a patient gives continuous excuses for why they can't follow certain parts of the diet plan, and I offer reasonable, realistic solutions that they turn down, then it tells me that they may not be truly motivated to improve their health and their skin.

So if for some reason you can't fully comply with the plan in this book, I suggest prioritizing what is most important. The focus of the diet plan is reducing sugar and sugar spikes, and this should be emphasized over everything else. This means ditching all sugars and anything made of flour.

If I had not been exposed to the many different intolerances and sensitivities in patients with acne, then yes, I could have summarized this entire book in five words: eliminate all sugars and flours. But the majority of the time, it is not that simple. Just cutting out sugars and flours will likely not be effective enough for the majority of people with acne to clear their skin for the long term.

I don't recommend sticking only to this simplified plan, but if it is all you are able to commit to or motivated to do at this time, it may provide enough of a change for you to start to see improvements. Everyone has different triggers for acne — which are often multifactorial — which is why I recommend a diet plan that covers all your bases. If your acne is tied primarily to glucose control, then you may see significant improvements just by limiting sugars and flours.

If it is the only option you can manage for now, start with just the basic change of eliminating all sugars and flours and see how your skin responds. If you see only mild improvements in your acne, consider following the full diet plan at a later point to maximize your results for clear skin.

Vibrant Skin Diet Plan to Settle Acne

This Vibrant Skin Diet Plan is designed to settle your acne and help you achieve sustained periods of clear skin.

When Will Your Skin Improve?

It is recommended that you follow the Vibrant Skin Diet Plan for a minimum of 3 months.

In many cases, I suggest following the plan as best as possible for 6 months. Six months is understandably a long commitment, but keep in mind that it can take 6 months or longer for antibiotics, birth control pills and Accutane regimens to take effect.

By the 6-month mark, there should be substantial improvements in your skin. There should be periods of sustained clear skin that last noticeably longer and are more frequent than you have seen since your acne started. Your skin may have completely cleared, or there should be at the very least dramatic improvements in your acne.

What If You Aren't Improving?

You may diligently follow the plan and still not see the improvements you were expecting. Everyone responds differently, and we all have varying constitutions and physiological responses. Unfortunately, there is no one health treatment that is guaranteed to work for every single person.

That being said, there are many additional acne treatment options recommended in the nutrient and herbal medicine section of this book (see Additional Nutrients to Support Clear Skin, page 182). If the diet alone is not giving you the results you want, you may want to consider adding on some nutrient or herbal medicines to your regimen.

If you are unsure of what types of support are best suited to improve your particular situation, I recommend getting an assessment from a licensed naturopathic doctor experienced in treating acne. They will provide you with guidance regarding which natural remedies may be most helpful to your individual situation and recommend an appropriate dose and schedule.

> **Did You Know?**
>
> **Stressful Outcomes**
>
> If stress is an ongoing concern, this may be the main factor that is impeding your skin's improvement. Consider talking to a qualified psychologist or psychotherapist to work through your emotional challenges. These health-care professionals are equipped to help you develop strategies to either overcome your stresses or improve your tolerance and ability to deal with stressful triggers.

Falling Off the Wagon

I must emphasize that if you happen to "slip" on the diet or consume a restricted food accidentally, do not beat yourself up over it or give up altogether. Just get back to the base of the program the next day. Many people have an all-or-nothing attitude with diets, and I stress with my patients that we have to keep things in perspective, make the diet plan manageable in the long term and always look at the big picture.

Physiologically, eating outside of the parameters of the diet plan will likely not re-aggravate your skin substantially. In the majority of cases, having an occasional "cheat" will not set you back and may not even be noticeable in your skin. In other cases, when people have very sensitive skin, a small slipup may lead to a noticeable breakout, especially during the first few months of the program.

It may be that you were at a friend's or family's house for dinner and they weren't able to properly accommodate your diet parameters. Or you may have been at your in-laws' home or out for a business meal and you didn't want to act "high maintenance" — perfectly understandable. In other instances, it may be that you had an extremely stressful day and you were just hankering for a chocolate bar to appease your feelings. No matter what the reason may be, if it happened, there is nothing you can do about it, so just keep calm and carry on. In the end, it is just a small step backward on your journey to clear skin, so keep moving forward.

After Your Skin Has Cleared

After your skin clears, it may stay clear. However, it is normal to experience some occasional minor pimples when eating foods that trigger your acne. You may also notice breakouts during periods of stress. These setbacks should be temporary, but be sure to monitor any dietary or stress triggers that may have re-aggravated your skin.

Once your skin has cleared for an extended period of time and after foods have been reintroduced successfully in moderation (see Vibrant Skin Maintenance Diet Plan, page 191), the goal is to achieve a more tolerant homeostasis so that reintroducing a few of the potential acne-trigger foods will not "rock the boat."

Relapses

Try not to get discouraged if your skin flares up after having been clear for an extended period of time; it can and does happen, in the same way that other health concerns can wax and wane. Our bodies do not have a black-or-white response to stimuli, and trying to fully understand which trigger brought back your acne can cause unneeded stress.

The goal is to eventually build up an increased tolerance to reintroduced foods. Once your diet has been optimized and your digestive function improves, your skin should be less prone to flare-ups, even with occasional deviations from your "safe" diet.

Keep in mind that even when you develop an improved tolerance to sensitizing foods, the big concern will always be sugar spikes. Physiologically, we are just not built to consume sugar and sugar derivatives on a regular basis. You will always need to be aware about controlling sugar in your diet. This is not just a benefit to your acne but also decreases your chances of developing chronic disease.

Vibrant Skin Maintenance Diet Plan

This second phase of the plan carefully expands your menu for long-term compliance and maintenance by reintroducing foods once your skin settles.

At this point, you are likely interested in adding restricted foods back to your normal diet. The Vibrant Skin Diet Plan has many parameters to optimize sugar control and limit potentially aggravating triggers to your acne. Following the regimen is manageable, but it takes a lot of effort and planning and is unrealistic to maintain forever.

Some people who have achieved clear skin for the first time in years may want to stick to the diet plan indefinitely. This is completely understandable because of the traumatic psychological effect that goes along with having suffered from acne.

Long-Term Goal

The long-term goal is to build tolerance to the dietary triggers of your acne.

After slowly reintroducing foods through the Maintenance Diet Plan phase, you will be more aware of food triggers and how they may affect you. You should be aware of foods that fall into one of three categories:

Did You Know?

Backup Plan
If acne does become chronic again, revert back to the diet plan and the nutrients and herbs that worked initially to clear your skin. Use the methods that you learned earlier and reset as needed. It usually will take less time to heal your skin (compared to the first time).

FAQ

Q Can I stick to the Vibrant Skin Diet Plan beyond 6 months if I find it helpful in controlling my acne?

A Sticking to a restrictive diet for too long can bring on other unhealthy conditions. It can lead to the following psychological and psychosocial ramifications:

- Alienating friends and family
- Developing an unhealthy relationship with food
- Experiencing stress related to meal preparation and eating
- Experiencing fears of potentially consuming the wrong food

For these reasons, I encourage patients to gradually expand their diet after their skin has settled down or cleared. Psychologically, it is helpful to know that this is not a "forever" commitment, but rather a defined interval of time set aside to improve your skin.

You can continue the diet up until the 6-month point, but I strongly recommend that beyond this point, you start to slowly reintroduce all foods. You may also reintroduce foods at an earlier point if you feel satisfied with the progress of your skin, and confident that your diet can be expanded.

- **Direct effect:** Your acne increases directly after consuming 1 serving; for example, drink a glass of milk, get pimples the following day.

  Avoid foods that have a direct effect on your acne. Approximately every 2 months, try to experiment with reintroducing a food that has a direct effect on your acne. At a certain point, your body may become more tolerant of that food. As your threshold improves, foods that previously had a direct effect on your acne may eventually move to the cumulative-effect category.

- **Cumulative effect:** These foods cause a breakout after being consumed regularly; for example, eat toast over 3 days and get pimples on the 4th day.

  Consume foods that have a cumulative effect on your acne on a rotational basis. They can be eaten once or twice a week at a maximum, if this does not aggravate your skin.

- **No effect:** These foods can be introduced on a daily basis with no return of acne; for example, eat a banana every day and it does not trigger acne.

  Foods that prove to have no effect on your skin may be eaten at your discretion. As with any aspect of your diet, always try to exert some degree of moderation with the frequency of consuming foods.

Protocol for Reintroducing Foods

The goal of this exercise is to divide newly introduced foods into categories. Introduce one restricted food item at a time. It will take anywhere from 3 to 8 days to completely determine if a new food has an effect on your skin.

Step One: 3-Day Cycle

(Refer to the 3-Day Cycle Food Reintroduction chart, page 195)

1. Consume moderate, normal serving sizes of the test food only on Day 1 of the 3-day cycle.
2. Observe if there are any perceptible acne breakouts over the 3-day interval and note your observations in the chart.
3. If there are no noticeable effects, proceed to Step Two.
4. If your acne returns on the second or third day (after consuming the test food on the first day), list this food in the Direct Effect column of the Categorization of Reintroduced Foods chart (see page 196).

Step Two: 5-Day Cycle

(Refer to the 5-Day Cycle Food Reintroduction chart, page 195)

1. Consume moderate, normal serving sizes of the test food only on the first 3 consecutive days of the 5-day cycle.
2. Observe if there are any perceptible acne breakouts over the 5-day interval and note your observations in the chart.
3. If there are no noticeable effects, this food item fits into the No Effect column of the Categorization of Reintroduced Foods chart (page 196).
4. If your acne returns at any point over the 5-day cycle after consuming the test food item on the first 3 consecutive days, categorize this food in the Cumulative Effect column of the Categorization of Reintroduced Foods chart.

Foods to Reintroduce

Be sure to reintroduce one item at a time (not a food that has a combination of ingredients, which makes it difficult to discern the ingredient that may have aggravated the acne). For example, eating a bowl of mango ice cream would likely mean that you are introducing eggs, sugar, tropical fruit and dairy all at once. Introduce eggs, mango and dairy individually.

Start with foods from the First Foods list. Sample one at a time (in any order you choose) according to the introduction schedule. Of course, introduce those foods you would normally eat. If you hate bananas and do not plan on eating them in the future, there is no need to reintroduce them.

Once you have introduced all the foods that you want from the first list and determined their effect, you can proceed to the Second Foods list, trying one food at a time. Alcohol and caffeine are included in this list as optional items. Introduce these fluids following the same reintroduction schedule as for the other foods on this list.

First Foods

- Starchy vegetables
- Pineapple
- Mango
- Banana
- Melons
- Grapes

Second Foods

- Dairy (hard aged cow's cheese, goat's cheese, sheep's cheese and fermented dairy, such as yogurt or kefir)
- Eggs
- Gluten (such as whole grains containing gluten, not in flour form)
- Dried fruit
- Caffeine (optional)
- Alcohol (optional; 1 cup/250 mL daily max.)

Foods to Keep Limited

These foods have no benefit but are okay to enjoy on special occasions if they are foods you truly enjoy.

- Natural sweeteners
- Artificial sweeteners, flavors, colors, preservatives and texturizers
- Processed foods
- Refined sugar
- Juice
- Soft drinks

Continue using the Vibrant Skin Diet Plan as your primary diet. Use the 80/20 rule — 80% of your meals should be similar to how you ate on the Vibrant Skin Diet Plan, while the other 20% can be more flexible and include the restricted foods.

Step One: 3-Day Cycle Food Reintroduction

Here is an example of a 3-day single-food reintroduction that measures if yogurt has a direct effect on acne.

Reintroduced Food: Yogurt

Day 1	Day 2	Day 3
Meal & form of reintroduced food: ¾ cup (175 mL) plain yogurt with berries and walnuts	*No reintroduced food*	*No reintroduced food*
Describe skin: Clear, nothing notable	*Describe skin:* Clear, nothing notable	*Describe skin:* Clear, nothing notable

Verdict: Yogurt does not appear to have a direct effect on acne.

Next steps: Yogurt must be tested in the 5-Day Cycle Food Reintroduction to determine if it has no effect or a cumulative effect on acne.

Step Two: 5-Day Cycle Food Reintroduction

Here is an example of a 5-day single-food reintroduction that measures if yogurt has a cumulative effect on acne.

Reintroduced Food: Yogurt

Day 1	Day 2	Day 3	Day 4	Day 5
Meal & form of reintroduced food: Lamb stew topped with 4 tbsp (60 mL) plain yogurt	*Meal & form of reintroduced food:* ¾ cup (175 mL) plain yogurt with berries and walnuts	*Meal & form of reintroduced food:* Mixed greens salad topped with olive oil, lemon juice and ¼ cup (60 mL) yogurt dressing	*No reintroduced food*	*No reintroduced food*
Describe skin: Clear, nothing notable	*Describe skin:* Clear, nothing notable	*Describe skin:* Two new small bumps on chin	*Describe skin:* One whitehead on chin	*Describe skin:* Continued enlargement of pimples and slight irritation of skin on chin

Verdict: Yogurt appears to have a cumulative effect that triggers your acne.

Next steps: List yogurt in the Cumulative Effect column. Because yogurt does not have a direct effect on your acne, you can eat it in moderation. Consume it once a week at a maximum to ensure that you can continue to enjoy it without having it lead to a breakout.

Categorization of Reintroduced Foods

No Effect	Direct Effect	Cumulative Effect

PART 4

Vibrant Skin Meal Plans and Recipes

Using the Meal Plans

The 4-week meal plans on pages 200–207 will help you take a step forward on your path to vibrant skin and improved health. They incorporate many of the recipes from this book and provide enough variety that you can rotate through them for several months without getting bored, but you can always sub in other appropriate recipes that are more to your taste. Keep in mind that the meal plans are simply templates you can use to help you plan for grocery shopping, food preparation and eating. You can use them as a rough guideline or you can follow them to the letter — it's up to you.

You may find that breakfast is the most challenging meal as you begin the Vibrant Skin Diet Plan. In North America, many of us are used to eating either greasy fried food (fried eggs and sausages) or quick, sweet, carb-laden meals (toast with jam or cereal with milk) for our first meal of the day. The meal plans include healthy versions of conventional breakfast options, such as Apple Cinnamon Hemp Porridge, Instant Coconut Flax Hot Cereal and various smoothies. But feel free to substitute lunch and dinner options for breakfast, to give you more flexibility.

Lunch or dinner foods for breakfast? This may be hard to wrap your head around, but it's the norm in many cultures. In Japan, for example, breakfast might feature miso soup, an assortment of pickles, fermented soybeans, fish and a small bowl of rice. When you're following a low-carb, high-protein meal plan such as the Vibrant Skin Diet Plan, you may ultimately find it easier to become accustomed to having typical lunch and dinner options for breakfast.

As you have learned in the previous chapters, protein is very important for skin repair, because your skin's collagen is a type of protein. The suggested meals provide adequate protein throughout the day, in both main meals and snacks.

Once you have been on the Vibrant Skin Diet for long enough to settle your skin, you can move into the maintenance phase. You can continue to use the meal plans as a guideline, if you wish, while introducing new foods as per the instructions on pages 193–196. As you determine which foods are "safe" for you, you can gradually expand your diet accordingly. Continue to monitor your skin as you allow new foods to have a more regular presence in your diet.

As you follow the meal plans, focus on savoring the tastes of the many options available to you instead of bemoaning the loss of comfort foods that may have been wreaking havoc on your skin. Once you find pleasure in foods you can enjoy without adverse reactions, you will gradually stop craving the less healthy foods you may have initially found difficult to let go.

Good luck on your journey, stay focused and persistent, and *bon appétit*!

Once you find pleasure in foods you can enjoy without adverse reactions, you will gradually stop craving the less healthy foods you may have initially found difficult to let go.

Week 1

Meal	Sunday	Monday	Tuesday	
Breakfast	Apple Cinnamon Hemp Porridge (page 211)	Green Gift smoothie (page 219)	Instant Coconut Flax Hot Cereal (page 210)	
Snack	Nori Pinwheels (page 222)	Brussels Sprouts Slaw (page 264)	Cauliflower Cocktail smoothie (page 217)	
Lunch	Caprese Salad with Tomatoes, Basil and Avocado (page 276) Eggplant Lentil Ragoût (page 288)	Roasted Cauliflower and Radicchio Salad (page 269) Basque Drumsticks (page 317)	Brined and Tender Lemon Roast Chicken (page 314) Citrus Fennel Slaw (page 262) Mushroom Tart (page 282)	
Snack	Multi-Seed Crackers (page 231) Olive Spread (page 232)	Salty Almonds with Thyme (page 229)	Nori Hand Rolls (page 223)	
Dinner	Bok Choy, Mushroom and Black Bean Stir-Fry (page 293) Peppery Red Onions (page 362)	Tomato Basil Soup (page 250) "Steak and Potatoes" (page 279)	BBQ Tarragon Mustard Turkey (page 332) Green Beans with Cashews (page 358)	
Beverage	Spearmint tea	Water with lemon slices	Fennel tea	

Wednesday	Thursday	Friday	Saturday
Green Tea and Blueberries smoothie (page 216)	Gingered Greens smoothie (page 219)	Tofu Scramble with Mushrooms and Peppers (page 212)	Rustproofer smoothie (page 220)
Roasted Chickpeas (page 228)	Curried Zucchini Strips (page 366)	Multi-Seed Crackers (page 231) Red Hot Hummus (page 235)	Radish and Cucumber Salad (page 272)
Celery Root Ravioli (page 285) Curried Zucchini Strips (page 366)	Herb-Roasted Salmon (page 301) Brussels Sprouts Slaw (page 264)	Avocado Cucumber Hand Rolls (page 224) Hearts of Palm and Mushroom Salad with Lemon Parsley Vinaigrette (page 271)	Souvlaki (page 348) Turkish Tomato, Pepper and Herb Salad (page 275)
Spicy Tamari Almonds (page 230)	Pea Tops with Pancetta and Tofu (page 361)	Green Tea and Blueberries smoothie (page 216)	Nori Pinwheels (page 222)
Baked Fish and Vegetables en Papillote (page 299) Slow-Cooked Sunchokes (page 364)	Zucchini Spaghetti with Lemon and Herbs (page 284) Chilled Avocado, Mint and Coconut Soup (page 246)	Beef and Chickpea Curry with Spinach (page 345) Veggie Kabobs (page 367)	Braised Chicken with Eggplant and Chickpeas (page 318) Stewed Okra (page 360)
Cucumber and Mint Coconut Water (page 215)	Dandelion tea	Water with lime slices	Ginger tea

Week 2

Meal	Sunday	Monday	Tuesday	
Breakfast	Kale, Apple and Walnut Slaw (page 263)	Instant Coconut Flax Hot Cereal (page 210)	Gingered Greens smoothie (page 219)	
Snack	Green Tea and Blueberries smoothie (page 216)	Green Beans with Cashews (page 358)	Fennel, Apple and Coconut Salad (page 266)	
Lunch	Smoked Tofu Gumbo (page 256) Marinated Kelp Noodles (page 283) Yellow Coconut Curry Sauce (page 241)	Tomato Dal with Spinach (page 289) Mega-Green Hemp Bowl (page 266)	Italian Sausage Patties (page 339) Herbed Mushroom Duxelles (page 233)	
Snack	Pea Tops with Pancetta and Tofu (page 361)	Nori Pinwheels (page 222)	Salty Almonds with Thyme (page 229)	
Dinner	Everyday Soup (page 251) Baked Pork Chops with Vegetable Rice (page 334)	Tofu Ratatouille (page 294) Gailan in Anchovy Garlic Butter (page 352)	Basil and Tomato Fillets (page 298) Creamed Greens with Pumpkin Seeds and Lemon (page 356)	
Beverage	Spearmint tea	Water with lemon slices	Fennel tea	

Wednesday	Thursday	Friday	Saturday
Apple Cinnamon Hemp Porridge (page 211)	Tofu Scramble with Mushrooms and Peppers (page 212)	Super-Seed Muffin (page 214)	Greek Tofu Scramble (page 213)
Roasted Chickpeas (page 228)	Mega-Green Hemp Bowl (page 266)	Green Gift smoothie (page 219)	Flaming Antibiotic smoothie (page 218)
Broiled Cilantro Ginger Salmon (page 302) Cauliflower "Mashed Potatoes" (page 353)	Avocado Cucumber Hand Rolls (page 224) Green Beans with Cashews (page 358)	Stir-Fried Scallops with Curried Sweet Peppers (page 310) Balsamic Tuna Salad in Avocado Halves (page 306)	Chipotle Pork "Tacos" (page 338) Garden Patch Spinach Salad (page 273)
Garden Patch Spinach Salad (page 273)	Nori Pinwheels (page 222)	Multi-Seed Crackers (page 231) Herbed Mushroom Duxelles (page 233)	Spicy Tamari Almonds (page 230)
Chickpea Tofu Stew (page 296) Asian Eggplant with Peppers and Peas (page 355)	Brined and Tender Lemon Roast Chicken (page 314) Fennel, Apple and Coconut Salad (page 266)	Black Bean Chili (page 292) Tangy Green Beans (page 357)	Caribbean Fish Stew (page 308) Stuffed Cucumber Cups (page 354)
Cucumber and Mint Coconut Water (page 215)	Dandelion tea	Water with lime slices	Ginger tea

Week 3

Meal	Sunday	Monday	Tuesday	
Breakfast	Apple Cinnamon Hemp Porridge (page 211)	Flaming Antibiotic smoothie (page 218)	Instant Coconut Flax Hot Cereal (page 210)	
Snack	Stuffed Cucumber Cups (page 354)	Multi-Seed Crackers (page 231) Olive Spread (page 232)	Roasted Chickpeas (page 228)	
Lunch	Black Bean Chili (page 292) Balsamic Tuna Salad in Avocado Halves (page 306)	Portobello Pot-au-Feu (page 249) Citrus Fennel Slaw (page 262)	Pesto-Stuffed Tomatoes (page 225) Fennel, Apple and Coconut Salad (page 266)	
Snack	Spicy Tamari Almonds (page 230)	Tangy Green Beans (page 357)	Multi-Seed Crackers (page 231) Perfect Guacamole (page 234)	
Dinner	Spelt-Stuffed Eggplant with Indian Spices (page 280) Citrus Fennel Slaw (page 262)	Cumin-Crusted Halibut Steaks (page 300) Pesto-Stuffed Tomatoes (page 225)	Indian-Style Chicken (page 322) Sesame, Hemp and Carrot Slaw (page 265)	
Beverage	Spearmint tea	Water with lemon slices	Fennel tea	

Wednesday	Thursday	Friday	Saturday
Gingered Greens smoothie (page 219)	Fennel, Apple and Coconut Salad (page 266)	Tofu Scramble with Mushrooms and Peppers (page 212)	Super-Seed Muffin (page 214)
Salty Almonds with Thyme (page 229)	Pea Tops with Pancetta and Tofu (page 361)	Spicy Tamari Almonds (page 230)	Pea Tops with Pancetta and Tofu (page 361)
Veggie Kabobs (page 367) Tuna and White Bean Salad (page 307)	Cumin-Crusted Halibut Steaks (page 300) Sesame, Hemp and Carrot Slaw (page 265)	Nori Hand Rolls (page 223) Spicy Chickpeas with Okra (page 291)	Simple Grilled Fish (page 298) Creamed Greens with Pumpkin Seeds and Lemon (page 356)
Nori Pinwheels (page 222)	Multi-Seed Crackers (page 231) Olive Spread (page 232)	Tuna and White Bean Salad (page 307)	Multi-Seed Crackers (page 231) Perfect Guacamole (page 234)
Portobello Pot-au-Feu (page 249) Spicy Chickpeas with Okra (page 291)	Roman-Style Oxtails with Celery (page 346) Creamed Greens with Pumpkin Seeds and Lemon (page 356)	Roast Chicken with Leeks (page 315) Roasted Cauliflower and Red Pepper Soup (page 248)	Asian-Style Baked Tofu (page 227) Summer Vegetable Ragoût (page 287)
Cucumber and Mint Coconut Water (page 215)	Dandelion tea	Water with lime slices	Ginger tea

Week 4

Meal	Sunday	Monday	Tuesday	
Breakfast	Instant Coconut Flax Hot Cereal (page 210)	Kale, Apple and Walnut Slaw (page 263)	Super-Seed Muffin (page 214)	
Snack	Fennel, Apple and Coconut Salad (page 266)	Salty Almonds with Thyme (page 229)	Green Tea and Blueberries smoothie (page 216)	
Lunch	Roast Chicken with Leeks (page 315) Curried Zucchini Strips (page 366)	Simple Grilled Fish (page 298) Pan-Fried Baby Bok Choy with Sesame Oil and Ginger (page 350)	Asian-Style Baked Tofu (page 227) Green Bean Salad with Toasted Hazelnuts (page 270)	
Snack	Slow-Cooked Sunchokes (page 364)	Multi-Seed Crackers (page 231) Perfect Guacamole (page 234)	Curried Zucchini Strips (page 366)	
Dinner	Roman-Style Oxtails with Celery (page 346) Tomato Basil Soup (page 250)	Marinated Kelp Noodles (page 283) Best-Ever Bolognese Sauce (page 242) Turkish Tomato, Pepper and Herb Salad (page 275)	Hemp and Sunflower Banquet Burger (page 278) Slow-Cooked Sunchokes (page 364)	
Beverage	Spearmint tea	Water with lemon slices	Fennel tea	

Wednesday	Thursday	Friday	Saturday
Gingered Greens smoothie (page 219)	Apple Cinnamon Hemp Porridge (page 211)	Flaming Antibiotic smoothie (page 218)	Tofu Scramble with Mushrooms and Peppers (page 212)
Turkish Tomato, Pepper and Herb Salad (page 275)	Multi-Seed Crackers (page 231) Olive Spread (page 232)	Spicy Tamari Almonds (page 230)	Green Gift smoothie (page 219)
Moroccan Lentil Soup (page 254) Hearts of Palm and Mushroom Salad with Lemon Parsley Vinaigrette (page 271)	Tuna and White Bean Salad (page 307)	Poached Jumbo Shrimp (page 311) Creamy Cherry Tomato Salad (page 274)	Chicken Breasts with Chili Butter (page 325) Herbed Mushroom Duxelles (page 233)
Cajun Cocktail smoothie (page 216)	Garden Patch Spinach Salad (page 273)	Nori Pinwheels (page 222)	Stuffed Cucumber Cups (page 354)
Braised Lamb Shanks with Lemon Gremolata (page 347) Pan-Fried Baby Bok Choy with Sesame Oil and Ginger (page 350)	Middle Eastern Chicken Soup (page 260) Roasted Cauliflower and Radicchio Salad (page 269)	Broiled Cilantro Ginger Salmon (page 302) Brussels Sprouts Slaw (page 264)	Sea Gumbo (page 258) Fennel, Orange and Olive Salad (page 267)
Cucumber and Mint Coconut Water (page 215)	Dandelion tea	Water with lime slices	Ginger tea

About the Nutrient Analyses

The nutrient analysis done on the recipes in this book was derived from the Food Processor SQL Nutrition Analysis software, version 10.9, ESHA Research (2011). Where necessary, data was supplemented using the following references: USDA National Nutrient Database for Standard Reference, Release #27 (2015). Retrieved April 2015 from the USDA Agricultural Research Service website: www.nal.usda.gov/fnic/foodcomp/search/; Coconut Secret Coconut Aminos Soy-Free Seasoning Sauce (2015). Retrieved April 2015 from the Vitacost website: http://www.vitacost.com/coconut-secret-coconut-aminos-soy-free-seasoning-sauce-8-fl-oz-12.

Recipes were evaluated as follows:

- The larger number of servings was used where there is a range.
- Where alternatives are given, the first ingredient and amount listed were used.
- Optional ingredients and ingredients that are not quantified were not included.
- Calculations were based on imperial measures and weights.
- Nutrient values were rounded to the nearest whole number for calories, fat, carbohydrate, protein, fiber, vitamin A, vitamin C and vitamin E.
- Nutrient values were rounded to one decimal point for iron, zinc and selenium.
- The smaller quantity of an ingredient was used where a range is provided.
- Calculations involving meat and poultry used lean portions.
- Recipes were analyzed prior to cooking.

It is important to note that the cooking method used to prepare the recipe may alter the nutrient content per serving, as may ingredient substitutions and differences among brand-name products.

Breakfasts and Beverages

Instant Coconut Flax Hot Cereal

This three-ingredient mix takes seconds to throw together, and preparing the porridge in the morning is as easy as adding boiling water and your favorite toppings.

Tips

This recipe works best with finely flaked coconut, but if you have large-flake coconut, you can still use it: simply crumble it into fine pieces (with your fingers) or chop before using.

You can use an equal amount of whole psyllium husks in place of the ground flax seeds.

If desired, replace half of the chia seeds with hemp hearts.

PORRIDGE MIX

2 cups	unsweetened finely flaked or shredded coconut	500 mL
1 cup	ground flax seeds (flaxseed meal)	250 mL
1 cup	chia seeds	250 mL

FOR 1 SERVING PORRIDGE

1/2 cup	porridge mix	125 mL
3/4 cup	boiling water	175 mL
2 tbsp	well-stirred coconut milk (full-fat)	30 mL
Pinch	fine sea salt (optional)	Pinch

SUGGESTED ACCOMPANIMENTS

Coconut sugar or coconut nectar

Chopped fresh fruit or berries

Toasted seeds (green pumpkin, sunflower, sesame)

1. *Porridge Mix:* In a large airtight container or sealable plastic bag, whisk together coconut, flax seeds and chia seeds. Store at room temperature for up to 1 month or in the refrigerator or freezer for up to 6 months.

2. *Porridge:* In a serving bowl or mug, stir porridge mix and boiling water until blended. Let stand for 3 to 4 minutes to thicken. Stir in coconut milk and salt (if using). Top with any of the suggested accompaniments, as desired.

Advice for Clear Skin

▶ When choosing fresh fruit for your accompaniments, avoid pineapples, bananas, mangos and grapes.

Nutrients per 1/2 cup (125 mL) porridge mix

Calories	249
Fat	19 g
Carbohydrate	16 g
Fiber	14 g
Protein	7 g
Vitamin A	0 IU
Vitamin C	1 mg
Iron	1.3 mg
Vitamin E	0 IU
Zinc	1.6 mg
Selenium	5.6 mcg

Apple Cinnamon Hemp Porridge

MAKES 2 SERVINGS

You don't need to wait for a chilly morning to savor this cozy apple breakfast. The combination of flax and hemp seeds provides a healthy dose of omega-3 fatty acids to improve the healing of your skin.

Tips

For the apple, try Braeburn, Gala or Golden Delicious.

Use an equal amount of chopped pear, mango, peaches or apricots in place of the apple.

An equal amount of raw sunflower seeds can be used in place of the hemp hearts.

For a different flavor, try ground ginger, cardamom or allspice in place of the cinnamon.

Nutrients per serving	
Calories	400
Fat	26 g
Carbohydrate	27 g
Fiber	5 g
Protein	16 g
Vitamin A	31 IU
Vitamin C	8 mg
Iron	6.1 mg
Vitamin E	0 IU
Zinc	0.7 mg
Selenium	4.5 mcg

- **Food processor**

½ cup	hemp hearts (hulled hemp seeds)	125 mL
⅔ cup	coconut water	150 mL
1⅓ cups	coarsely chopped peeled tart-sweet apple	325 mL
2 tbsp	ground flax seeds (flaxseed meal)	30 mL
1 tbsp	golden or dark raisins	15 mL
¾ tsp	ground cinnamon	3 mL
Pinch	fine sea salt	Pinch
¼ cup	well-stirred coconut milk (full-fat)	60 mL
1 tbsp	coconut sugar (optional)	15 mL

1. In a small bowl, combine hemp hearts and coconut water. Cover and refrigerate for at least 4 hours or overnight.

2. Drain hemp hearts, reserving coconut water. In food processor, combine hemp hearts, apple, flax seeds, raisins, cinnamon and salt; pulse until finely chopped.

3. In a small saucepan, combine the reserved coconut water and coconut milk. Bring to a simmer over medium-low heat. Add hemp heart mixture and cook, stirring, for 4 to 5 minutes or until warmed through.

4. Divide porridge between two bowls and sprinkle with coconut sugar, if desired.

Advice for Clear Skin

▶ Omit the raisins and coconut sugar.

Tofu Scramble with Mushrooms and Peppers

Bronzed in a hot skillet with mushrooms and peppers, crumbled tofu absorbs a delectable blend of flavors. It's an excellent source of protein, which means you'll feel satisfied for hours, and iron, providing 33.8% of the daily value per 4-oz (125 g) serving.

Tips

An equal amount of organic, non-GMO, gluten-free soy sauce can be used in place of the liquid coconut amino acids.

Other colors of bell pepper can be used in place of the red pepper.

2 tbsp	virgin coconut oil	30 mL
1	large red bell pepper, chopped	1
12 oz	mushrooms, chopped	375 g
1	package (16 oz/500 g) extra-firm or firm tofu, drained and coarsely mashed with a fork	1
¼ cup	chopped green onions	60 mL
2 tbsp	well-stirred coconut milk (full-fat)	30 mL
1 tbsp	gluten-free liquid coconut amino acids	15 mL
Pinch	freshly ground black pepper	Pinch

1. In a large skillet, melt coconut oil over medium heat. Add red pepper and mushrooms; increase heat to medium-high and cook, stirring, for 4 to 5 minutes or until softened.

2. Add tofu, green onions, coconut milk and liquid amino acids; cook, stirring, for 5 to 6 minutes or until flavors are blended and tofu is golden brown. Season with pepper.

> ### Advice for Clear Skin
> ▶ Use organic, non-GMO tofu.

Nutrients per serving	
Calories	222
Fat	15 g
Carbohydrate	9 g
Fiber	4 g
Protein	15 g
Vitamin A	1388 IU
Vitamin C	56 mg
Iron	2.6 mg
Vitamin E	1 IU
Zinc	0.6 mg
Selenium	8.5 mcg

Greek Tofu Scramble

This vivid scramble features vegetables likely found in many Greek dishes. The addition of the Greek Herbed Soy Feta elevates the taste to another level.

3 tbsp	olive oil, divided	45 mL
1/2	red onion, finely chopped	1/2
1	green bell pepper, finely chopped	1
2	cloves garlic, minced	2
1 lb	firm tofu, drained and crumbled	500 g
1 tbsp	ground turmeric	15 mL
1 tbsp	fresh oregano	15 mL
2 cups	packed baby spinach	500 mL
1	tomato, seeded and chopped	1
1/2 cup	chopped kalamata olives	125 mL
3/4 tsp	freshly ground black pepper	3 mL
3/4 cup	drained and crumbled Greek Herbed Soy Feta in Olive Oil (page 226) or store-bought soy feta	175 mL

1. Place a large skillet over medium heat and let pan get hot. Add 1 tbsp (15 mL) oil and tip pan to coat. Add red onion, bell pepper and garlic and cook, stirring occasionally, until just beginning to soften, 5 to 6 minutes.

2. Push vegetables to sides of pan, add the remaining oil to center and heat for 30 seconds. Add tofu, turmeric and oregano, stir in vegetables and cook, stirring frequently, until tofu starts to slightly brown, 6 to 8 minutes. Add spinach, tomato, olives and black pepper and cook, stirring frequently, until spinach is wilted and tomatoes and olives are heated through, 3 to 5 minutes.

3. Top with soy feta and serve immediately.

Advice for Clear Skin

▶ Use organic, non-GMO tofu and soy feta.

Nutrients per serving

Calories	488
Fat	45 g
Carbohydrate	10 g
Fiber	4 g
Protein	13 g
Vitamin A	1906 IU
Vitamin C	36 mg
Iron	3.8 mg
Vitamin E	9 IU
Zinc	0.4 mg
Selenium	0.8 mcg

Super-Seed Muffins

The array of seeds adds terrific crunch and flavor to these muffins, not to mention healthy fats, fiber and a kick of protein, too.

Tips

If you're in a hurry, you can skip resting the batter in step 3. The results are superior with the resting time, but even without it, the muffins are extremely good.

Store the cooled muffins, wrapped in foil or plastic wrap, in the refrigerator for up to 3 days. Alternatively, wrap them in plastic wrap, then foil, completely enclosing them, and freeze for up to 3 months. Let thaw at room temperature for 1 to 2 hours before serving.

- **Food processor**
- **12-cup muffin pan, greased with coconut oil**

3 tbsp	psyllium husk	45 mL
1½ cups	coconut water or water	375 mL
1¾ cups	green pumpkin seeds (pepitas)	425 mL
1 cup	sunflower seeds	250 mL
⅔ cup	flaked unsweetened coconut	150 mL
½ cup	sesame seeds	125 mL
⅓ cup	ground flax seeds (flaxseed meal)	75 mL
1 tsp	fine sea salt	5 mL
3 tbsp	virgin coconut oil, melted	45 mL

1. In a small bowl, whisk together psyllium and coconut water. Let stand for 5 minutes to thicken.
2. Meanwhile, in food processor, combine pumpkin seeds, sunflower seeds, coconut and sesame seeds. Pulse five or six times, until coarsely chopped.
3. Add seed mixture to psyllium mixture, along with flax seeds, salt and coconut oil. Stir until blended. Let stand for 1 hour.
4. Meanwhile, preheat oven to 350°F (180°C).
5. Divide batter equally among prepared muffin cups.
6. Bake for 28 to 33 minutes or until a toothpick inserted in the center comes out clean. Let cool in pan on a wire rack for 10 minutes, then transfer to the rack to cool completely.

Variation

Seeded Power Muffins: Add 1 cup (250 mL) coarsely shredded beets, apples, pears, zucchini or carrots with the flax seeds.

Nutrients per muffin	
Calories	295
Fat	26 g
Carbohydrate	10 g
Fiber	6 g
Protein	10 g
Vitamin A	72 IU
Vitamin C	1 mg
Iron	3.6 mg
Vitamin E	7 IU
Zinc	2.8 mg
Selenium	11.9 mcg

Cucumber and Mint Coconut Water

MAKES 8 SERVINGS

This is a spa-style drink, if ever there was one. Coconut water contains a wealth of nutrients, including vitamins, minerals, amino acids and antioxidants. It is also considered the second purest liquid after water, so it's an excellent choice for hydration in general and skin hydration in particular. Cucumber is high in silica, a mineral that provides strength to your skin.

Tips

Give the lemon and cucumber a vigorous scrub before use to remove any wax or dirt.

Whenever possible, use organic fruits and vegetables to avoid pesticide residue.

Nutrients per serving	
Calories	47
Fat	1 g
Carbohydrate	9 g
Fiber	3 g
Protein	2 g
Vitamin A	14 IU
Vitamin C	8 mg
Iron	0.7 mg
Vitamin E	0 IU
Zinc	0.3 mg
Selenium	2.4 mcg

8 cups	coconut water	2 L
1	small lemon, quartered	1
1/2	English cucumber, sliced	1/2
1/2 cup	packed fresh mint leaves	125 mL

1. In a pitcher, combine coconut water, lemon, cucumber and mint. Refrigerate for at least 12 hours to blend the flavors. Strain, discarding solids.
2. Store in the refrigerator for up to 2 days.

Variation

Orange and Basil Coconut Water: Replace the lemon with 1/2 navel orange, cut into 4 pieces, and replace the mint with an equal amount of fresh basil leaves.

Green Tea and Blueberries

MAKES 2 SERVINGS

This tea is packed with antioxidant compounds that support the skin.

Nutrients per serving	
Calories	104
Fat	1 g
Carbohydrate	25 g
Fiber	6 g
Protein	2 g
Vitamin A	422 IU
Vitamin C	29 mg
Iron	0.8 mg
Vitamin E	2 IU
Zinc	0.6 mg
Selenium	0.4 mcg

- **Blender**

½ cup	steeped green tea, chilled	125 mL
1 cup	blueberries	250 mL
1 cup	blackberries	250 mL
2	black plums, halved	2

1. In blender, combine green tea, blueberries, blackberries and plums. Secure lid and blend (from low to high if using a variable-speed blender) until smooth.

Cajun Cocktail

MAKES 2 SERVINGS

This tasty cocktail packs a zippy punch.

Nutrients per serving	
Calories	58
Fat	1 g
Carbohydrate	12 g
Fiber	3 g
Protein	3 g
Vitamin A	2342 IU
Vitamin C	78 mg
Iron	1.1 mg
Vitamin E	2 IU
Zinc	0.6 mg
Selenium	0.8 mcg

- **Blender**

½ cup	tomato juice	125 mL
	Juice of 1 lime	
2	tomatoes, quartered	2
1	small zucchini, cut into chunks	1
1	clove garlic	1
1	sprig parsley	1
1	chile pepper, chopped	1
½ tsp	prepared horseradish	2 mL
¼ tsp	dill seeds	1 mL

1. In blender, combine tomato juice, lime juice, tomatoes, zucchini, garlic, parsley, chile pepper, horseradish and dill seeds. Secure lid and blend (from low to high if using a variable-speed blender) until smooth.

Cauliflower Cocktail

MAKES 2 SERVINGS

MAKES 2 SERVINGS

This drinkable salad is nutritious and delicious.

Nutrients per serving	
Calories	80
Fat	1 g
Carbohydrate	18 g
Fiber	4 g
Protein	2 g
Vitamin A	29,814 IU
Vitamin C	27 mg
Iron	1.1 mg
Vitamin E	3 IU
Zinc	0.5 mg
Selenium	1.2 mcg

- **Blender**

1 cup	carrot juice	250 mL
1/4 cup	cooked chopped cauliflower	60 mL
1	tomato, quartered	1
1/2 cup	cooked chopped carrot	125 mL
1	stalk celery, cut into chunks	1
1 tsp	flaked kelp	5 mL
1/4 tsp	ground turmeric	1 mL

1. In blender, combine carrot juice, cauliflower, tomato, carrot, celery, kelp and turmeric. Secure lid and blend (from low to high if using a variable-speed blender) until smooth.

Celery Cream

MAKES 1 SERVING

Curry powder, turmeric and cumin have acne-fighting properties.

Nutrients per serving	
Calories	84
Fat	2 g
Carbohydrate	12 g
Fiber	3 g
Protein	5 g
Vitamin A	1373 IU
Vitamin C	18 mg
Iron	1.4 mg
Vitamin E	2 IU
Zinc	0.6 mg
Selenium	3.1 mcg

- **Blender**

1/2 cup	soy or rice milk	125 mL
1/4 cup	chopped celery	60 mL
1/4 cup	chopped fennel bulb or celeriac (optional)	60 mL
1	tomato, quartered	1
1/2 tsp	curry powder	2 mL
1/4 tsp	ground turmeric	1 mL
Pinch	ground cumin	Pinch

1. In blender, combine soy milk, celery, fennel (if using), tomato, curry powder, turmeric and cumin. Secure lid and blend (from low to high if using a variable-speed blender) until smooth.

Advice for Clear Skin

▶ Use organic, non-GMO soy milk.

Creamy Fennel

This savory concoction features fennel seeds.

Nutrients per serving

Calories	202
Fat	15 g
Carbohydrate	20 g
Fiber	5 g
Protein	2 g
Vitamin A	109 IU
Vitamin C	11 mg
Iron	1.6 mg
Vitamin E	0 IU
Zinc	0.6 mg
Selenium	4.0 mcg

- **Blender**

1/2 cup	coconut milk	125 mL
1 cup	chopped fennel bulb	250 mL
1	apple, quartered	1
1 tsp	fennel seeds	5 mL

1. In blender, combine coconut milk, chopped fennel, apple and fennel seeds. Secure lid and blend (from low to high if using a variable-speed blender) until smooth.

Flaming Antibiotic

This zingy smoothie offers phytochemicals with antibacterial activity.

Nutrients per serving

Calories	113
Fat	1 g
Carbohydrate	27 g
Fiber	6 g
Protein	3 g
Vitamin A	8948 IU
Vitamin C	75 mg
Iron	1.3 mg
Vitamin E	2 IU
Zinc	0.6 mg
Selenium	0.8 mcg

- **Blender**

1/2 cup	tomato juice	125 mL
2	tomatoes, quartered	2
1	apple, quartered	1
1/2 cup	cooked chopped carrots	125 mL
1/2	cucumber, cut into chunks	1/2
1/2	clove garlic	1/2
1	chile pepper, chopped	1
2 tsp	fresh thyme	10 mL

1. In blender, combine tomato juice, tomatoes, apple, carrots, cucumber, garlic, chile pepper and thyme. Secure lid and blend (from low to high if using a variable-speed blender) until smooth.

Gingered Greens

This quick green sipper contains power ingredients to improve your acne.

Nutrients per serving	
Calories	71
Fat	1 g
Carbohydrate	14 g
Fiber	6 g
Protein	6 g
Vitamin A	3143 IU
Vitamin C	65 mg
Iron	2.2 mg
Vitamin E	6 IU
Zinc	1.4 mg
Selenium	12.2 mcg

- **Blender**

¼ cup	ready-to-use vegetable or chicken broth	60 mL
1 cup	cooked chopped asparagus	250 mL
½ cup	cooked chopped broccoli	125 mL
1 tsp	grated gingerroot	5 mL

1. In blender, combine broth, asparagus, broccoli and ginger. Secure lid and blend (from low to high if using a variable-speed blender) until smooth.

Advice for Clear Skin

▶ Choose gluten-free broth until the reintroduction phase of the diet plan, when you can test to see if gluten-containing products are safe for your skin.

Green Gift

This refreshing drink contains a pop of parsley.

Nutrients per serving	
Calories	48
Fat	0 g
Carbohydrate	11 g
Fiber	2 g
Protein	2 g
Vitamin A	5877 IU
Vitamin C	63 mg
Iron	1.0 mg
Vitamin E	0 IU
Zinc	0.3 mg
Selenium	0.9 mcg

- **Blender**

⅔ cup	steeped green tea, chilled	150 mL
1 cup	chopped kale	250 mL
½ cup	broccoli florets	125 mL
½ cup	green grapes	125 mL
4	sprigs parsley	4

1. In blender, combine green tea, kale, broccoli, grapes and parsley. Secure lid and blend (from low to high if using a variable-speed blender) until smooth.

Rustproofer

This vibrant drink is high in carotenoids — important antioxidants that support the health of the skin — thanks to its ample supply of carrots and tomatoes.

- **Blender**

⅓ cup	carrot juice	75 mL
1 cup	cooked chopped carrots	250 mL
2	tomatoes, quartered	2
1	sprig parsley	1
1	apple, quartered	1

1. In blender, combine carrot juice, carrots, tomatoes, parsley and apple. Secure lid and blend (from low to high if using a variable-speed blender) until smooth.

Nutrients per serving

Calories	113
Fat	1 g
Carbohydrate	27 g
Fiber	6 g
Protein	2 g
Vitamin A	21,924 IU
Vitamin C	28 mg
Iron	0.9 mg
Vitamin E	3 IU
Zinc	0.5 mg
Selenium	0.8 mcg

Appetizers,
Snacks, Dips
and Sauces

Nori Pinwheels

Working with raw nori sheets is easier than you might think. Make these delicious pinwheels ahead so you can enjoy them on busy days when you are on the go.

Tips

If you have a sushi mat, feel free to use it for this recipe.

Nori, a deep purple alga, and dulse, a red seaweed, are often referred to as "sea vegetables." They are among the best sources of natural iodine and also contain an appreciable amount of potassium. Iodine is essential for proper functioning of the thyroid gland, which produces hormones needed to support healthy skin.

- **Food processor**

3	sheets raw nori, divided	3
1 cup	raw sunflower seeds	250 mL
1/2 cup	chopped celery	125 mL
1/4 cup	filtered water	60 mL
1/4 cup	freshly squeezed lemon juice	60 mL
1 tbsp	chopped gingerroot	15 mL
1/2 tsp	fine sea salt	2 mL

1. In food processor, combine 1 sheet nori, sunflower seeds, celery, water, lemon juice, ginger and salt. Process until smooth, stopping motor to scrape down sides of work bowl as necessary. Transfer to a bowl.

2. Lay the remaining nori sheets side by side on a flat surface. Divide sunflower seed mixture into two equal parts and spread evenly on each sheet. Starting at the bottom of the sheet, roll each up to form a cylinder. Cut each roll into 8 equal pieces. Serve immediately or cover and refrigerate for up to 2 days.

Variation

Pumpkin Red Pepper Nori Pinwheels: Substitute pumpkin seeds for the sunflower seeds, chopped red bell pepper for the celery and 2 cloves garlic for the ginger.

Nutrients per roll	
Calories	53
Fat	5 g
Carbohydrate	2 g
Fiber	1 g
Protein	2 g
Vitamin A	44 IU
Vitamin C	2 mg
Iron	0.5 mg
Vitamin E	5 IU
Zinc	0.5 mg
Selenium	4.7 mcg

Nori Hand Rolls

These hand rolls are an easy and delicious way to consume protein along with nutrient-dense seaweed.

Tips

To soak the sunflower seeds for this recipe, place in a bowl and add ½ cup (125 mL) water. Cover and set aside for 30 minutes. Drain, discarding soaking water and any shells or unwanted particles. Rinse under cold running water until the water runs clear.

Tahini, or sesame seed paste/butter, has a wonderful creamy texture and provides calcium, phosphorus, vitamin E and mono- and polyunsaturated fats.

• **Food processor**

¼ cup	raw sunflower seeds, soaked (see tip, at left)	60 mL
2 tbsp	filtered water	30 mL
1 tbsp	freshly squeezed lemon juice	15 mL
1 tsp	chopped gingerroot	5 mL
¼ tsp	dried dill weed	1 mL
¼ tsp	fine sea salt	1 mL
2 tbsp	tahini	30 mL
2	nori sheets, cut in half	2

1. In food processor, process soaked sunflower seeds, water, lemon juice, ginger, dill and salt until smooth. Add tahini and process until creamy.

2. Place nori, shiny side down, in your left hand, long edge facing you. Arrange filling on a diagonal on the left side of the nori. Fold bottom left corner of nori over the filling and roll into a cone shape. Enjoy immediately.

Variation

Nori hand rolls are an easy way to combine a favorite dip or pâté and nutrient-dense nori. Before rolling, top the filling with ¼ cup (60 mL) each thinly sliced red pepper and cucumber and a few avocado slices.

Nutrients per roll

Calories	97
Fat	9 g
Carbohydrate	4 g
Fiber	1 g
Protein	3 g
Vitamin A	81 IU
Vitamin C	3 mg
Iron	0.9 mg
Vitamin E	5 IU
Zinc	0.8 mg
Selenium	7.2 mcg

Avocado Cucumber Hand Rolls

These hand rolls are refreshing, healthy and packed with protein.

Tips

To soak the sunflower seeds, place in a bowl and add 2 cups (500 mL) warm water. Cover and set aside for 10 minutes. Drain, discarding soaking water and any bits of shell or unwanted particles. Rinse under cold running water until the water runs clear.

Be sure to purchase high-quality nori from a reputable source, such as your favorite raw foods retailer, health food store or well-stocked grocery store.

- **Food processor**

1 cup	raw sunflower seeds, soaked (see tip, at left)	250 mL
1/4 cup	freshly squeezed lemon juice	60 mL
1/4 cup	filtered water	60 mL
1/4 tsp	fine sea salt	1 mL
1	sheet raw nori, cut in half lengthwise (see tip, at left)	1
1/2	cucumber, seeded and thinly sliced lengthwise	1/2
1/2	avocado, thinly sliced lengthwise	1/2

1. In food processor, process soaked sunflower seeds, lemon juice, water and salt until smooth.

2. Place 1 piece of nori, shiny side down, in the palm of your left hand (if you are right-handed), long edge facing you. Place half the sunflower mixture on a diagonal starting from the upper left corner. Top with half the cucumber and avocado slices. Fold bottom left corner of nori over filling and roll into a cone shape. Repeat with second piece of nori. Enjoy immediately.

Variations

Substitute an equal quantity of finely sliced red bell pepper for the cucumber.

For some added crunch, add 1 tsp (5 mL) raw white sesame seeds to each roll.

Nutrients per serving	
Calories	502
Fat	44 g
Carbohydrate	22 g
Fiber	10 g
Protein	16 g
Vitamin A	214 IU
Vitamin C	20 mg
Iron	4.1 mg
Vitamin E	38 IU
Zinc	3.9 mg
Selenium	37.4 mcg

Pesto-Stuffed Tomatoes

*Pumpkin seeds are a
unique alternative to
pine nuts in the pesto
that fills these yummy
hors d'oeuvres. Moreover,
they contain zinc, a
mineral that supports
hormone balance,
thereby contributing
to the healing of acne.*

Tips

If you need a last-minute
appetizer, use purchased
basil pesto to make these
super-easy appetizers.

Green pumpkin seeds are
also known as pepitas.
They are often toasted
to bring out their nutty
flavor. Be sure to use
hulled pumpkin seeds
in this recipe.

- **Food processor or blender**
- **Piping bag with medium-size round tip**

2	cloves garlic, minced	2
1 cup	packed fresh basil leaves	250 mL
1/3 cup	green pumpkin seeds (pepitas), toasted and cooled	75 mL
1/4 tsp	salt	1 mL
1/4 tsp	freshly ground black pepper	1 mL
3 tbsp	extra virgin olive oil	45 mL
24	cherry tomatoes, cored	24

1. In food processor, combine garlic, basil, pumpkin seeds, salt, pepper and oil; process until smooth.

2. Transfer pesto to piping bag and pipe into cherry tomatoes; do not overfill. Cover and refrigerate until chilled, for up to 4 hours.

Variation

To give these appetizers a cheesy twist, combine half the pesto with 1/4 cup (60 mL) softened goat cheese. Pipe into cored tomatoes. Cover and refrigerate the remaining pesto for up to 2 days for another use.

This recipe courtesy of dietitian Heather McColl.

Nutrients per
3 appetizers

Calories	87
Fat	8 g
Carbohydrate	3 g
Fiber	1 g
Protein	2 g
Vitamin A	706 IU
Vitamin C	8 mg
Iron	0.8 mg
Vitamin E	2 IU
Zinc	0.6 mg
Selenium	0.6 mcg

Greek Herbed Soy Feta in Olive Oil

Salty soy feta cubes swirl in rich olive oil with intense red and green jewels of flavor. Choose a lovely jar to complete the stunning presentation. A gorgeous addition to an appetizer platter, these spicy, salty little pillows are scrumptious on crackers or grilled slices of focaccia.

Tip

Vary the saltiness of the soy feta by increasing or decreasing the salt brine soaking time.

4 oz	extra-firm tofu	125 g
¼ cup	kosher salt	60 mL
1 tbsp	white wine vinegar	15 mL
2 cups	water	500 mL
1 cup	olive oil	250 mL
1 tbsp	drained oil-packed sun-dried tomato strips	15 mL
1	large clove garlic, slivered	1
1	bay leaf, crumbled	1
1½ tsp	drained capers	7 mL
½ tsp	mixed whole black and red peppercorns	2 mL
¼ tsp	hot pepper flakes	1 mL
¼ tsp	dried oregano	1 mL

1. Drain tofu, wrap in a clean thick kitchen towel or paper towels and place on a dinner plate. Place a second dinner plate on top, place a heavy can on top of plate and set aside for 1 hour. Transfer tofu to a resealable freezer bag and freeze for at least 12 hours.

2. Let frozen tofu thaw at room temperature and cut into 1-inch (2.5 cm) cubes. In a bowl, combine salt, vinegar and water. Add tofu cubes and immerse in liquid. Cover and refrigerate for 4 to 6 hours (see tip, at left). Remove tofu from brine and carefully pat dry. Discard brine.

3. In a glass jar with a tight-fitting lid, combine oil, sun-dried tomatoes, garlic, bay leaf, capers, peppercorns, hot pepper flakes and oregano. Add tofu and gently stir to distribute ingredients. Store in refrigerator for up to 1 week. Before serving, let mixture stand at room temperature for 30 minutes to allow oil to re-liquefy.

Advice for Clear Skin

▸ Use organic, non-GMO tofu.

Nutrients per ¼ cup (60 mL)

Calories	341
Fat	37 g
Carbohydrate	1 g
Fiber	0 g
Protein	2 g
Vitamin A	57 IU
Vitamin C	1 mg
Iron	0.6 mg
Vitamin E	8 IU
Zinc	0 mg
Selenium	0.1 mcg

Asian-Style Baked Tofu

MAKES 4 SERVINGS

This tasty tofu can be eaten as a snack, as an appetizer or in an Asian stir-fry. It can be served hot or cold. Organic tofu can have a regulating effect on hormones in the body, making it a good choice for treating acne that results from imbalanced hormones.

Tip

To drain tofu, place the cubes on a plate lined with a double layer of paper towels. Cover with another paper towel and another plate and place a weight on top of the plate to press the water from the tofu. Let stand for 30 minutes. Drain off water.

- **Preheat oven to 350°F (180°C)**
- **8-inch (20 cm) square glass baking dish**

1/4 cup	low-sodium soy sauce	60 mL
1/4 cup	vegan teriyaki sauce	60 mL
2 tbsp	freshly squeezed lime juice	30 mL
1 tbsp	finely grated gingerroot	15 mL
2	cloves garlic, minced (about 2 tsp/10 mL)	2
1 lb	firm or extra-firm tofu, cut in 1-inch (2.5 cm) cubes and drained (see tip, at left)	500 g

1. In a small bowl, whisk together soy sauce, teriyaki sauce, lime juice, ginger and garlic.

2. Arrange tofu evenly over the bottom of baking dish. Add sauce and stir until cubes are completely covered with sauce. Marinate for 1 hour at room temperature or in the refrigerator for at least 2 hours or for up to 8 hours.

3. Bake, uncovered, in preheated oven, for 35 to 40 minutes, stirring and turning pieces over after 20 minutes, or until tofu is firm and liquid is absorbed.

Advice for Clear Skin

▸ Use organic, non-GMO soy sauce and tofu, and make sure the soy sauce you choose is gluten-free.

Nutrients per serving

Calories	125
Fat	5 g
Carbohydrate	8 g
Fiber	1 g
Protein	12 g
Vitamin A	4 IU
Vitamin C	3 mg
Iron	2.0 mg
Vitamin E	0 IU
Zinc	0.1 mg
Selenium	0.6 mcg

Roasted Chickpeas

*Roasted chickpeas make
a nice savory snack
alternative to chips. Kids
love the crunch, but be
sure they're old enough
that these do not pose a
choking hazard.*

Tips

Be sure to drain and
rinse the chickpeas to
remove excess sodium.
Pat them dry so the
coating adheres.

These can be stored in
an airtight container at
room temperature for
1 week, but they likely
won't last that long!

- **Preheat oven to 350°F (180°C)**
- **Baking sheet, lined with foil**

1	can (19 oz/540 mL) chickpeas, rinsed, drained and patted dry	1
1 tbsp	canola oil	15 mL
¹/₂ tsp	chili powder	2 mL
¹/₄ tsp	garlic powder	1 mL
¹/₄ tsp	ground cumin	1 mL

1. In a small bowl, combine chickpeas, oil, chili powder,
garlic powder and cumin. Stir to coat well. Spread evenly
on preparing baking sheet.

2. Bake in preheated oven, stirring occasionally, for 60 to
75 minutes or until crisp. Let cool on pan on a wire rack.

Variation

Vary the spices to your liking; added cayenne pepper will
give them a hot kick.

This recipe courtesy of dietitian Jaclyn Pritchard.

Advice for Clear Skin

▶ Substitute extra virgin olive oil for the canola oil.

Nutrients per 2 tbsp (30 mL)

Calories	59
Fat	2 g
Carbohydrate	10 g
Fiber	2 g
Protein	2 g
Vitamin A	40 IU
Vitamin C	2 mg
Iron	0.6 mg
Vitamin E	0 IU
Zinc	0.5 mg
Selenium	1.2 mcg

Salty Almonds with Thyme

When entertaining in winter, light a fire and place small bowls full of these tasty nibblers where they are easily accessible to guests.

Tips

Use a small to medium slow cooker so the nuts are less likely to burn. You can make them in a larger slow cooker (about 5 quarts) but watch carefully and stir every 15 minutes, because the nuts will cook quite quickly (in just over an hour).

Sea salt is available in most supermarkets. It is much sweeter than table salt and is much better for you.

Nutrients per ¼ cup (60 mL)	
Calories	238
Fat	21 g
Carbohydrate	8 g
Fiber	4 g
Protein	8 g
Vitamin A	29 IU
Vitamin C	1 mg
Iron	1.4 mg
Vitamin E	15 IU
Zinc	1.1 mg
Selenium	0.9 mcg

- **Small (maximum 3½-quart) slow cooker**

2 cups	unblanched almonds	500 mL
½ tsp	freshly ground white pepper	2 mL
1 tbsp	fine sea salt (or to taste)	15 mL
2 tbsp	extra virgin olive oil	30 mL
2 tbsp	fresh thyme	30 mL

1. In slow cooker stoneware, combine almonds and white pepper. Cover and cook on High for 1½ hours, stirring every 30 minutes, until nuts are nicely toasted.

2. In a bowl, combine salt, olive oil and thyme. Add to hot almonds in stoneware and stir thoroughly to combine. Spoon mixture into a small serving bowl and serve hot or let cool.

Spicy Tamari Almonds

MAKES ABOUT 2 CUPS (500 ML)

These tasty tidbits are great as pre-dinner nibbles paired with a cold beverage. Tamari is a wheat-free soy sauce, so you can happily serve these as a gluten-free snack.

Tip

For a holiday gift, make up a batch or two and package in pretty jars. If well sealed, the nuts will keep for 10 days.

- **Small (2- to 3½-quart) slow cooker**

2 cups	whole almonds	500 mL
¼ tsp	cayenne pepper	1 mL
2 tbsp	reduced-sodium tamari or coconut amino acids	30 mL
1 tbsp	extra virgin olive oil	15 mL
	Fine sea salt	

1. In slow cooker stoneware, combine almonds and cayenne. Place a clean tea towel folded in half (so you will have 2 layers) over top of stoneware to absorb moisture. Cover and cook on High for 45 minutes.

2. In a small bowl, combine tamari and olive oil. Add to hot almonds and stir thoroughly to combine. Replace tea towel. Cover and cook on High for 1½ hours, until nuts are hot and fragrant, stirring every 30 minutes and replacing towel each time. Sprinkle with salt to taste. Store in an airtight container.

> ### Advice for Clear Skin
> ▸ Use organic, non-GMO tamari.

Nutrients per ¼ cup (60 mL)

Calories	223
Fat	19 g
Carbohydrate	8 g
Fiber	4 g
Protein	8 g
Vitamin A	24 IU
Vitamin C	0 mg
Iron	1.4 mg
Vitamin E	14 IU
Zinc	1.1 mg
Selenium	0.9 mcg

Multi-Seed Crackers

**MAKES
2 DOZEN MEDIUM
CRACKERS**

With their crispy crunch and toasty flavor, these little numbers are especially delectable. Spread them with seed butter in the morning, top them with hummus at lunch or serve them with soup at supper. They make a great snack, too.

Tips

Do not bother trying to separate the cracker dough before baking; it is tricky and the dough is prone to tearing. Once baked, it is easy to separate the crackers along the score lines.

Store the cooled crackers in a tin at room temperature for up to 3 days.

Nutrients per 3 crackers

Calories	163
Fat	14 g
Carbohydrate	8 g
Fiber	4 g
Protein	4 g
Vitamin A	109 IU
Vitamin C	0 mg
Iron	1.8 mg
Vitamin E	5 IU
Zinc	1.3 mg
Selenium	12.7 mcg

- **Preheat oven to 325°F (160°C)**
- **Parchment paper**
- **Food processor**
- **Large baking sheet**

¾ cup	sunflower seeds	175 mL
3 tbsp	psyllium husk	45 mL
¼ tsp	fine sea salt	1 mL
¼ tsp	baking soda	1 mL
¼ tsp	garlic powder	1 mL
½ cup	sesame seeds	125 mL
2 tbsp	melted virgin coconut oil	30 mL
2 to 3 tbsp	coconut water or water	30 to 45 mL

1. Cut two pieces of parchment paper, each large enough to line baking sheet. In food processor, pulse sunflower seeds until finely ground. Add psyllium, salt, baking soda and garlic powder; pulse two or three times to combine. Add sesame seeds and coconut oil; pulse two or three times, until just blended. Add coconut water, 1 tbsp (15 mL) at a time, until the mixture begins to come together as a cohesive dough.

2. Place one piece of parchment paper on a flat surface. Transfer dough to parchment and cover with second piece of parchment. Using a rolling pin, roll dough into a ⅛-inch (3 mm) thick rectangle. Remove top piece of parchment and use your fingers to patch any small tears in the dough.

3. Using a knife or a pizza cutter, score dough into 2 dozen squares or rectangles (do not separate crackers). Slide the piece of parchment paper, with the dough, onto baking sheet.

4. Bake in preheated oven for 18 to 22 minutes or until golden brown. Using the parchment paper, slide the crackers (on the paper) onto a wire rack; let cool completely. Once cool, carefully snap crackers apart along score lines.

Olive Spread

Serve this spread on crackers as a tasty hors d'oeuvre.

Tips

Dry-cured black olives are often heavily salted, although the salt content varies from brand to brand and even between batches of the same brand. If you're trying to restrict your salt intake, use a brand of canned black olives that contains less salt.

This spread is very strong in flavor, so a little goes a long way. It keeps well in the refrigerator for up to 1 week.

1½ tbsp	olive oil	22 mL
2	cloves garlic, minced (about 2 tsp/10 mL)	2
1 tbsp	finely chopped fresh flat-leaf (Italian) parsley	15 mL
¾ tsp	finely grated lemon zest	3 mL
½ tsp	dried thyme (or 1½ tsp/7 mL fresh)	2 mL
¾ cup	pitted dry-cured black olives, finely chopped	175 mL
¼ tsp	freshly ground black pepper	1 mL

1. In a small skillet, heat olive oil with garlic over low heat. Cook for about 30 seconds or until garlic is soft and fragrant but not browned. Remove from heat and stir in parsley, lemon zest and thyme. Transfer to a small bowl, scraping the pan with a spatula to capture all the flavorings.

2. Add olives and pepper to bowl and stir well. Cover and refrigerate for at least 2 hours to allow the flavors to develop.

Variation

To turn this spread into a sauce, combine ¼ cup (60 mL) Olive Spread; ¼ cup (60 mL) olive oil; 4 plum tomatoes, seeded and chopped; and ¼ cup (60 mL) finely chopped fresh flat-leaf (Italian) parsley. Serve over steamed cauliflower as a pasta substitute.

Nutrients per 1 tbsp (15 mL)	
Calories	18
Fat	2 g
Carbohydrate	1 g
Fiber	0 g
Protein	0 g
Vitamin A	44 IU
Vitamin C	1 mg
Iron	0.3 mg
Vitamin E	0 IU
Zinc	0 mg
Selenium	0.1 mcg

Herbed Mushroom Duxelles

**MAKES
3 CUPS (750 ML)**

This dip is a take on a classic French stuffing. It is delicious served with fresh cauliflower and broccoli florets.

Tip

Never clean mushrooms by washing them in running water, or they will become gray and soggy. Use a damp towel to lightly brush the surface. This will remove any dirt.

- **Electric food dehydrator**
- **Food processor**

2 cups	sliced white mushrooms	500 mL
1 cup	sliced shiitake mushrooms	250 mL
1 cup	sliced oyster mushrooms	250 mL
1/4 cup	cold-pressed (extra virgin) olive oil	60 mL
1 tsp	fine sea salt	5 mL
3 tbsp	tamari	45 mL
2 tbsp	chopped fresh thyme leaves	30 mL

1. In a bowl, toss together white, shiitake and oyster mushrooms, olive oil, salt and tamari. Ladle onto a nonstick dehydrator sheet and spread evenly. Dehydrate at 115°F (46°C) for 45 to 60 minutes or until mushrooms appear sautéed.

2. Transfer mushrooms to food processor. Add thyme and process until smooth. Transfer to a serving bowl and serve immediately or cover and refrigerate for up to 4 days.

Variation

Use any kind of mushrooms for this recipe. If using portobello mushrooms, which are denser than other varieties, increase the amount of olive oil and tamari to compensate.

Advice for Clear Skin

▶ Use organic, non-GMO tamari.

Nutrients per 1/4 cup (60 mL)

Calories	55
Fat	5 g
Carbohydrate	3 g
Fiber	1 g
Protein	1 g
Vitamin A	22 IU
Vitamin C	1 mg
Iron	0.4 mg
Vitamin E	1 IU
Zinc	0.3 mg
Selenium	4.3 mcg

Perfect Guacamole

This simple, classic dip is one of the best flavor combinations possible, as well as being very nutritious. Avocado contains glutathione, which helps to neutralize free-radical compounds that may damage the skin.

Tip

The key is not to purée the avocado but to retain its texture so the guacamole is somewhat chunky.

3	avocados	3
1/4 cup	freshly squeezed lemon juice	60 mL
2 tbsp	finely diced red onion	30 mL
3	cloves garlic, minced	3
1 tsp	fine sea salt	15 mL
Pinch	freshly ground black pepper	Pinch

1. In a bowl, combine avocados, lemon juice, onion, garlic, salt and pepper. Using a wire whisk, fork or potato masher, mix until the avocado is crushed and the ingredients are evenly distributed. Serve immediately or cover and refrigerate for up to 3 days.

Variation

Add 1/4 cup (60 mL) chopped fresh cilantro, 2 tbsp (30 mL) chopped tomatoes and a pinch of cayenne pepper or some minced fresh chile pepper for some heat.

Nutrients per 1/4 cup (60 mL)

Calories	83
Fat	7 g
Carbohydrate	5 g
Fiber	3 g
Protein	1 g
Vitamin A	74 IU
Vitamin C	7 mg
Iron	0.3 mg
Vitamin E	2 IU
Zinc	0.3 mg
Selenium	0.3 mcg

Red Hot Hummus

Go easy on the chili paste until you get the heat just the way you like it. Substitute 1 to 2 tsp (5 to 10 mL) powdered chile pepper or hot pepper flakes for the paste. Chia seeds contain omega-3 oils that support hydration of the epidermis.

Tip

You can use 2 cups (500 mL) cooked chickpeas instead of canned.

- **Food processor**

	Juice of 1 lime or lemon	
2 tbsp	whole chia seeds	30 mL
½ cup	coarsely chopped sun-dried tomatoes	125 mL
1 cup	hot water	250 mL
1	can (14 to 19 oz/398 to 540 mL) chickpeas, drained and rinsed	1
2	cloves garlic	2
1 tbsp	toasted sesame oil	15 mL
¼ cup	olive oil	60 mL
1 to 2 tbsp	chili paste	15 to 30 mL
	Sea salt and freshly ground pepper	

1. In a bowl, combine lemon juice and chia seeds. In a separate bowl, combine sun-dried tomatoes and hot water. Set both aside for at least 20 minutes or until chia seeds are gelatinous.

2. In food processor, combine chickpeas, garlic and sesame oil. Process for 20 seconds. With the motor running, add lemon juice and chia seed mixture and sun-dried tomato mixture through the feed tube. Keep the motor running and slowly add olive oil through the opening. Process until well blended, about 20 seconds. Add chili paste, salt and pepper to taste and process for 5 seconds to blend into the hummus.

3. Transfer mixture to a clean container with lid. Store hummus in the refrigerator for up to 3 days.

Nutrients per ¼ cup (60 mL)

Calories	106
Fat	7 g
Carbohydrate	10 g
Fiber	3 g
Protein	2 g
Vitamin A	36 IU
Vitamin C	3 mg
Iron	0.7 mg
Vitamin E	1 IU
Zinc	0.5 mg
Selenium	1.1 mcg

Piquant White Bean and Parsley Dip

If you're looking for a snack with some heat, this is it! This piquant dip also works as a healthy alternative to mayonnaise. The jalapeño peppers and garlic have antibacterial properties that will help combat acne.

Tip

It's best to start by adding just one pepper to the dip; then you can add more to taste.

- **Food processor or blender**

2	green onions, coarsely chopped	2
2	cloves garlic, minced	2
1 to 2	jalapeño peppers, seeded and coarsely chopped	1 to 2
1	can (19 oz/540 mL) white kidney beans, drained and rinsed	1
¹⁄₂ cup	loosely packed chopped fresh parsley	125 mL
¹⁄₄ cup	freshly squeezed lemon juice	60 mL
1 tbsp	canola oil	15 mL
1 tsp	ground cumin	5 mL

1. In food processor, combine green onions, garlic, jalapeños to taste, beans, parsley, lemon juice, oil and cumin; process until smooth.

2. Transfer to a bowl, cover and refrigerate for at least 1 hour, until chilled, or for up to 1 day.

Variation

For Asian flair, add a few drops of sesame oil and garnish this dip with sesame seeds.

This recipe courtesy of dietitian Mary Sue Waisman.

Advice for Clear Skin

▶ Substitute extra virgin olive oil for the canola oil.

Nutrients per 2 tbsp (30 mL)

Calories	48
Fat	1 g
Carbohydrate	7 g
Fiber	2 g
Protein	2 g
Vitamin A	219 IU
Vitamin C	7 mg
Iron	0.8 mg
Vitamin E	0 IU
Zinc	0.2 mg
Selenium	0.5 mcg

Cashew Scallion Cream Cheese

This take on traditional cream cheese is rich and spreadable. Use it virtually anytime you want a spread, as a replacement for store-bought hummus or as a dip for carrot sticks and broccoli florets.

Tip

To soak the cashews for this recipe, place in a bowl and cover with 4 cups (1 L) water. Cover and set aside for 30 minutes. Drain, discarding soaking water, and rinse under cold running water until the water runs clear.

- **High-powered blender**

2 cups	raw cashews, soaked (see tip, at left)	500 mL
1 cup	chopped green onions, white and green parts, divided	250 mL
¼ cup	filtered water	60 mL
1 tbsp	freshly squeezed lemon juice	15 mL
1 tsp	fine sea salt	5 mL

1. In blender, blend ½ cup (125 mL) green onions, water, lemon juice and salt on high speed until smooth. Add soaked cashews and blend on high speed until smooth, stopping the motor once and stirring the mixture with a rubber spatula.

2. Transfer to a serving bowl and stir in the remaining green onions. Serve immediately or cover and refrigerate for up to 3 days.

Variation

This recipe can be enhanced with a variety of herbs and spices or seasonings. For instance, try substituting parsley leaves for half of the green onion and adding a clove of garlic.

Nutrients per 2 tbsp (30 mL)	
Calories	77
Fat	6 g
Carbohydrate	5 g
Fiber	1 g
Protein	2 g
Vitamin A	19 IU
Vitamin C	1 mg
Iron	0.9 mg
Vitamin E	0 IU
Zinc	0.7 mg
Selenium	1.5 mcg

Herbed Golden Tofu Spread

This versatile golden spread flecked with fresh herbs is a rich addition to any menu. Serve with crudités for a light but filling midday snack or slather on baked wild-caught salmon piled with tomatoes and red onion for a sumptuous meal.

1 lb	firm tofu, drained	500 g
½ cup	vegan mayonnaise	125 mL
2 tsp	Dijon mustard	10 mL
4 tsp	freshly squeezed lemon juice	20 mL
2 tbsp	finely chopped green onion, white part only	30 mL
1 tbsp	finely chopped fresh parsley	15 mL
1 tbsp	finely chopped fresh dill	15 mL
1½ tsp	ground turmeric	7 mL
½ tsp	garlic powder	2 mL
½ tsp	salt	2 mL
½ tsp	freshly ground black pepper	2 mL

1. In a bowl, using a potato masher, mash tofu into medium crumbs. Stir in mayonnaise, mustard, lemon juice, green onion, parsley, dill, turmeric, garlic powder, salt and pepper and mash into a semi-smooth and slightly chunky mixture or to desired consistency. Cover and refrigerate for at least 30 minutes or up to overnight. Taste and adjust seasonings, adding additional lemon juice, mustard, garlic powder, salt or pepper, if needed, before serving.

Variation

Finely shredded cabbage, grated carrot and minced celery are all great additions.

Advice for Clear Skin

▶ Use organic, non-GMO tofu.

Nutrients per 2 tbsp (30 mL)

Calories	30
Fat	2 g
Carbohydrate	2 g
Fiber	0 g
Protein	2 g
Vitamin A	22 IU
Vitamin C	1 mg
Iron	0.3 mg
Vitamin E	0 IU
Zinc	0 mg
Selenium	0.1 mcg

Sardine and Pesto Spread

MAKES
1/2 CUP (125 ML)

Three simple ingredients give big taste to this chunky spread. Serve with crudités or as a topper for grilled organic chicken. Sardines contain omega-3 oils to support skin healing.

Tips

Don't mash the sardines too much, or you'll end up with more of a paste than a spread.

Try Mediterranean-style or lemon-flavored sardines.

1	can (3½ oz/106 g) sardines, drained	1
2 tbsp	basil pesto	30 mL
1 tbsp	freshly squeezed lime juice	15 mL

1. In a small bowl, mash sardines with a fork. Stir in pesto and lime juice until just blended.

This recipe courtesy of dietitian Claude Gamache.

Nutrients per 1 tbsp (15 mL)

Calories	46
Fat	3 g
Carbohydrate	0 g
Fiber	0 g
Protein	4 g
Vitamin A	51 IU
Vitamin C	1 mg
Iron	0.5 mg
Vitamin E	1 IU
Zinc	0.2 mg
Selenium	6.5 mcg

Creamy Mayonnaise

*This creamy and
absolutely delicious
spread has the
consistency and taste of
mayonnaise and uses dry
mustard powder to give
it a little snap. It is easily
infused with roasted
garlic, chopped herbs,
curry or a multitude
of flavorings. Thin
with water for a quick
dressing or sauce.*

• **Immersion blender or small food processor**

4 oz	firm or extra-firm silken tofu	125 g
2 oz	extra-firm tofu, drained	60 g
4¾ tsp	freshly squeezed lemon juice	23 mL
4 tsp	olive oil	20 mL
¼ tsp	Dijon mustard	1 mL
⅛ tsp	salt (approx.)	0.5 mL
⅛ tsp	dry mustard (approx.)	0.5 mL

1. In a small, deep bowl, combine silken and extra-firm tofu, lemon juice, oil, Dijon mustard, salt and dry mustard. Use an immersion blender to thoroughly blend ingredients into a very creamy, smooth mixture with the texture of mayonnaise, 2 to 3 minutes. Taste and adjust seasoning, adding a pinch each of dry mustard and salt, if desired. Store mayonnaise in an airtight container in the refrigerator for up to 1 week.

Advice for Clear Skin

▸ Use organic, non-GMO tofu.

Nutrients per 1 tbsp (15 mL)	
Calories	27
Fat	2 g
Carbohydrate	1 g
Fiber	0 g
Protein	1 g
Vitamin A	2 IU
Vitamin C	1 mg
Iron	0.2 mg
Vitamin E	0 IU
Zinc	0 mg
Selenium	0.1 mcg

Yellow Coconut Curry Sauce

**MAKES
4 CUPS (1 L)**

This smooth and rich curry sauce is as delicious as any traditional yellow curry, but with none of the hidden unhealthy fats found in refined oils. It is slightly spicy and great served on cold nights when the body is craving warmth. Serve it over spiralized zucchini or roasted cauliflower.

Tip

To soak the cashews for this recipe, place in a bowl and add 2 cups (500 mL) water. Cover and set aside for 20 minutes. Drain, discarding any remaining water. Rinse under cold running water until water runs clear.

Blender

1 cup	raw cashews, soaked (see tip, at left)	250 mL
2 cups	water	500 mL
¼ cup	chopped tomato	60 mL
3 tbsp	coconut butter	45 mL
2 to 3 tbsp	curry powder	30 to 45 mL
1 tbsp	ground cumin	15 mL
1 tbsp	chopped gingerroot	15 mL
2	cloves garlic	2
1	wild lime leaf	1
2 tsp	fine sea salt	10 mL
1 tsp	freshly squeezed lemon juice	5 mL

1. In blender, combine soaked cashews, water, tomato, coconut butter, curry powder to taste, cumin, ginger, garlic, lime leaf, salt and lemon juice. Blend at high speed until smooth. Serve immediately or cover and refrigerate for up to 3 days.

Nutrients per ½ cup **(125 mL)**

Calories	95
Fat	9 g
Carbohydrate	3 g
Fiber	0 g
Protein	1 g
Vitamin A	3 IU
Vitamin C	1 mg
Iron	0.6 mg
Vitamin E	0 IU
Zinc	0.5 mg
Selenium	1.1 mcg

Best-Ever Bolognese Sauce

**MAKES ABOUT
15 CUPS (3.75 L)**

This version of the hearty Italian meat sauce combines beef, pork and pancetta with traditional vegetables and robust porcini mushrooms. Traditionally the sauce develops flavor from long, slow simmering, making it perfect for the slow cooker. This makes a large batch and the servings are generous. It is wonderful to have on hand. If it is too large, freeze half or make half a batch. Serve it over roasted spaghetti squash, and add some steamed broccoli to maximize the nutritional punch.

Nutrients per 1¼ cups (300 mL)

Calories	153
Fat	5 g
Carbohydrate	10 g
Fiber	2 g
Protein	15 g
Vitamin A	2277 IU
Vitamin C	9 mg
Iron	2.6 mg
Vitamin E	1 IU
Zinc	2.6 mg
Selenium	14.1 mcg

- **Medium to large (3½- to 5-quart) slow cooker**

1	package (½ oz/14 g) dried porcini mushrooms	1
1 cup	hot water	250 mL
1 tbsp	olive oil (approx.)	15 mL
2 oz	chunk pancetta, diced	60 g
1 lb	lean ground beef	500 g
8 oz	ground pork or chicken	250 g
2	onions, diced	2
2	stalks celery, diced	2
2	carrots, peeled and diced	2
4	cloves garlic, minced	4
1 tbsp	dried Italian seasoning	15 mL
2	bay leaves	2
½ tsp	salt	2 mL
½ tsp	cracked black peppercorns	2 mL
½ tsp	ground cinnamon	2 mL
1 cup	dry red wine	250 mL
1	can (28 oz/796 mL) no-salt added tomatoes, with juice, coarsely chopped	1
¼ cup	tomato paste	60 mL

1. In a bowl, combine dried mushrooms and hot water. Let stand for 30 minutes. Drain through a fine sieve, reserving liquid. Pat mushrooms dry with paper towels and chop finely. Set liquid and mushrooms aside.

2. Meanwhile, in a large skillet, heat oil over medium-high heat. Add pancetta and cook, stirring, until browned, about 3 minutes. Using a slotted spoon, transfer to slow cooker stoneware. Add more oil to pan if necessary. (You should have about 1 tbsp/15 mL.) Add beef, pork, onions, celery and carrots and cook, stirring, until carrots have softened and meat is no longer pink, about 7 minutes.

Tips

If you choose to halve this recipe, use a small (2- to 3½-quart) slow cooker.

Bolognese sauce should be thick. Placing the tea towels over the top of the slow cooker absorbs generated moisture that would dilute the sauce.

Make Ahead

Complete steps 1, 2 and 3. Cover mixture, ensuring that it cools promptly, and refrigerate for up to 2 days. When you're ready to cook, complete the recipe.

3. Add garlic, Italian seasoning, bay leaves, salt, peppercorns, cinnamon and the reserved soaked mushrooms and cook, stirring, for 1 minute. Add wine, bring to a boil and boil, stirring and scraping up brown bits from bottom of pan, for 2 minutes. Add the reserved mushroom liquid.

4. Transfer to stoneware. Add tomatoes and stir well. Stir in tomato paste. Place two clean tea towels, each folded in half (so you will have four layers), over top of stoneware to absorb moisture. Cover and cook on Low for 6 hours or on High for 3 hours.

Advice for Clear Skin

▹ Replace the red wine with an equal amount of gluten-free ready-to-use beef broth.

Turkey, Mushroom and Chickpea Sauce

**MAKES ABOUT
10½ CUPS
(2.625 L)**

Kids always want seconds of this lip-smacking sauce, which is delicious over roasted spaghetti squash. This makes a very generous serving, so you don't need to add anything else.

Tips

If you don't have hot paprika, use regular paprika instead with a pinch of cayenne.

If you don't have a mortar or a spice grinder, place the toasted fennel seeds on a cutting board and use the bottom of a wine bottle or measuring cup to grind them.

Nutrients per
1¾ cups (425 mL)

Calories	276
Fat	10 g
Carbohydrate	28 g
Fiber	7 g
Protein	22 g
Vitamin A	2180 IU
Vitamin C	42 mg
Iron	3.9 mg
Vitamin E	2 IU
Zinc	2.5 mg
Selenium	21.3 mcg

- **Medium to large (3½- to 5-quart) slow cooker**

½ tsp	fennel seeds	2 mL
1 tbsp	olive oil	15 mL
1 lb	ground turkey	500 g
2	onions, minced	2
4	stalks celery, diced	4
2	cloves garlic, minced	2
1 tsp	dried oregano, crumbled	5 mL
1 tsp	sea salt	5 mL
½ tsp	cracked black peppercorns	2 mL
8 oz	cremini mushrooms, trimmed and quartered	250 g
1	can (28 oz/796 mL) tomatoes, with juice, coarsely chopped	1
1 cup	ready-to-use vegetable, chicken or turkey broth	250 mL
2 cups	cooked chickpeas, drained and rinsed	500 mL
2 tsp	hot paprika (see tip, at left), dissolved in 1 tbsp (15 mL) lemon juice	10 mL
1	red bell pepper, diced	1

1. In a dry skillet over medium heat, toast fennel seeds, stirring, until fragrant, about 3 minutes. Immediately transfer to a mortar or a spice grinder and grind (see tip, at left). Set aside.

2. In same skillet, heat oil over medium heat. Add turkey, onions and celery and cook, stirring, until celery is softened and no hint of pink remains in the turkey, about 6 minutes. Add fennel seeds, garlic, oregano, salt and peppercorns and cook, stirring, for 1 minute. Add mushrooms and toss to coat. Add tomatoes and broth and bring to a boil. Transfer to slow cooker stoneware. Add chickpeas and stir well.

3. Cover and cook on Low for 6 hours or on High for 3 hours, until mixture is hot and bubbly. Add paprika solution and stir well. Add bell pepper and stir well. Cover and cook on High for 20 minutes, until pepper is tender.

Soups

Chilled Avocado, Mint and Coconut Soup

This cooling soup is a refreshing way to treat your body as a temple.

Tip

An equal amount of fresh cilantro or basil leaves can be used in place of the mint.

- **Food processor or blender**

2	small ripe Hass avocados, pitted and peeled	2
1	green onion, coarsely chopped	1
1/2	large English cucumber, peeled and coarsely chopped	1/2
1/4 cup	fresh mint leaves	60 mL
1 1/2 cups	coconut water	375 mL
1/2 cup	well-stirred coconut milk (full-fat)	125 mL
1 tbsp	freshly squeezed lemon juice	15 mL
1 tsp	fine sea salt	5 mL
	Additional fresh mint leaves	

1. In food processor, working in batches, purée avocados, green onion, cucumber, mint, coconut water, coconut milk, lemon juice and salt until smooth. Transfer to a large bowl. Stir to combine. Cover and refrigerate for at least 1 hour, until cold, or for up to 4 hours.

2. Stir soup, divide among bowls and garnish with mint leaves.

Nutrients per serving

Calories	414
Fat	37 g
Carbohydrate	24 g
Fiber	16 g
Protein	6 g
Vitamin A	399 IU
Vitamin C	26 mg
Iron	2.0 mg
Vitamin E	6 IU
Zinc	1.7 mg
Selenium	3.6 mcg

Bok Choy and Mushroom Soup

Bok choy has a light, sweet flavor and crisp texture that comes from its high water content, which makes it perfect for fast, flavorful soups because it takes just minutes to wilt. As for nutrition, bok choy is very high in vitamin A, vitamin C, calcium and fiber, and very low in calories.

Tip

Store the cooled soup in an airtight container in the refrigerator for up to 2 days. Warm soup in a medium saucepan over medium-low heat.

3	cloves garlic, minced	3
1 tbsp	minced gingerroot	15 mL
6 cups	reduced-sodium ready-to-use chicken or vegetable broth	1.5 L
2 tbsp	reduced-sodium tamari or soy sauce	30 mL
2 tbsp	unseasoned rice vinegar	30 mL
1 tbsp	toasted sesame oil	15 mL
1 lb	cremini or button mushrooms, trimmed and sliced	500 g
8 oz	firm tofu, drained and cut into $\frac{1}{2}$-inch (1 cm) cubes	250 g
6 cups	sliced bok choy	1.5 L
$\frac{2}{3}$ cup	thinly sliced green onions	150 mL

1. In a large saucepan, combine garlic, ginger, broth, tamari, vinegar and oil. Bring to a boil over medium-high heat. Stir in mushrooms, reduce heat and simmer, stirring occasionally, for 5 minutes or until mushrooms are tender. Stir in tofu, bok choy and green onions; simmer for 3 to 4 minutes or until bok choy is wilted and tofu is heated through.

Advice for Clear Skin

▶ Choose gluten-free broth until the reintroduction phase of the diet plan, when you can test to see if gluten-containing products are safe for your skin.

▶ Use organic, non-GMO tamari or soy sauce, and make sure soy sauce is gluten-free.

Nutrients per serving

Calories	188
Fat	9 g
Carbohydrate	14 g
Fiber	3 g
Protein	19 g
Vitamin A	4539 IU
Vitamin C	33 mg
Iron	3.6 mg
Vitamin E	0 IU
Zinc	1.3 mg
Selenium	11.5 mcg

Roasted Cauliflower and Red Pepper Soup

MAKES 6 SERVINGS

This soup offers great flavor and attractive colors and textures. The red peppers and carrots supply carotenoids, and the garlic and thyme provide antibacterial compounds to heal acne.

Tip

To roast red peppers, quarter peppers and remove seeds. Place skin side up on a rimmed baking sheet in a 450°F (230°C) oven and roast for 10 minutes. Turn peppers over and roast for 10 to 15 minutes or until skins are blackened. Transfer peppers to a small bowl, cover tightly and let stand for about 15 minutes. When cool enough to handle, peel off blackened skin.

Nutrients per serving

Calories	90
Fat	4 g
Carbohydrate	12 g
Fiber	4 g
Protein	4 g
Vitamin A	4854 IU
Vitamin C	99 mg
Iron	1.1 mg
Vitamin E	2 IU
Zinc	0.5 mg
Selenium	4.2 mcg

- **Preheat oven to 425°F (220°C)**
- **Rimmed baking sheet, lined with foil**

5 cups	bite-size cauliflower florets	1.25 L
4 tsp	canola oil, divided	20 mL
1 cup	finely chopped onion	250 mL
1 cup	finely chopped carrots	250 mL
2	cloves garlic, minced	2
4 cups	ready-to-use reduced-sodium chicken or vegetable broth	1 L
2	roasted red bell peppers (see tip, at left), finely chopped	2
2	sprigs fresh thyme	2
	Freshly ground black pepper	

1. Place cauliflower on prepared baking sheet and drizzle with 2 tsp (10 mL) oil. Roast in preheated oven, turning once, for 20 to 25 minutes or until florets start to caramelize and are lightly browned.

2. Meanwhile, in a large pot, heat the remaining oil over medium heat. Sauté onion and carrots for 3 to 4 minutes or until softened. Add garlic and sauté for 30 seconds. Stir in caramelized cauliflower, broth, roasted peppers and thyme; increase heat to high and bring to a boil. Reduce heat and simmer for 10 minutes to blend the flavors. Discard thyme sprigs. Season to taste with pepper.

Variation

Use a combination of cauliflower and broccoli, keeping the total amount at 5 cups (1.25 L).

This recipe courtesy of dietitian Mary Sue Waisman.

Advice for Clear Skin

▶ Substitute olive oil for the canola oil.

▶ Choose gluten-free broth until the reintroduction phase of the diet plan, when you can test to see if gluten-containing products are safe for your skin.

Portobello Pot-au-Feu

MAKES 4 SERVINGS

The French term pot-au-feu literally means "pot on fire" and is a dish of meat and vegetables slowly cooked in water. The broth is served as a first course and the meat and vegetables make up the entrée. This is a vegan take on the traditional dish, with two ways to serve it.

- **Preheat oven to 375°F (190°C)**
- **Rimmed baking sheet, lightly oiled**

4	carrots, halved lengthwise	4
4	white baby turnips, halved	4
8	asparagus spears	8
3 tbsp	olive oil, divided	45 mL
4	large portobello mushrooms, stems removed	4
	Sea salt and freshly ground pepper	
3 cups	ready-to-use vegetable broth or water	750 mL
20	fresh fiddleheads or green beans	20
4	green onions, sliced	4
2 cups	packed baby spinach	500 mL
1/4 cup	chopped fresh chives (optional)	60 mL

1. On prepared baking sheet, combine carrots, turnips and asparagus. Toss with 2 tbsp (30 mL) oil. Roast in preheated oven for 10 minutes. Stir vegetables. Add mushrooms, gills facing down. Drizzle the remaining oil over mushrooms. Season vegetables and mushrooms with salt and pepper to taste. Roast for 20 minutes or until vegetables are easily pierced with the tip of a knife.

2. Meanwhile, in a saucepan over high heat, bring broth to a gentle boil. Add fiddleheads. Reduce heat and simmer for 8 minutes. Add green onions and spinach and simmer for 2 minutes.

3. Divide roasted vegetables evenly among 4 large soup bowls. Spoon broth and simmered vegetables over roasted vegetables. Garnish each bowl with chives, if using.

Nutrients per serving

Calories	177
Fat	11 g
Carbohydrate	19 g
Fiber	5 g
Protein	5 g
Vitamin A	12,867 IU
Vitamin C	28 mg
Iron	2.2 mg
Vitamin E	4 IU
Zinc	1.2 mg
Selenium	17.2 mcg

Advice for Clear Skin

▶ Choose gluten-free broth until the reintroduction phase of the diet plan, when you can test to see if gluten-containing products are safe for your skin.

▶ Fiddleheads are a good source of iron, which is beneficial for supporting your energy, immune system and skin.

Tomato Basil Soup

This very quick version of the classic tomato soup is just right for a refreshingly light supper. Serve it hot in winter or cold in summer. Look to the fresh tomato variation below for even more flavor when tomatoes are in season.

• **Food processor or blender**

3 cups	ready-to-use chicken broth	750 mL
3	cloves garlic, minced	3
1	can (28 oz/798 mL) diced tomatoes	1
1 cup	fresh basil leaves, thinly sliced	250 mL
	Salt and freshly ground black pepper	

1. In a large saucepan over high heat, bring broth, garlic and tomatoes to a boil. Reduce heat. Cover and cook slowly for 20 minutes.

2. Remove from heat. Cool slightly before puréeing half of the soup in food processor until smooth. Repeat with the remaining soup.

3. Return to saucepan. Add basil and reheat to serving temperature. Season with salt and pepper to taste.

Variation

Replace canned tomatoes with 6 large peeled and diced tomatoes. Add $\frac{1}{4}$ cup (60 mL) tomato paste during the cooking and then follow the method, using all the ingredients.

Advice for Clear Skin

▶ Choose gluten-free broth until the reintroduction phase of the diet plan, when you can test to see if gluten-containing products are safe for your skin.

Nutrients per serving

Calories	78
Fat	1 g
Carbohydrate	14 g
Fiber	3 g
Protein	6 g
Vitamin A	1557 IU
Vitamin C	17 mg
Iron	2.7 mg
Vitamin E	0 IU
Zinc	0.7 mg
Selenium	1.2 mcg

Everyday Soup

MAKES 4 SERVINGS

Simple soups are standard on the weeknight menu in homes all over Asia. This soup can accompany a main course of fish or chicken.

Tip

Because this soup is simple and quick, you can make it just before serving, allowing only enough time to heat everything up. You could also prepare it ahead up to step 4, adding tofu but reserving spinach, and then remove it from the heat. When you are ready to serve, heat it to a gentle boil and add spinach and green onions, then sesame oil. Serve hot.

3 cups	ready-to-use chicken or vegetable broth	750 mL
4	shiitake mushrooms or large button mushrooms	4
1/2 cup	shredded carrots	125 mL
4 oz	firm tofu, chopped into 1/2-inch (1 cm) chunks	125 g
1 cup	fresh baby spinach	250 mL
1/4 cup	thinly sliced green onions	60 mL
2 tsp	Asian sesame oil	10 mL

1. In a saucepan, bring broth to a boil over medium-high heat.
2. Meanwhile, remove stems from shiitake mushrooms and discard. Slice caps into thin strips. If using button mushrooms, slice them thinly.
3. When broth is boiling, add mushrooms and carrots and cook until carrots have brightened in color and are tender-crisp, about 2 minutes.
4. Add tofu, spinach and green onions and stir gently. Cook for 1 minute more.
5. Transfer to serving bowls and pour sesame oil over the top of the soup. Serve hot.

Variations

Add diced cooked chicken, shrimp or ham instead of tofu.

Add shredded napa cabbage instead of spinach.

Add frozen shredded collard greens or turnip greens instead of spinach and carrot shreds, and cook until they are tender, 2 to 3 minutes.

Add cooked salmon instead of tofu. Then add chopped fresh hot green chiles along with the green onions and top the soup with a generous squeeze of lime juice and a handful of cilantro leaves just before serving.

Advice for Clear Skin

▸ Choose gluten-free broth until the reintroduction phase of the diet plan, when you can test to see if gluten-containing products are safe for your skin.

Nutrients per serving

Calories	83
Fat	5 g
Carbohydrate	5 g
Fiber	1 g
Protein	7 g
Vitamin A	3063 IU
Vitamin C	4 mg
Iron	1.1 mg
Vitamin E	1 IU
Zinc	0.3 mg
Selenium	0.7 mcg

Chunky Southwest Vegetable Soup

A touch of heat from the jalapeño gives this soup Southwest flair. Serve with Red Hot Hummus (page 235) and crudités.

Tip

If you prefer your vegetables sautéed in oil, add 1 tbsp (15 mL) extra virgin olive oil to the saucepan and heat over medium heat, then sauté the celery, onion, mushrooms, green pepper and jalapeño with the chili powder.

1 cup	chopped celery	250 mL
1 cup	chopped onion	250 mL
1 cup	chopped mushrooms	250 mL
1/2 cup	chopped green bell pepper	125 mL
1 tbsp	minced jalapeño pepper	15 mL
1 tsp	chili powder	5 mL
1	can (19 oz/540 mL) diced tomatoes (about 2$\frac{1}{3}$ cups/575 mL)	1

1. In a large saucepan, over medium heat, combine celery, onion, mushrooms, green pepper, jalapeño and chili powder. Add tomatoes, then fill can twice with water and add to saucepan; bring to a boil. Reduce heat, cover and simmer for 25 minutes.

Variation

If your family does not like heat, substitute 1 tbsp (15 mL) chopped fresh parsley for the jalapeño.

This recipe courtesy of Eileen Campbell.

Nutrients per serving

Calories	57
Fat	1 g
Carbohydrate	13 g
Fiber	3 g
Protein	3 g
Vitamin A	1051 IU
Vitamin C	22 mg
Iron	1.7 mg
Vitamin E	1 IU
Zinc	0.5 mg
Selenium	2.3 mcg

Country Lentil Soup

This hearty soup can be satisfying for lunch or dinner. Soups made with legumes are sources of protein and fiber.

Tip

If you prefer, when puréeing soups, you can use a stick blender and blend the soup right in the pot. This will save you some cleanup time, but the result will be less smooth.

- **Blender**

1 tbsp	vegetable oil	15 mL
1 cup	diced onion	250 mL
1/2 cup	diced carrot	125 mL
1/2 cup	diced celery	125 mL
4 cups	ready-to-use vegetable or chicken broth	1 L
1 cup	dried red lentils, well rinsed	250 mL
1/4 tsp	dried thyme	1 mL
	Salt and freshly ground black pepper	
1/2 cup	chopped fresh flat-leaf (Italian) parsley	125 mL

1. In a large saucepan, heat oil over medium heat. Sauté onion, carrot and celery until softened, about 5 minutes. Add broth, lentils and thyme; bring to a boil. Reduce heat, cover and simmer for 20 minutes or until lentils are soft. Remove from heat.

2. Working in batches, transfer soup to blender. Purée on high speed until creamy. Add up to 1 cup (250 mL) water if purée is too thick. Season with salt and pepper to taste. Return to saucepan to reheat, if necessary.

3. Ladle into bowls and garnish with parsley.

Variations

Substitute green lentils, well rinsed and drained, canned chickpeas or white kidney beans for the red lentils. Decrease the simmering time to 15 minutes if using canned legumes.

To make this a heartier soup, add 1 cup (250 mL) diced cooked lean ham after puréeing.

This recipe courtesy of Eileen Campbell.

Advice for Clear Skin

▶ Substitute extra virgin olive oil for the vegetable oil.

▶ Choose gluten-free broth until the reintroduction phase of the diet plan, when you can test to see if gluten-containing products are safe for your skin.

Nutrients per serving

Calories	118
Fat	2 g
Carbohydrate	19 g
Fiber	3 g
Protein	6 g
Vitamin A	1951 IU
Vitamin C	8 mg
Iron	2.2 mg
Vitamin E	1 IU
Zinc	1.0 mg
Selenium	2.1 mcg

Moroccan Lentil Soup

This lentil and chickpea soup is a wonderful addition to vegetarian meals. You can replace the vegetable broth with beef or chicken broth for non-vegetarians.

Tip

Turmeric, paprika, cumin and cayenne pepper are frequently added to this soup to provide a more authentic North African flavor. Add the spices to the onions while they soften. At serving time, garnish with chopped cilantro for color.

1	large onion, chopped	1
1 cup	red lentils	250 mL
4 cups	ready-to-use vegetable broth	1 L
1	can (19 oz/540 mL) chickpeas, drained and rinsed	1
	Salt and freshly ground black pepper	

1. In a large saucepan over medium heat, sauté onion with a little water or oil until softened. Add lentils and broth.

2. Bring to a boil over high heat. Reduce heat, cover and cook slowly, stirring occasionally, for 30 minutes or until lentils are soft.

3. Stir in chickpeas. Season with salt and pepper to taste.

Advice for Clear Skin

▶ Choose gluten-free broth until the reintroduction phase of the diet plan, when you can test to see if gluten-containing products are safe for your skin.

Nutrients per serving

Calories	282
Fat	2 g
Carbohydrate	52 g
Fiber	9 g
Protein	15 g
Vitamin A	446 IU
Vitamin C	7 mg
Iron	4.4 mg
Vitamin E	0 IU
Zinc	2.7 mg
Selenium	6.3 mcg

Minestrone

Advice for Clear Skin

▶ Choose gluten-free broth until the reintroduction phase of the diet plan, when you can test to see if gluten-containing products are safe for your skin.

• **Blender**

1½ cups	ready-to-use vegetable or chicken broth, divided	375 mL
½	clove garlic	½
1	sprig parsley	1
½	onion	½
2	stalks celery, cut into chunks	2
1	carrot, cut into chunks	1
2 tbsp	fresh oregano	30 mL
1	tomato, quartered	1
¾ cup	sliced cabbage	175 mL
½ cup	cooked chickpeas (optional)	125 mL
¼ tsp	salt, or to taste	1 mL

1. In blender, combine ½ cup (125 mL) broth, garlic, parsley, onion, celery and carrot. Secure lid and blend on low speed for 30 seconds. Pour into a saucepan; heat over medium heat until vegetables are soft.

2. Meanwhile, in blender, combine ½ cup (125 mL) broth, oregano, tomato and cabbage. Secure lid and blend on low speed for 30 seconds. Add chickpeas, if using. Secure lid and blend on high speed for 30 seconds or until smooth. Add to saucepan. Bring to a boil, reduce heat to low and simmer for 2 to 3 minutes or until heated through.

3. Stir in enough of the remaining broth to make desired consistency. Season with salt. Serve hot or cold.

Nutrients per serving

Calories	21
Fat	0 g
Carbohydrate	5 g
Fiber	1 g
Protein	1 g
Vitamin A	2086 IU
Vitamin C	8 mg
Iron	0.4 mg
Vitamin E	1 IU
Zinc	0.1 mg
Selenium	0.2 mcg

Smoked Tofu Gumbo

MAKES 6 SERVINGS

If you periodically get cravings for smoked food, here's a recipe that will provide satisfaction and save you the trouble of heating up the smoker.

Tips

Look for smoked organic tofu in well-stocked natural foods stores.

Use any kind of chile pepper here, but taste the broth before adding and adjust the quantity to ensure the spiciness meets your taste.

Filé powder is ground sassafras leaves. It is a traditional Cajun seasoning used to thicken and add flavor to gumbo.

Nutrients per serving

Calories	151
Fat	6 g
Carbohydrate	18 g
Fiber	3 g
Protein	8 g
Vitamin A	4659 IU
Vitamin C	41 mg
Iron	1.7 mg
Vitamin E	2 IU
Zinc	0.4 mg
Selenium	0.6 mcg

- **Medium to large (4- to 5-quart) slow cooker**

1 tbsp	vegetable oil	15 mL
2	onions, finely chopped	2
4	stalks celery, diced	4
2	carrots, peeled and diced	2
4	cloves garlic, minced	4
1 to 2 tsp	Cajun seasoning	5 to 10 mL
1 tsp	salt	5 mL
1 tsp	cracked black peppercorns	5 mL
1 tsp	dried thyme	5 mL
2	bay leaves	2
1/4 cup	short-grain brown rice	60 mL
5 cups	ready-to-use vegetable broth, divided	1.25 L
2 cups	cubed smoked tofu (1/2-inch/1 cm cubes)	500 mL
1	red bell pepper, finely chopped	1
1	fresh chile pepper, finely chopped (see tip, at left)	1
1 tsp	filé powder (optional)	5 mL
	Finely chopped green onions	
	Hot pepper sauce	

1. In a skillet, heat oil over medium heat. Add onions, celery and carrots and cook, stirring, until softened, about 7 minutes. Add garlic, Cajun seasoning to taste, salt, peppercorns, thyme and bay leaves and cook, stirring, for 1 minute. Add rice and toss to coat. Add 2 cups (500 mL) broth and bring to a boil. Boil for 2 minutes. Transfer to slow cooker stoneware.

2. Add the remaining broth. Cover and cook on Low for 6 hours or High for 3 hours, until rice is tender.

3. Add smoked tofu, bell pepper, and chile pepper. Cover and cook on High for 20 minutes, until pepper is tender and tofu is heated through. Discard bay leaves. Stir in filé powder (if using). Ladle into bowls and garnish with green onions. Pass the hot pepper sauce at the table.

Advice for Clear Skin

▶ Substitute extra virgin olive oil for the vegetable oil.

Curried Tomato and Shellfish Broth

Mustard greens, which are available in Chinese markets, give this broth an interesting bite. The combination of tomatoes and curry provides a fabulous complement to the seafood.

6	scallops, thinly sliced	6
8	prawns, peeled and deveined	8
	Salt and freshly ground white pepper	
2 tsp	vegetable oil	10 mL
1	small onion, sliced	1
1 tbsp	curry powder, preferably Madras	15 mL
5 cups	ready-to-use chicken broth	1.25 L
4	small tomatoes, seeded and quartered	4
12	clams, scrubbed	12
2 cups	thinly sliced mustard greens or napa cabbage	500 mL

1. Season scallops and prawns with salt and pepper; set aside.

2. In a large saucepan or soup pot, heat oil over medium heat for 30 seconds. Add onion and curry powder; sauté for 1 minute. Add chicken broth; bring to a boil. Add tomatoes and cook for 3 minutes. Add clams; cook until they open, about 2 to 5 minutes, depending on size. Skim off any impurities that rise to the top.

3. Add scallops, prawns and mustard greens or cabbage; bring to a boil. Remove from heat. Season to taste with salt and pepper. Cover and let steep for 2 minutes. Serve immediately.

Advice for Clear Skin

▶ Substitute extra virgin olive oil for the vegetable oil.

▶ Choose gluten-free broth until the reintroduction phase of the diet plan, when you can test to see if gluten-containing products are safe for your skin.

Nutrients per serving

Calories	110
Fat	4 g
Carbohydrate	9 g
Fiber	3 g
Protein	11 g
Vitamin A	3824 IU
Vitamin C	34 mg
Iron	2.0 mg
Vitamin E	3 IU
Zinc	0.8 mg
Selenium	21.7 mcg

Sea Gumbo

This nourishing soup contains seaweed, which is rich in vitamins and minerals and has a balancing effect on your skin.

Tip

The arame lends a taste of the sea to this dish. You can also add 1 lb (500 g) fresh shrimp or scallops in step 3 and simmer for 5 to 10 minutes. For a Louisiana-style gumbo, add 1 tbsp (15 mL) Old Bay seasoning or 2 tsp (10 mL) cayenne pepper and a couple of drops of a hot sauce such as Tabasco.

3 tbsp	olive oil	45 mL
1 cup	chopped onions	250 mL
1¾ cups	sliced leeks (white and light green parts only)	425 mL
3	cloves garlic, minced	3
½ cup	chopped celery	125 mL
½ cup	chopped green bell pepper	125 mL
½ cup	chopped red bell pepper	125 mL
1	can (28 oz/796 mL) diced tomatoes, with juice	1
1 cup	chopped okra or zucchini	250 mL
1 cup	ready-to-use vegetable broth	250 mL
1	bay leaf	1
3 tbsp	chopped fresh thyme	45 mL
1 cup	arame or hijiki	250 mL
½ cup	shredded fresh basil	125 mL

1. In a large saucepan, heat oil over medium heat. Add onions and cook for 5 minutes or until soft. Add leeks and garlic; cook for 3 minutes. Add celery, green pepper and red pepper; cook for another 5 minutes.

2. Stir in tomatoes, okra, broth, bay leaf, thyme and arame. If desired, season to taste with salt. Cover and simmer, stirring occasionally, for 35 minutes or until vegetables are tender. Stir in basil. Serve hot.

Advice for Clear Skin

▶ Choose gluten-free broth until the reintroduction phase of the diet plan, when you can test to see if gluten-containing products are safe for your skin.

Nutrients per serving

Calories	204
Fat	11 g
Carbohydrate	26 g
Fiber	6 g
Protein	5 g
Vitamin A	2645 IU
Vitamin C	54 mg
Iron	4.0 mg
Vitamin E	4 IU
Zinc	1.0 mg
Selenium	2.1 mcg

Big-Batch Chicken Vegetable Soup

Freeze this big-batch soup in microwave-safe glass containers for fast lunches or weeknight meals.

Tip

When you're going to be freezing meal-sized portions of soup, ladle hot soup into airtight containers, leaving at least 1 inch (2.5 cm) headspace, and let it cool slightly. Refrigerate until completely cold, then freeze for up to 3 months.

8 to 10	skinless chicken drumsticks (about 2 lbs/1 kg total)	8 to 10
12	mushrooms, sliced	12
4	stalks celery, diced	4
4	leeks (white and light green parts only), chopped	4
4	carrots, diced	4
3	large tomatoes, chopped	3
1	large onion, chopped	1
1	can (5$\frac{1}{2}$ oz/156 mL) tomato paste	1
10 cups	ready-to-use chicken broth	2.5 L
$\frac{1}{4}$ cup	chopped fresh parsley	60 mL
	Salt and freshly ground black pepper (optional)	

1. In a large pot, combine drumsticks, mushrooms, celery, leeks, carrots, tomatoes, onion, tomato paste, broth, parsley and salt and pepper to taste (if using). Bring to a boil over high heat. Reduce heat, cover and simmer for 30 minutes or until chicken is falling off the bone and vegetables are soft.

2. Remove drumsticks and debone. Discard bones and return chicken to saucepan. Bring back to a boil for a few minutes to reheat chicken.

This recipe courtesy of Candice Wilke.

Advice for Clear Skin

▶ Choose gluten-free broth until the reintroduction phase of the diet plan, when you can test to see if gluten-containing products are safe for your skin.

Nutrients per serving

Calories	67
Fat	1 g
Carbohydrate	8 g
Fiber	2 g
Protein	7 g
Vitamin A	2795 IU
Vitamin C	11 mg
Iron	1.2 mg
Vitamin E	1 IU
Zinc	0.8 mg
Selenium	6.9 mcg

Middle Eastern Chicken Soup

A little leftover chicken and canned broth make a quick and wholesome main-course soup. Serve with a splash of fresh lemon juice if you wish.

1	can (10 oz/284 mL) chicken broth	1
1	can (19 oz/540 mL) chickpeas, drained and rinsed	1
1 cup	chopped or shredded cooked chicken	250 mL
1	small onion, chopped	1
1	carrot, chopped	1
1	clove garlic, chopped	1
1 tsp	dried oregano	5 mL
1 tsp	ground cumin	5 mL
$\frac{1}{2}$	package (10 oz/300 g) spinach, stemmed and coarsely chopped	$\frac{1}{2}$
	Salt and freshly ground black pepper	

1. In a medium saucepan, combine broth, $1\frac{1}{2}$ broth cans water, chickpeas, chicken, onion, carrot, garlic, oregano and cumin. Bring to a boil, reduce heat and simmer, covered, for 15 minutes.

2. Stir in the spinach and cook, uncovered, for 2 minutes. Season to taste with salt and pepper.

Variation

Chunky Vegetable Chicken Soup: Omit the chickpeas and spinach. Substitute $\frac{1}{2}$ tsp (2 mL) dried thyme for the cumin. Add another carrot and 1 coarsely chopped potato. Add 1 coarsely chopped red bell pepper and 1 coarsely chopped zucchini halfway through the cooking time.

Advice for Clear Skin

▶ Choose gluten-free broth until the reintroduction phase of the diet plan, when you can test to see if gluten-containing products are safe for your skin.

Nutrients per serving

Calories	246
Fat	3 g
Carbohydrate	36 g
Fiber	8 g
Protein	19 g
Vitamin A	5918 IU
Vitamin C	18 mg
Iron	3.8 mg
Vitamin E	2 IU
Zinc	2.1 mg
Selenium	15.6 mcg

Salads

Citrus Fennel Slaw

The fennel and citrus combination is a natural in this crunchy twist on coleslaw. Kids enjoy the citrus flavors. The grated lemon and orange rind not only provide a nice tangy flavor but also help to support liver function, which is important for normalizing acne.

Tips

To get thin, even slices, use a mandoline to cut the fennel bulb.

Instead of serving it on top of the greens on individual plates, you can also simply pass the slaw.

1	large fennel bulb	1
¼	red onion, very thinly sliced	¼
	Grated zest and juice of 1 lemon	
	Grated zest of 1 orange	
2 tbsp	freshly squeezed orange juice	30 mL
1 tbsp	canola oil	15 mL
Pinch	salt	Pinch
	Freshly ground black pepper	
6 cups	mesclun mix	1.5 L
3 tbsp	toasted pine nuts (see tip, page 312)	45 mL

1. Remove the stalks and tough outer leaves of the fennel bulb and discard. Cut bulb in half lengthwise and trim out core. Cut bulb crosswise into very thin slices.

2. Place fennel slices and red onion in a large bowl. Stir in lemon zest, lemon juice, orange zest and orange juice. Drizzle with oil and sprinkle with salt and pepper to taste.

3. Divide mesclun mix evenly among six small plates. Mound one-sixth of the fennel slaw on each plate and garnish with pine nuts.

Variation

Substitute toasted unsalted sunflower seeds for the pine nuts.

This recipe courtesy of dietitian Jaclyn Pritchard.

Advice for Clear Skin

▶ This recipe contains only a minimal amount of fresh orange juice, which should not cause any issues.

▶ Substitute extra virgin olive oil for the canola oil.

Nutrients per serving

Calories	81
Fat	5 g
Carbohydrate	8 g
Fiber	3 g
Protein	2 g
Vitamin A	2730 IU
Vitamin C	11 mg
Iron	0.9 mg
Vitamin E	1 IU
Zinc	0.4 mg
Selenium	0.6 mcg

Kale, Apple and Walnut Slaw

MAKES 4 SERVINGS

This refreshing salad provides a nice combination of flavors and ample crunch. The walnuts contain omega-3s to assist with normalizing skin.

1½ tbsp	extra virgin olive oil	22 mL
2 tsp	sherry vinegar	10 mL
½ tsp	Dijon mustard	2 mL
¼ tsp	fine sea salt	1 mL
1	large bunch kale, stems and ribs removed, leaves very thinly sliced crosswise (about 5 cups/1.25 L)	1
1	large tart-sweet apple (such as Gala, Braeburn or Golden Delicious), halved, cored and very thinly sliced crosswise	1
½ cup	thinly sliced green onions	125 mL
3 tbsp	chopped toasted walnuts (see tip, page 312)	45 mL

1. In a small bowl, whisk together oil, vinegar, mustard and salt.

2. In a large bowl, combine kale, apple and green onions. Add dressing and gently toss to coat. Sprinkle with walnuts.

Nutrients per serving	
Calories	157
Fat	9 g
Carbohydrate	18 g
Fiber	4 g
Protein	5 g
Vitamin A	13,034 IU
Vitamin C	106 mg
Iron	1.9 mg
Vitamin E	2 IU
Zinc	0.6 mg
Selenium	1.8 mcg

Brussels Sprouts Slaw

Brussels sprouts look like tiny cabbages; as such, they are ideal for a fresh slaw. Their natural nuttiness pairs perfectly with the fresh lemon-coconut dressing. They also contain a compound called indole-3-carbinol, which helps your body metabolize hormones via the liver.

Tips

Trim the root end from Brussels sprouts and cut off any loose, thick outer leaves, then rinse well to remove any grit that may have gathered under loose leaves.

If using a mandoline to slice the Brussels sprouts, leave the stem ends on, hold each sprout by the stem end and slice crosswise instead of lengthwise.

Nutrients per serving	
Calories	154
Fat	11 g
Carbohydrate	13 g
Fiber	6 g
Protein	5 g
Vitamin A	856 IU
Vitamin C	99 mg
Iron	2.1 mg
Vitamin E	2 IU
Zinc	0.9 mg
Selenium	2.7 mcg

1½ lbs	Brussels sprouts, trimmed	750 g
2 tbsp	melted virgin coconut oil	30 mL
1 tsp	finely grated lemon zest	5 mL
2 tbsp	freshly squeezed lemon juice	30 mL
1 tsp	Dijon mustard	5 mL
¼ tsp	fine sea salt	1 mL
¼ tsp	freshly cracked black pepper	1 mL
⅓ cup	unsweetened flaked or shredded coconut, toasted	75 mL
¼ cup	hemp hearts or sunflower seeds, toasted	60 mL

1. Using a very sharp knife, very thinly slice Brussels sprouts lengthwise. Use your fingers to separate the leaves and place in a large bowl.

2. In a small bowl, whisk together coconut oil, lemon zest, lemon juice, mustard, salt and pepper.

3. Finely chop coconut until it has the texture of grated Parmesan cheese.

4. Add coconut and hemp hearts to Brussels sprouts. Add dressing and gently toss to coat.

Sesame, Hemp and Carrot Slaw

This take on classic coleslaw has virtually all the same flavors and textures but is much more nutritious. The healthy fats in the hemp seeds and hemp oil support your skin.

Tips

Be sure to zest your lemon before juicing. For this quantity of zest you will need 2 to 3 lemons.

Hemp oil provides omega fatty acids, which your body needs. It has a good balance of omega-3 and omega-6 essential fatty acids and also provides omega-9 fatty acids and a small amount of vitamin E, all beneficial nutrients for achieving clear skin.

3 cups	shredded carrots	750 mL
1 cup	shredded red cabbage	250 mL
1/4 cup	cold-pressed hemp oil	60 mL
2 tbsp	finely grated lemon zest	30 mL
3 tbsp	freshly squeezed lemon juice	45 mL
1/2 tsp	fine sea salt	2 mL
1/4 cup	chopped parsley leaves	60 mL
3 tbsp	sesame seeds	45 mL
3 tbsp	raw shelled hemp seeds (hemp hearts)	45 mL
2 tbsp	caraway seeds	30 mL

1. In a bowl, toss together carrots, red cabbage, hemp oil, lemon juice and salt. Set aside for 15 to 20 minutes, until softened.

2. Add parsley, sesame, hemp and caraway seeds and lemon zest and toss well. Taste for seasoning, adding more salt if necessary. Serve immediately.

Variation

You can give this slaw an Asian spin by substituting rice wine vinegar for the lemon juice and sesame oil for the hemp oil. Add a sprinkle of dried dulse flakes.

Nutrients per serving	
Calories	261
Fat	21 g
Carbohydrate	15 g
Fiber	5 g
Protein	6 g
Vitamin A	14,365 IU
Vitamin C	32 mg
Iron	3.1 mg
Vitamin E	5 IU
Zinc	1.0 mg
Selenium	3.0 mcg

Mega-Green Hemp Bowl

MAKES 4 SERVINGS

2 cups	chopped spinach leaves	500 mL
1 cup	thinly sliced kale (see tip, at left)	250 mL
1 cup	thinly sliced chard	250 mL
1/2 cup	arugula	125 mL
3 tbsp	raw shelled hemp seeds (hemp hearts)	45 mL
1/2 cup	cold-pressed hemp oil	125 mL
1/4 cup	freshly squeezed lemon juice	60 mL
1 tsp	fine sea salt	5 mL

1. In a bowl, toss together spinach, kale, chard, arugula and hemp seeds. Add hemp oil, lemon juice and salt and toss well. Set aside for 15 minutes to soften the greens. Serve immediately or transfer to an airtight container and refrigerate for up to 2 days.

Nutrients per serving

Calories	300
Fat	31 g
Carbohydrate	5 g
Fiber	1 g
Protein	4 g
Vitamin A	4593 IU
Vitamin C	34 mg
Iron	1.8 mg
Vitamin E	7 IU
Zinc	0.2 mg
Selenium	0.4 mcg

Fennel, Apple and Coconut Salad

MAKES 6 SERVINGS

2 tbsp	melted virgin coconut oil	30 mL
1 tsp	finely grated lemon zest	5 mL
2 tsp	freshly squeezed lemon juice	10 mL
1/8 tsp	fine sea salt	0.5 mL
1/8 tsp	cracked black pepper	0.5 mL
1	large bulb fennel, halved lengthwise (see tip, page 267), cored and very thinly sliced crosswise, fronds reserved	1
1	large Granny Smith apple, peeled, cored and thinly sliced	1
3 tbsp	unsweetened shredded or flaked coconut, toasted	45 mL

1. In a small bowl, whisk together coconut oil, lemon zest, lemon juice, salt and pepper.

2. Chop enough of the reserved fennel fronds to measure 2 tbsp (30 mL).

3. In a large bowl, combine fennel fronds, fennel bulb and apple. Add dressing and gently toss to coat. Let stand for 10 minutes to blend the flavors. Sprinkle with coconut.

Nutrients per serving

Calories	88
Fat	6 g
Carbohydrate	9 g
Fiber	3 g
Protein	1 g
Vitamin A	73 IU
Vitamin C	8 mg
Iron	0.4 mg
Vitamin E	0 IU
Zinc	0.2 mg
Selenium	0.7 mcg

Fennel, Orange and Olive Salad

Unmistakable for its delicate crunch and licorice undertones, fresh fennel becomes even more enticing when paired with fresh oranges and topped with sweet-hot red onion, cooling mint and briny olives.

Tip

To prepare the fennel bulb, trim off the tough stalks from the top and the root end before cutting the bulb in half. Chop any feathery fronds from the stalks and sprinkle on top of the salad with the olives, if desired. If the outer layers of the bulb are tough and stringy, you can discard them or peel off the outer layer with a sharp vegetable peeler.

2	large oranges	2
1	large bulb fennel, halved lengthwise, cored and very thinly sliced crosswise	1
½ cup	very thinly sliced red onion	125 mL
⅓ cup	packed fresh mint leaves, torn	75 mL
⅛ tsp	fine sea salt	0.5 mL
⅛ tsp	cracked black pepper	0.5 mL
2 tbsp	extra virgin olive oil	30 mL
½ cup	pitted brine-cured black olives (such as kalamata), quartered	125 mL

1. Using a sharp knife, cut peel and pith from oranges. Working over a large bowl, cut between membranes to release segments. Squeeze the membranes to release any remaining juice into the bowl.

2. To the oranges, add fennel, red onion, mint, salt, pepper and oil, gently tossing to combine. Sprinkle with olives.

Nutrients per serving	
Calories	99
Fat	6 g
Carbohydrate	12 g
Fiber	3 g
Protein	1 g
Vitamin A	296 IU
Vitamin C	39 mg
Iron	0.8 mg
Vitamin E	1 IU
Zinc	0.2 mg
Selenium	0.7 mcg

Avocado Melissa Sue Anderson

This is one of those salads you put together during a sunny day on the patio, slicing lovely things into a large bowl, adding layer upon layer of color. At the end, you toss it all together gently and offer it to your assembled friends. Avocado provides healthy fats and contains a compound called glutathione that supports your body's detoxification processes.

2 tbsp	freshly squeezed lime juice	30 mL
2	ripe avocados	2
1	Granny Smith apple, peeled and thinly sliced	1
2	peaches, peeled and cut into chunks	2
5	green onions, cut into $1/2$-inch (1 cm) pieces	5
3 cups	sliced mushrooms	750 mL
2	sticks celery, chopped	2
$3/4$ cup	unpeeled, diced English cucumber	175 mL
2	tomatoes, cubed	2
$1/3$ cup	toasted cashew pieces (see tip, page 312)	75 mL
3 tbsp	finely chopped fresh coriander	45 mL
2 tbsp	vegetable oil	30 mL
1 tbsp	sesame oil	15 mL
1 tbsp	raspberry or white wine vinegar	15 mL
1 tsp	salt	5 mL
1 tsp	cayenne pepper (optional)	5 mL
	Alfalfa sprouts	

1. Put lime juice in a large bowl. Peel avocado and cut into slices (or scoop out with a small spoon) and add to the lime juice. Toss gently until well coated. Add apple slices and toss again. Add peaches, green onions, mushrooms, celery, cucumber, tomatoes and cashew pieces.

2. In a small bowl, whisk together coriander, vegetable oil, sesame oil, vinegar, salt and cayenne (if using) until emulsified. Drizzle half of the dressing over the salad. Fold in the dressing, mixing the various ingredients of the salad. Do this gently but thoroughly. Add the rest of the dressing, and fold in 5 or 6 more times.

3. Transfer to a serving bowl and garnish with alfalfa sprouts for that final California touch. Serve immediately or keep up to 1 hour, covered and unrefrigerated.

Nutrients per serving

Calories	198
Fat	16 g
Carbohydrate	15 g
Fiber	5 g
Protein	4 g
Vitamin A	516 IU
Vitamin C	15 mg
Iron	1.0 mg
Vitamin E	3 IU
Zinc	0.9 mg
Selenium	3.4 mcg

Advice for Clear Skin

▶ Substitute extra virgin olive oil for the vegetable oil.

Roasted Cauliflower and Radicchio Salad

MAKES 6 SERVINGS

A zesty sherry vinegar and mustard dressing brings out the best in nutty roasted cauliflower and bitter radicchio. In traditional herbal medicine, parsley is considered a blood purifier that is important for normalizing skin conditions.

- **Preheat oven to 450°F (230°C)**
- **Large rimmed baking sheet, lined with parchment paper or foil**

4 cups	small cauliflower florets (about 1 medium head)	1 L
1/2 tsp	fine sea salt, divided	2 mL
1/4 tsp	freshly ground black pepper	1 mL
2 tbsp	extra virgin olive oil, divided	30 mL
1 tbsp	sherry vinegar	15 mL
1/2 tsp	whole-grain Dijon mustard	2 mL
1	large head radicchio, cut crosswise into 1/4-inch (0.5 cm) wide strips	1
1 cup	packed fresh flat-leaf (Italian) parsley leaves, roughly chopped	250 mL
3 tbsp	chopped toasted walnuts (see tip, page 312)	45 mL

1. In a large bowl, toss cauliflower with half the salt, pepper and half the oil. Spread in a single layer on prepared baking sheet. Roast in preheated oven for 35 to 40 minutes, stirring once or twice, until tender and golden brown. Let cool slightly in pan on a wire rack.

2. In a small bowl, whisk together the remaining salt, the remaining oil, vinegar and mustard.

3. In a large bowl, combine warm cauliflower, radicchio and parsley. Add dressing and gently toss to coat. Sprinkle with walnuts.

Nutrients per serving	
Calories	87
Fat	7 g
Carbohydrate	5 g
Fiber	2 g
Protein	2 g
Vitamin A	855 IU
Vitamin C	48 mg
Iron	1.1 mg
Vitamin E	1 IU
Zinc	0.4 mg
Selenium	0.7 mcg

Green Bean Salad with Toasted Hazelnuts

MAKES 6 SERVINGS

Simply prepared with a short list of ingredients, this salad is a case study in understated elegance.

- **Steamer basket**

12 oz	green beans, trimmed and halved crosswise	375 g
	Ice water	
1 tbsp	extra virgin olive oil	15 mL
1 tsp	whole-grain Dijon mustard	5 mL
1 tsp	sherry vinegar or white wine vinegar	5 mL
$\frac{1}{8}$ tsp	fine sea salt	0.5 mL
$\frac{1}{4}$ cup	finely chopped red onion	60 mL
2 tbsp	chopped toasted hazelnuts (see tip, page 312)	30 mL

1. Place green beans in a steamer basket set over a large pot of boiling water. Cover and steam for 4 to 6 minutes or until tender. Transfer to a large bowl of ice water to stop the cooking. Drain and pat dry with paper towels.

2. In a small bowl, whisk together oil, mustard, vinegar and salt.

3. In a large bowl, combine green beans and red onion. Add dressing and gently toss to coat. Cover and refrigerate for at least 30 minutes, until chilled, or for up to 2 hours. Sprinkle with hazelnuts just before serving.

Nutrients per serving	
Calories	56
Fat	4 g
Carbohydrate	5 g
Fiber	2 g
Protein	2 g
Vitamin A	392 IU
Vitamin C	8 mg
Iron	0.7 mg
Vitamin E	1 IU
Zinc	0.2 mg
Selenium	0.4 mcg

Hearts of Palm and Mushroom Salad with Lemon Parsley Vinaigrette

Look for white mushrooms to complement the creamy colors and flecks of vibrant green that swirl through this delightful salad. Hearts of palm are a nutritious part of this salad, providing vitamin C, calcium, iron and several B vitamins, including folate.

1 lb	white mushrooms, thinly sliced	500 g
1	can (14 oz/398 mL) hearts of palm, drained and sliced into bite-size pieces	1
¾ cup	chopped toasted walnuts (see tip, page 312)	175 mL
3	green onions, white and green parts, finely chopped	3
⅔ cup	olive oil	150 mL
½ cup	freshly squeezed lemon juice	125 mL
½ cup	finely chopped parsley	125 mL
½ tsp	salt	2 mL
½ tsp	freshly ground black pepper	2 ml

1. In a large serving bowl, gently toss together mushrooms, hearts of palm, walnuts and green onions.

2. In a pint jar or other jar with a tight-fitting lid, place oil, lemon juice, parsley, salt and pepper and shake vigorously to blend. Pour over salad. Cover and refrigerate salad for 20 minutes. Toss to refresh and serve.

Nutrients per serving

Calories	255
Fat	25 g
Carbohydrate	8 g
Fiber	3 g
Protein	4 g
Vitamin A	454 IU
Vitamin C	22 mg
Iron	3.0 mg
Vitamin E	5 IU
Zinc	1.2 mg
Selenium	7.5 mcg

Radish and Cucumber Salad

Radishes and cucumbers are available throughout the winter, which means you can make this lively salad as a refreshing counterpoint to hearty dishes all season long. Cucumbers have a high water content and are a source of silica, so they work to support the strength and hydration of your skin.

Tips

You can replace the fresh tarragon with 1 tsp (5 mL) dried.

A large field cucumber can be used in place of the English cucumber. Peel the cucumber, slice it in half lengthwise and scrape out the seeds with a spoon before slicing crosswise.

Nutrients per serving	
Calories	74
Fat	7 g
Carbohydrate	3 g
Fiber	1 g
Protein	1 g
Vitamin A	157 IU
Vitamin C	9 mg
Iron	0.3 mg
Vitamin E	0 IU
Zinc	0.2 mg
Selenium	0.3 mcg

2 tsp	minced fresh tarragon	10 mL
¼ tsp	fine sea salt	1 mL
2 tbsp	melted virgin coconut oil	30 mL
1 tbsp	freshly squeezed lemon juice	15 mL
1	large English cucumber, peeled and sliced	1
1 cup	thinly sliced (crosswise) red radishes	250 mL
3 tbsp	chopped chives	45 mL

1. In a small bowl, whisk together tarragon, salt, coconut oil and lemon juice.

2. In a large bowl, combine cucumber, radishes and chives. Add dressing and gently toss to coat.

Garden Patch Spinach Salad

Full of good things, this colorful salad is scrumptious and supports your skin by providing a good supply of carotenoids, folate, iron and lycopene.

1	avocado, peeled, pitted and diced	1
4 cups	baby spinach	1 L
1 cup	grated carrot	250 mL
1 cup	julienned red bell pepper	250 mL
1 cup	grape tomatoes, halved	250 mL
1 cup	canned chickpeas, drained and rinsed	250 mL
1/2 cup	sunflower seeds	125 mL
1/4 to 1/2 cup	lower-fat dressing of your choice	60 to 125 mL

1. In a large salad bowl, combine avocado, spinach, carrot, red pepper, tomatoes, chickpeas and sunflower seeds. Serve with dressing on the side.

This recipe courtesy of Eileen Campbell.

Advice for Clear Skin

▶ Avoid commercially available low-fat dressings and opt for a "healthy-fat" homemade dressing using extra virgin olive oil combined with vinegar or citrus juice.

Nutrients per serving	
Calories	148
Fat	9 g
Carbohydrate	15 g
Fiber	5 g
Protein	5 g
Vitamin A	4273 IU
Vitamin C	26 mg
Iron	1.6 mg
Vitamin E	6 IU
Zinc	1.1 mg
Selenium	5.8 mcg

Creamy Cherry Tomato Salad

Add some healthy fat to your diet with this salad, which combines the sweet, juicy pop of cherry tomatoes with smooth, creamy avocado.

Tips

To ripen avocados, place them in a brown paper bag with a tomato or an apple. If your avocado is ripe and won't be consumed within a day or two, place it in the coolest part of the refrigerator to lengthen its life by 3 to 4 days.

Once you take an avocado out of the fridge, do not put it back in — it will turn black.

You can substitute ¼ cup (60 mL) fresh basil leaves for the dried basil.

- **Food processor**

2	avocados, divided	2
¼ cup	freshly squeezed lemon juice	60 mL
2 tbsp	cold-pressed (extra virgin) olive oil	30 mL
¼ cup	filtered water	60 mL
1 tbsp	dried basil	15 mL
½ tsp	fine sea salt	2 mL
2 cups	halved cherry tomatoes	500 mL

1. In food processor, combine 1 avocado, lemon juice, olive oil, water, basil and salt. Process until smooth.

2. Cut the remaining avocado into 1-inch (2.5 cm) cubes and place in a bowl. Add tomatoes and avocado purée. Toss well to coat. Serve immediately or cover and refrigerate for up to 1 day.

Nutrients per serving	
Calories	239
Fat	22 g
Carbohydrate	13 g
Fiber	8 g
Protein	3 g
Vitamin A	772 IU
Vitamin C	26 mg
Iron	1.3 mg
Vitamin E	5 IU
Zinc	0.8 mg
Selenium	0.4 mcg

Turkish Tomato, Pepper and Herb Salad

MAKES 6 SERVINGS

A familiar offering of Turkish cafés and street vendors, this lively play of fresh, smoky, citrusy and peppery is a celebration of summer produce.

1/2 tsp	hot smoked paprika	2 mL
1/4 tsp	fine sea salt	1 mL
2 tbsp	extra virgin olive oil	30 mL
2 tsp	finely grated lemon zest	10 mL
2 tbsp	freshly squeezed lemon juice	30 mL
1	cucumber, peeled, seeded and thinly sliced	1
2 cups	halved cherry or grape tomatoes	500 mL
1 cup	packed arugula, roughly chopped	250 mL
1 cup	packed fresh flat-leaf (Italian) parsley leaves, roughly chopped	250 mL
1/2 cup	roughly chopped drained roasted red bell peppers	125 mL
1/2 cup	chopped green onions	125 mL
1/4 cup	packed fresh mint leaves, roughly chopped	60 mL
2 tbsp	drained capers (optional)	30 mL

1. In a small bowl, whisk together paprika, salt, oil, lemon zest and lemon juice.

2. In a large bowl, combine cucumber, tomatoes, arugula, parsley, roasted peppers, green onions, mint and capers (if using). Add dressing and gently toss to coat. Cover and refrigerate for at least 30 minutes, until chilled, or for up to 2 hours.

Nutrients per serving

Calories	66
Fat	5 g
Carbohydrate	6 g
Fiber	2 g
Protein	1 g
Vitamin A	1927 IU
Vitamin C	46 mg
Iron	1.2 mg
Vitamin E	2 IU
Zinc	0.3 mg
Selenium	0.2 mcg

Caprese Salad with Tomatoes, Basil and Avocado

A fresh play on a classic Caprese, perfectly ripe avocado is a creamy stand-in for buffalo mozzarella. Ripe tomatoes are essential to making this refreshing summer salad.

4	large ripe tomatoes, sliced 1/4 inch (0.5 cm) thick	4
1/2 cup	fresh basil leaves	125 mL
2	large ripe avocados, sliced 1/2 inch (1 cm) thick	2
3 tbsp	good-quality olive oil	45 mL
	Salt and freshly ground black pepper	

1. On a large platter or 4 individual plates, arrange ingredients in an overlapping pattern, placing slices of tomato between basil and avocado in the following order: tomato, basil, tomato, avocado, tomato, basil, etc. Drizzle with oil and sprinkle with salt and pepper to taste. Serve immediately.

Variation

If basil is unavailable, use arugula, mâche or baby spinach.

Nutrients per serving	
Calories	284
Fat	25 g
Carbohydrate	16 g
Fiber	9 g
Protein	4 g
Vitamin A	1942 IU
Vitamin C	36 mg
Iron	1.3 mg
Vitamin E	7 IU
Zinc	1.0 mg
Selenium	0.4 mcg

Vegetarian Dishes

Hemp and Sunflower Banquet Burgers

MAKES 4 BURGERS

Thanks to the hemp oil and seeds, these burgers are packed with skin-friendly omega-3s.

Tips

To soak the sunflower seeds, cover with 2 cups (500 mL) water. Set aside for 30 minutes. Drain and rinse under cold water until the water runs clear.

Do not over-dehydrate the burgers. Keeping the inside a bit soft gives the mouth feel of a real burger. To check for doneness, stick a toothpick into the middle of a burger. If it comes out clean, the patty is ready to be removed from the dehydrator.

Nutrients per burger	
Calories	452
Fat	38 g
Carbohydrate	18 g
Fiber	8 g
Protein	14 g
Vitamin A	1446 IU
Vitamin C	54 mg
Iron	4.3 mg
Vitamin E	23 IU
Zinc	2.6 mg
Selenium	22.8 mcg

- **Food processor**
- **Electric food dehydrator**

1 cup	raw sunflower seeds, soaked (see tip, at left)	250 mL
1 cup	chopped red bell pepper	250 mL
1/2 cup	chopped celery	125 mL
1/4 cup	chopped onion	60 mL
1/2 cup	filtered water	125 mL
3 tbsp	cold-pressed hemp oil	45 mL
2 tbsp	freshly squeezed lemon juice	30 mL
1 tsp	fine sea salt	5 mL
1 tsp	dried oregano	5 mL
1 tsp	chili powder	5 mL
4	cloves garlic	4
1/4 cup	raw shelled hemp seeds (hemp hearts)	60 mL
1/2 cup	ground flax seeds (flaxseed meal)	125 mL

1. In food processor, process red pepper, celery, onion, water, hemp oil, lemon juice, salt, oregano, chili powder and garlic, until smooth. Add soaked sunflower seeds and hemp seeds and process until smooth, stopping the motor and scraping down the sides of the work bowl as necessary. Transfer to a bowl.

2. Add flax seeds and mix well. Set aside for 10 minutes so the flax can absorb the liquid and swell.

3. Divide into 4 equal portions and, using your hands, flatten into patties. Place on a nonstick dehydrator sheet at least 2 inches (5 cm) apart. Dehydrate at 105°F (41°C) for 3 to 4 hours or until firm enough to handle. Flip and transfer to mesh sheet. Return to dehydrator and dehydrate for 1 to 2 hours or until firm on the outside but still soft in the middle. Serve immediately with the accompaniments of your choice.

Variation

Replace the hemp seeds with 1/4 cup (60 mL) sesame seeds.

"Steak and Potatoes"

This is a comforting recipe when you're craving something hearty and rich. Nutritional yeast is a good source of B vitamins to support proper metabolism of hormones, which is important for healing acne.

Tip

To slice the mushrooms, use a sharp chef's knife and cut them on a slight bias. You want to expose as much surface area as possible so the marinade can penetrate the mushrooms and soften them.

- Food processor
- Blender

2	portobello mushrooms, thinly sliced (see tip, at left)	2
¼ cup	cold-pressed (extra virgin) olive oil	60 mL
3 tbsp	tamari	45 mL
1½ cups	whole raw almonds	375 mL
2 tbsp	nutritional yeast	30 mL
¼ tsp	fine sea salt	1 mL
½ cup	filtered water	125 mL

1. In a bowl, toss mushrooms with olive oil and tamari, until well coated. Cover and set aside for 12 to 13 minutes, until softened.

2. In food processor, process almonds, nutritional yeast and salt until combined and no large pieces remain. With the motor running, slowly drizzle water through the feed tube to create a paste. Process for 20 to 30 seconds.

3. Transfer almond mixture to blender. Blend at high speed until smooth and creamy, stopping motor to scrape down sides of jar as necessary.

4. Place almond mixture in the middle of a serving plate and top with marinated mushrooms. Serve immediately or cover and refrigerate for up to 3 days.

Variation

If you have more time, try replacing the almond mixture (step 2) in this recipe with 1 cup (250 mL) Cauliflower "Mashed Potatoes" (page 353).

Advice for Clear Skin

▶ Use organic, non-GMO tamari.

Nutrients per serving	
Calories	919
Fat	80 g
Carbohydrate	30 g
Fiber	15 g
Protein	32 g
Vitamin A	1 IU
Vitamin C	0 mg
Iron	5.7 mg
Vitamin E	48 IU
Zinc	4.3 mg
Selenium	21.8 mcg

Spelt-Stuffed Eggplant with Indian Spices

Eggplant is native to India and has been cultivated in eastern Asia since prehistory. This spicy Indian-inspired dish is made heartier with the addition of nutty spelt berries.

- **8-inch (20 cm) glass baking dish, lightly oiled**

1/2 cup	spelt berries, rinsed and soaked 6 hours or overnight	125 mL
1 1/2 cups	ready-to-use vegetable broth	375 mL
2	small eggplants (each about 12 oz/375 g)	2
2 1/2 tsp	salt, divided	12 mL
2 tbsp	olive oil	30 mL
1/2 cup	chopped onion	125 mL
1 tbsp	minced gingerroot	15 mL
2 tsp	minced garlic	10 mL
2 tsp	ground turmeric	10 mL
1 tsp	ground cumin (see tip, opposite)	5 mL
1/8 tsp	hot pepper flakes	0.5 mL
1/8 tsp	freshly ground black pepper	0.5 mL
1/2 cup	water	125 mL
1 1/2 cups	seeded and chopped tomatoes	375 mL

1. Drain spelt. In a saucepan, combine spelt and broth and bring to a boil over high heat. Cover, reduce heat to low and simmer until spelt is tender and most of the liquid is absorbed, about 1 1/2 hours. Drain and set aside. This may be done up to 2 days ahead of time.

2. Cut eggplants in half, lengthwise. Run a small knife around cut edge of flesh, 1/4 to 1/2 inch (0.5 to 1 cm) inside skin. Then make two lengthwise cuts through eggplant halves, being careful not to cut through to the bottom. Gently pull and cut lengthwise sections away from shell to hollow out, leaving 1/4- to 1/2-inch (0.5 to 1 cm) thick walls, reserving flesh. Place hollowed out shells in prepared baking dish and set aside.

3. Coarsely chop the reserved eggplant flesh and place in a colander. Toss with 2 tsp (10 mL) salt and let stand for 20 minutes to sweat. Rinse thoroughly, drain and pat dry with a clean kitchen towel.

Nutrients per serving

Calories	208
Fat	8 g
Carbohydrate	32 g
Fiber	10 g
Protein	6 g
Vitamin A	829 IU
Vitamin C	15 mg
Iron	2.5 mg
Vitamin E	3 IU
Zinc	1.2 mg
Selenium	3.5 mcg

Tip

For the best flavor, toast cumin seeds and grind them yourself. To toast seeds, place them in a dry skillet over medium heat and cook, stirring, until fragrant, about 3 minutes. Immediately transfer to a spice grinder or mortar and grind finely.

4. Preheat oven to 350°F (180°C). Place a large skillet over medium heat and let pan get hot. Add oil and tip pan to coat. Add onion, ginger and garlic and cook, stirring, until softened, 6 to 8 minutes. Stir in chopped eggplant, turmeric, cumin, $\frac{1}{2}$ tsp (2 mL) salt, hot pepper flakes, black pepper and water. Reduce heat to low, cover and cook, stirring occasionally, until eggplant is soft, about 10 minutes. Remove from heat and stir in cooked spelt and tomatoes.

5. Fill eggplant shells with spelt mixture. Cover with foil and bake until filling is hot and eggplant shells are tender, 40 to 50 minutes. Serve immediately.

Variation

Add diced zucchini or carrots to the vegetable sauté mixture with the chopped eggplant.

Advice for Clear Skin

▶ Substitute quinoa or millet for the spelt berries.

▶ Choose gluten-free broth until the reintroduction phase of the diet plan, when you can test to see if gluten-containing products are safe for your skin.

Mushroom Tart

MAKES 2 SERVINGS

This tart's dense shell and creamy mushroom filling will be sure to fulfill your cravings for something hearty and rich.

- **Food processor**
- **Two 4-inch (10 cm) quiche molds, lined with plastic wrap**

4 cups	thinly sliced button mushrooms	1 L
1/4 cup	tamari	60 mL
2 tbsp	cold-pressed (extra virgin) olive oil	30 mL
1 cup	whole raw almonds	250 mL
1/4 tsp	fine sea salt	1 mL
6 tbsp	filtered water, divided	90 mL
1 cup	whole raw cashews	250 mL

1. In a bowl, toss mushrooms, tamari and olive oil until well combined. Cover and set aside for 10 minutes, until softened.

2. In food processor, combine almonds and salt and process until flour-like in consistency. Transfer to a bowl. Add 3 tbsp (45 mL) water and mix well. Divide mixture into 2 equal parts and press into prepared quiche molds.

3. In food processor, combine marinated mushrooms, the remaining water and cashews. Process until smooth, stopping motor to scrape down sides of work bowl as necessary. Divide mixture in half and spread in each prepared crust. Serve immediately or cover and refrigerate for up to 2 days.

Variations

Add 1/2 cup (125 mL) baby spinach, 2 tbsp (30 mL) nutritional yeast and 1 tbsp (15 mL) chopped fresh thyme to the food processor in step 3.

Substitute an equal amount of thinly sliced shiitake mushrooms, stems removed, for the button mushrooms.

Advice for Clear Skin

▸ Use organic, non-GMO tamari.

Nutrients per serving

Calories	976
Fat	81 g
Carbohydrate	45 g
Fiber	13 g
Protein	34 g
Vitamin A	1 IU
Vitamin C	3 mg
Iron	8.4 mg
Vitamin E	32 IU
Zinc	6.9 mg
Selenium	23.1 mcg

Marinated Kelp Noodles

Kelp noodles are thin, spaghetti-like noodles that are translucent and have a neutral flavor. They are great to use in recipes because they absorb whatever flavors they are matched with. This is a very simple way to prepare them that manipulates the texture to make them soft. Kelp noodles are a skin-friendly, low-carbohydrate substitute for flour noodles.

Tip

Kelp noodles have a long shelf life and do not need to be refrigerated until opened. Once opened, transfer to an airtight container and store in the refrigerator for up to one week.

1	bag (16 oz/454 g) kelp noodles	1
3 tbsp	cold-pressed (extra virgin) olive oil	45 mL
2 tsp	freshly squeezed lemon juice	10 mL
1/4 tsp	fine sea salt	1 mL

1. Using your hands, separate the noodles until none are stuck together, transferring to a bowl as completed.

2. In a small bowl, whisk olive oil, lemon juice and salt. Add to noodles and toss well. Set aside for at least 30 minutes or overnight, until softened.

Nutrients per serving	
Calories	185
Fat	14 g
Carbohydrate	15 g
Fiber	2 g
Protein	3 g
Vitamin A	176 IU
Vitamin C	6 mg
Iron	4.4 mg
Vitamin E	5 IU
Zinc	1.9 mg
Selenium	1.1 mcg

Zucchini Spaghetti with Lemon and Herbs

MAKES 2 SERVINGS

In this dish, zucchini noodles are tossed with rich olive oil, aromatic fresh herbs and zesty lemon. Spiralized vegetables are a skin-safe alternative to carb-laden pasta.

- **Spiral vegetable slicer, fitted with the smallest blade**
- **Food processor**

2	large zucchini	2
2	bunches flat-leaf (Italian) parsley, stems removed, roughly chopped	2
¼ cup	cold-pressed (extra virgin) olive oil	60 mL
1 tbsp	lemon zest	15 mL
¼ cup	freshly squeezed lemon juice	60 mL
½ tsp	fine sea salt	2 mL

1. Using a sharp chef's knife, remove a small portion from each end of the zucchini to create a flat surface. Using spiralizer fitted with the smallest blade, secure zucchini on prongs. Rotate crank while gently pushing zucchini toward blade to create long strands of "pasta." Transfer noodles to a bowl.

2. In food processor, combine parsley, olive oil, lemon zest and juice and salt. Process until smooth, stopping motor to scrape down sides of work bowl as necessary. Add to zucchini noodles and toss until well coated. Serve immediately.

Variations

Try spiralizing other vegetables or fruits — such as carrots, parsnips, beets, apples or squash — in place of the zucchini in this recipe.

Substitute 3 bunches of fresh cilantro, roughly chopped, for the parsley and add other vegetables, such as broccoli florets, cauliflower florets or shredded carrot.

For a boost of protein, add ¼ cup (60 mL) raw shelled hemp seeds.

Nutrients per serving	
Calories	302
Fat	28 g
Carbohydrate	13 g
Fiber	3 g
Protein	4 g
Vitamin A	734 IU
Vitamin C	75 mg
Iron	1.5 mg
Vitamin E	6 IU
Zinc	1.1 mg
Selenium	0.7 mcg

Celery Root Ravioli

Here's a simple way to create delicious ravioli using only a few ingredients. Celery root gives this dish a deep, rich flavor.

Tips

You may replace the olive oil with any organic cold-pressed oil such as flax, hemp, chia, pumpkin or avocado oil.

To soak the cashews, place in a bowl and cover with 2 cups (500 mL) water. Cover and set aside for 10 minutes. Drain, discarding soaking water, and rinse under cold running water until the water runs clear.

- **Mandoline**
- **Food processor**

1	celery root, peeled	1
1/4 cup	cold-pressed (extra virgin) olive oil	60 mL
1/4 cup	freshly squeezed lemon juice, divided	60 mL
3/4 tsp	fine sea salt, divided	3 mL
1 cup	whole raw cashews, soaked (see tip, at left)	250 mL
1/4 cup	filtered water	60 mL
2 tbsp	nutritional yeast	30 mL

1. Using mandoline, slice celery root crosswise approximately $\frac{1}{16}$ inch (2 mm) thick. Transfer slices to a bowl.

2. Add olive oil, 2 tbsp (30 mL) lemon juice and $\frac{1}{4}$ tsp (1 mL) salt to celery root slices. Toss until well combined. Cover and set aside for 10 minutes, until softened.

3. In food processor, combine soaked cashews, water, nutritional yeast and the remaining lemon juice and salt. Process until nuts are roughly chopped (you want to retain some texture). Set aside.

4. Place half of the celery root slices on a flat work surface. Spoon 1 to 2 tbsp (15 to 30 mL) cashew filling in center of each. Top with another slice of celery root. Using your hands, gently push down edges around filling to squeeze out any excess air and form a ravioli shape. Serve immediately or cover and refrigerate for up to 4 days.

Nutrients per serving	
Calories	366
Fat	30 g
Carbohydrate	21 g
Fiber	3 g
Protein	9 g
Vitamin A	1 IU
Vitamin C	12 mg
Iron	3.0 mg
Vitamin E	4 IU
Zinc	2.4 mg
Selenium	6.2 mcg

Mixed Vegetable Coconut Curry

Here's a great weeknight meal that can be made with ingredients you're likely to have on hand. The culinary herbs and spices support healing of the skin, thanks to their antibacterial and antioxidant properties. Serve over hot steamed rice.

Tips

For the best flavor, toast the cumin and coriander seeds and grind them yourself. To toast seeds: Place in a dry skillet over medium heat and cook, stirring, until fragrant, about 3 minutes. Immediately transfer to a spice grinder or mortar and grind finely.

If you choose to halve this recipe, use a small (about 2-quart) slow cooker.

Nutrients per serving

Calories	244
Fat	13 g
Carbohydrate	32 g
Fiber	8 g
Protein	6 g
Vitamin A	13,438 IU
Vitamin C	67 mg
Iron	3.9 mg
Vitamin E	2 IU
Zinc	1.2 mg
Selenium	4.3 mcg

- **Medium to large (4- to 5-quart) slow cooker**

1 tbsp	vegetable oil or virgin coconut oil	15 mL
3 cups	cubed ($\frac{1}{2}$ inch/1 cm) peeled carrots (about 4 medium)	750 mL
2	onions, finely chopped	2
2	stalks celery, diced	2
4	cloves garlic, minced	4
1 tbsp	minced gingerroot	15 mL
2 tsp	ground cumin (see tip, at left)	10 mL
2 tsp	ground coriander	10 mL
1 tsp	salt	5 mL
1 tsp	cracked black peppercorns	5 mL
$\frac{1}{2}$ tsp	ground turmeric	2 mL
1	bay leaf	1
1	can (28 oz/796 mL) diced tomatoes, with juice	1
4 cups	cubed (1 inch/2.5 cm) peeled winter squash	1 L
1 cup	coconut milk	250 mL
1	red bell pepper, seeded and diced	1
1	long red or green chile pepper, seeded and minced	1

1. In a skillet, heat oil over medium heat. Add carrots, onions and celery and cook, stirring, until softened, about 7 minutes. Add garlic, ginger, cumin, coriander, salt, peppercorns, turmeric and bay leaf and cook, stirring, for 1 minute. Add tomatoes and bring to a boil. Transfer to stoneware.

2. Stir in squash. Cover and cook on Low for 6 hours or on High for 3 hours. Add coconut milk, bell pepper and chile pepper and stir well. Cover and cook on High for 15 minutes, until peppers are tender.

Advice for Clear Skin

▶ Substitute extra virgin olive oil for the vegetable oil.

Summer Vegetable Ragoût

*Summer vegetables,
especially fresh peas,
zucchini and tomatoes,
combine to lend a
distinctly summertime
taste to this stew.*

3 tbsp	olive oil, divided	45 mL
1	onion, chopped	1
1	leek, white and green parts, sliced	1
1 cup	sliced stemmed shiitake mushrooms	250 mL
2	small zucchini, sliced	2
2	carrots, sliced	2
2	tomatoes, chopped	2
3 cups	ready-to-use vegetable broth or water	750 mL
1 tbsp	tamari	15 mL
1 cup	fresh or frozen green peas	250 mL
2 tbsp	shredded fresh basil	30 mL
	Sea salt and freshly ground pepper	

1. In a saucepan, heat 2 tbsp (30 mL) oil over medium heat. Add onion and leek. Cover, reduce heat to low and sweat, stirring once or twice, for 10 minutes or until soft. Add the remaining oil and increase heat to medium-high. Add mushrooms and cook, stirring frequently, for 6 to 8 minutes or until mushrooms are reduced by about half.

2. Add zucchini, carrots, tomatoes, broth and tamari. Simmer for 10 minutes or until vegetables are almost tender. Add peas and basil and cook for 3 to 5 minutes or until peas are tender. Season to taste with salt and pepper.

Advice for Clear Skin

▶ Choose gluten-free broth until the reintroduction phase of the diet plan, when you can test to see if gluten-containing products are safe for your skin.

▶ Use organic, non-GMO tamari.

Nutrients per serving

Calories	209
Fat	11 g
Carbohydrate	26 g
Fiber	6 g
Protein	5 g
Vitamin A	6820 IU
Vitamin C	40 mg
Iron	1.9 mg
Vitamin E	4 IU
Zinc	1.4 mg
Selenium	10.2 mcg

Eggplant Lentil Ragoût

Lentils are a great ally for healing acne: they are a good source of protein, zinc, iron, B vitamins (including folate), manganese and magnesium.

Tip

To sweat eggplant, place cubed eggplant in a colander, sprinkle liberally with salt, toss well and set aside for 30 minutes to 1 hour. If time is short, blanch the pieces for a minute or two in heavily salted water. In either case, rinse thoroughly in fresh cold water and, using your hands, squeeze out excess moisture. Pat dry with paper towels and it's ready for cooking.

- **Medium (about 4-quart) slow cooker**

1	eggplant (about 1 lb/500 g) peeled, cut into 2-inch (5 cm) cubes and sweated (see tip, at left)	1
2 tbsp	olive oil (approx.)	30 mL
2	onions, finely chopped	2
4	cloves garlic, minced	4
1 tbsp	ground cumin	15 mL
1 tsp	finely grated lemon zest	5 mL
1 tsp	salt	5 mL
1/2 tsp	cracked black peppercorns	2 mL
1 cup	brown or green lentils, rinsed	250 mL
3 cups	ready-to-use vegetable broth	750 mL
1 tbsp	freshly squeezed lemon juice	15 mL
1/2 cup	finely chopped dill	125 mL

1. In a skillet, heat oil over medium-high heat. Add eggplant, in batches, and cook until browned, adding more oil as necessary. Transfer to slow cooker stoneware.

2. Add onions to pan, adding more oil, if necessary, and cook, stirring, until softened, about 3 minutes. Add garlic, cumin, lemon zest, salt and peppercorns and cook, stirring, for 1 minute. Add lentils and toss until coated. Transfer to stoneware. Stir in broth.

3. Cover and cook on Low for 6 to 8 hours or on High for 3 to 4 hours, until lentils are tender. Stir in lemon juice and dill.

Nutrients per serving

Calories	197
Fat	6 g
Carbohydrate	30 g
Fiber	7 g
Protein	10 g
Vitamin A	361 IU
Vitamin C	8 mg
Iron	3.5 mg
Vitamin E	1 IU
Zinc	1.5 mg
Selenium	3.4 mcg

Advice for Clear Skin

▶ Choose gluten-free broth until the reintroduction phase of the diet plan, when you can test to see if gluten-containing products are safe for your skin.

Tomato Dal with Spinach

This mildly spiced but tasty dal is delicious over steamed cauliflower or as a substantial side dish.

Tip

For the best flavor, toast cumin and coriander seeds and grind them yourself. To toast seeds, place them in a dry skillet over medium heat and cook, stirring, until fragrant, about 3 minutes. Immediately transfer to a spice grinder or mortar and grind finely.

Make Ahead

Complete steps 1 and 2. Cover and refrigerate for up to 2 days. When you're ready to cook, complete the recipe.

Nutrients per serving

Calories	519
Fat	6 g
Carbohydrate	93 g
Fiber	34 g
Protein	31 g
Vitamin A	22,666 IU
Vitamin C	45 mg
Iron	10.1 mg
Vitamin E	4 IU
Zinc	4.2 mg
Selenium	4.4 mcg

- **Large (about 5-quart) slow cooker**

2 cups	yellow split peas, rinsed	500 mL
1 tbsp	vegetable oil	15 mL
1	onion, finely chopped	1
6	carrots, peeled and diced	6
6	cloves garlic, finely chopped	6
1 tbsp	minced gingerroot	15 mL
1 tbsp	ground cumin (see tip, at left)	15 mL
1 tbsp	ground coriander	15 mL
1 tsp	salt	5 mL
1 tsp	cracked black peppercorns	5 mL
1	can (28 oz/796 mL) tomatoes, with juice, coarsely chopped	1
4 cups	ready-to-use vegetable broth	1 L
1 tsp	curry powder, dissolved in 1 tbsp (15 mL) freshly squeezed lemon juice	5 mL
8 cups	trimmed fresh spinach leaves	2 L
	Vegan yogurt alternative (optional)	

1. In a large saucepan, combine split peas with 8 cups (2 L) cold water. Bring to a boil. Reduce heat and boil for 25 minutes or until peas are just tender. Drain.

2. Meanwhile, in a skillet, heat oil over medium heat. Add onion and carrots and cook, stirring, until softened, about 7 minutes. Add garlic, ginger, cumin, coriander, salt and peppercorns and cook, stirring, for 1 minute. Add tomatoes and bring to a boil, breaking up with a spoon. Transfer to slow cooker stoneware. Add broth and the reserved split peas and stir to combine.

3. Cover and cook on Low for 8 hours or on High for 4 hours, until peas are soft. Stir in curry powder solution. Add spinach, in batches, stirring to submerge each before adding the next. Cover and cook on High for 20 minutes, until spinach is cooked and mixture is bubbly. Ladle into bowls and drizzle with vegan yogurt (if using).

Advice for Clear Skin

▶ Substitute extra virgin olive oil for the vegetable oil.

Cumin-Laced Lentils with Sun-Dried Tomatoes and Roasted Peppers

MAKES 6 SERVINGS

This luscious dish is underscored by slightly Middle Eastern flavors. It is very forgiving. If you don't have sun-dried tomatoes, substitute tomato paste.

Tips

If you don't have sun-dried tomatoes, substitute 1 tbsp (15 mL) tomato paste.

If you don't have harissa, dissolve ½ tsp (2 mL) cayenne pepper in 1 tbsp (15 mL) freshly squeezed lemon juice and stir in along with the roasted peppers.

Nutrients per serving

Calories	245
Fat	4 g
Carbohydrate	41 g
Fiber	8 g
Protein	14 g
Vitamin A	2043 IU
Vitamin C	62 mg
Iron	5.3 mg
Vitamin E	2 IU
Zinc	2.3 mg
Selenium	4.9 mcg

• **Medium (about 4-quart) slow cooker**

1 tbsp	olive oil	15 mL
1	onion, finely chopped	1
2	stalks celery, diced	2
4	cloves garlic, minced	4
1 tbsp	ground cumin	15 mL
1 tbsp	ground coriander	15 mL
1 tsp	salt	5 mL
1 tsp	cracked black peppercorns	5 mL
1 cup	brown or green lentils, rinsed	250 mL
½ cup	dried red lentils, rinsed	125 mL
1	can (14 oz/398 mL) diced tomatoes, with juice	1
2	finely chopped sun-dried tomatoes	2
2 cups	ready-to-use vegetable broth	500 mL
2	roasted red peppers, thinly sliced	2
1 to 2 tsp	harissa (see tip, at left)	5 to 10 mL
	Finely chopped cilantro	

1. In a skillet, heat oil over medium heat. Add onion and celery and cook, stirring, until softened, about 5 minutes. Add garlic, cumin, coriander, salt and peppercorns and cook, stirring, for 1 minute. Add brown and red lentils and toss until well coated with mixture. Add diced tomatoes and sun-dried tomatoes. Transfer to slow cooker stoneware.

2. Stir in broth. Cover and cook on Low for 6 hours or on High for 3 hours, until lentils are tender. Add roasted peppers and harissa and stir well. Cover and cook on High for 15 minutes to meld flavors. Garnish with cilantro.

Advice for Clear Skin

▶ Choose gluten-free broth until the reintroduction phase of the diet plan, when you can test to see if gluten-containing products are safe for your skin.

Spicy Chickpeas with Okra

This tasty combination, which is Moroccan-inspired, makes a nice main course accompanied by salad or a side. It is also a great dish for a buffet. The flavors are deep and deliciously different: hints of cumin and ginger and a sparkle of harissa-induced heat.

Tips

For this quantity of chickpeas, use 2 cans (14 to 19 oz/398 to 540 mL), drained and rinsed, reserving the excess, or cook $1\frac{1}{2}$ cups (375 mL) dried chickpeas.

Harissa is a North African condiment made from hot peppers and various seasonings. It is available in specialty food stores.

Nutrients per serving

Calories	191
Fat	5 g
Carbohydrate	30 g
Fiber	8 g
Protein	9 g
Vitamin A	333 IU
Vitamin C	14 mg
Iron	3.4 mg
Vitamin E	1 IU
Zinc	1.6 mg
Selenium	3.8 mcg

- **Medium to large ($3\frac{1}{2}$- to 5-quart) slow cooker**

1 tbsp	olive oil	15 mL
2	onions, finely chopped	2
4	cloves garlic, minced	4
1 tbsp	minced gingerroot	15 mL
1 tbsp	ground cumin	15 mL
1 tsp	salt	5 mL
1 tsp	crushed black peppercorns	5 mL
1 cup	ready-to-use vegetable broth	250 mL
3 cups	drained cooked chickpeas (see tip, at left)	750 mL
2 cups	sliced trimmed okra ($\frac{1}{2}$-inch/1 cm slices)	500 mL
1 tsp	harissa (see tip, at left)	5 mL

1. In a skillet, heat oil over medium heat. Add onions and cook, stirring, until softened, about 3 minutes. Add garlic, ginger, cumin, salt and peppercorns and cook, stirring, for 1 minute. Add broth and bring to a boil. Transfer to slow cooker stoneware.

2. Stir in chickpeas. Cover and cook on Low for 6 hours or on High for 3 hours. Stir in okra and harissa. Cover and cook on High for 20 minutes, until okra is tender.

Advice for Clear Skin

▶ Choose gluten-free broth until the reintroduction phase of the diet plan, when you can test to see if gluten-containing products are safe for your skin.

Black Bean Chili

Serve this robust chili with a fresh chopped salad on the side.

2 tbsp	olive oil	30 mL
1 cup	chopped onions	250 mL
3	cloves garlic, minced	3
1½ cups	chopped red bell peppers	375 mL
2	fresh chile peppers, finely chopped	2
2 tsp	ground cumin	10 mL
1	can (28 oz/796 mL) tomatoes, with juice	1
1	can (19 oz/540 mL) black beans, with liquid	1
1	can (19 oz/540 mL) chickpeas, with liquid	1
2 tbsp	dried thyme	30 mL
1 tbsp	dried savory	15 mL
2 tbsp	chopped fresh parsley	30 mL

1. In a large skillet, heat oil over medium heat. Add onions, garlic, bell peppers and chiles; cook for 5 minutes or until soft.

2. Stir in cumin, tomatoes, black beans, chickpeas, thyme and savory. Bring to a boil; simmer for 5 minutes. Stir in parsley and serve.

Nutrients per serving	
Calories	449
Fat	9 g
Carbohydrate	75 g
Fiber	22 g
Protein	18 g
Vitamin A	2930 IU
Vitamin C	145 mg
Iron	7.7 mg
Vitamin E	3 IU
Zinc	2.6 mg
Selenium	6.3 mcg

Bok Choy, Mushroom and Black Bean Stir-Fry

With just the right amount of crisp, chewy and soft textures, this stir-fry is perfectly balanced. It is a drier mixture than other stir-fry dishes and teams well with puréed vegetables. Shiitake mushrooms are considered to be "medicinal" mushrooms. They are a good source of iron, zinc, selenium and B vitamins, which all contribute to skin repair.

2 tbsp	olive oil	30 mL
2	cloves garlic, finely chopped	2
1 tbsp	Chinese five-spice powder	15 mL
1/4 cup	sunflower seeds or pine nuts	60 mL
1 cup	sliced shiitake mushroom caps	250 mL
6 tbsp	tamari, divided	90 mL
1	head bok choy, thinly sliced	1
1	can (6 oz/175 g) water chestnuts, drained and thinly sliced	1
2 tsp	toasted sesame oil	10 mL
4	green onions, thinly sliced	4
1 cup	cooked black beans	250 mL
1/4 cup	shredded Thai basil	60 mL

1. In a wok or saucepan, heat oil over medium-high heat. Add garlic, five-spice seasoning and sunflower seeds. Stir-fry for 1 minute or until garlic begins to color. Increase heat to high, add mushrooms and stir-fry for 2 minutes. Add 3 tbsp (45 mL) tamari, bok choy and water chestnuts and stir-fry for 1 to 2 minutes or until bok choy is wilted. Add the remaining tamari, sesame oil, green onions and black beans. Stir-fry for 1 to 2 minutes or until onions are al dente. Toss basil with vegetables.

> **Advice for Clear Skin**
>
> ▶ Use organic, non-GMO tamari.

Nutrients per serving	
Calories	254
Fat	14 g
Carbohydrate	25 g
Fiber	6 g
Protein	10 g
Vitamin A	353 IU
Vitamin C	6 mg
Iron	2.4 mg
Vitamin E	7 IU
Zinc	1.4 mg
Selenium	7.6 mcg

Tofu Ratatouille

Although it is time-consuming, sautéing the vegetables individually ensures that their unique flavors aren't lost when the dish is complete. The results are worth the extra effort. Serve this to your most discriminating guests and expect requests for seconds.

Advice for Clear Skin

▶ Substitute extra virgin olive oil for the vegetable oil.

▶ Use organic, non-GMO tofu.

• **Large (about 5-quart) slow cooker**

1	large eggplant, peeled, cut into 1-inch (2.5 cm) cubes and sweated (see tip, page 288)	1
3 tbsp	vegetable oil (approx.), divided	45 mL
8 oz	mushrooms, stems removed, quartered	250 g
2	small zucchini, thinly sliced	2
1	large onion, finely chopped	1
3	cloves garlic, minced	3
½ tsp	cracked black peppercorns	2 mL
½ tsp	dried thyme	2 mL
½ tsp	ground cinnamon	2 mL
1	can (28 oz/796 mL) tomatoes, with juice, coarsely chopped	1
	Salt	
8 oz	firm tofu with fine herbs, cut into 1-inch (2.5 cm) cubes	250 g
	Freshly ground black pepper	

1. In a skillet, heat 1 tbsp (15 mL) oil over medium heat. Add mushrooms and cook, stirring, just until they begin to lose their liquid. Using a slotted spoon, transfer to slow cooker stoneware. Return pan to element and add more oil, if needed.

2. Add zucchini, in batches, and cook, stirring, until it softens and begins to brown. Using a slotted spoon, transfer to a bowl. Cover and refrigerate.

3. Add eggplant to pan, in batches, and sauté until lightly browned, adding more oil as needed. Transfer to slow cooker. Add onion to pan and cook, stirring, until softened. Add garlic, peppercorns, thyme and cinnamon and cook, stirring, for 1 minute. Add tomatoes and bring to a boil. Add salt to taste. Pour into slow cooker. Stir to blend.

4. Cover and cook on Low for 6 hours or High for 3 hours, until hot and bubbly. Add the reserved zucchini and cook on High for 15 minutes, until heated through.

5. Season tofu with salt and pepper to taste. In a skillet, heat 1 tbsp (15 mL) oil over medium heat. Add tofu and cook, stirring, until lightly browned, about 15 minutes. Spread tofu over top of eggplant mixture and serve immediately.

Nutrients per serving

Calories	182
Fat	9 g
Carbohydrate	20 g
Fiber	7 g
Protein	8 g
Vitamin A	1029 IU
Vitamin C	24 mg
Iron	2.9 mg
Vitamin E	2 IU
Zinc	0.9 mg
Selenium	5.0 mcg

Sweet Chili Tofu Stir-Fry

Stir-frying is a fast and easy way to prepare a meal without a lot of added fat. Vegetables and lean protein form the basis for this dish, with a little added sauce and seasoning for flavor. It's a flavorful way to introduce your family to tofu.

	Nonstick cooking spray	
5 oz	firm tofu, cut into thin strips	150 g
3/4 cup	sliced Spanish onion	175 mL
1 cup	broccoli florets	250 mL
1 cup	baby carrots, cut into bite-size pieces	250 mL
3/4 cup	sugar snap peas, trimmed	175 mL
1/2 cup	julienned red bell pepper	125 mL
1/2 cup	ready-to-use vegetable broth or water	125 mL
1/4 cup	sweet chili sauce	60 mL
1 tsp	grated orange zest	5 mL
1 tbsp	chopped fresh cilantro (optional)	15 mL

1. Heat a wok or large skillet over medium-high heat. Spray with vegetable cooking spray. Brown tofu on both sides, then remove from pan and set aside.

2. Add onion to wok and sauté for 1 minute. Add broccoli, carrots, peas and red pepper; stir-fry until tender-crisp, about 5 minutes. Return tofu to wok and stir in broth, chili sauce and orange zest. Heat until bubbling.

This recipe courtesy of Eileen Campbell.

Advice for Clear Skin

▶ Use olive oil cooking spray or substitute 1 tbsp (15 mL) extra virgin olive oil.

▶ Use organic, non-GMO tofu.

▶ Choose gluten-free broth until the reintroduction phase of the diet plan, when you can test to see if gluten-containing products are safe for your skin.

Nutrients per serving

Calories	85
Fat	2 g
Carbohydrate	14 g
Fiber	3 g
Protein	5 g
Vitamin A	6466 IU
Vitamin C	45 mg
Iron	1.2 mg
Vitamin E	1 IU
Zinc	0.3 mg
Selenium	1.0 mcg

Chickpea Tofu Stew

A filling and flavorful winter dish, this stew is bolstered by the addition of super-nutritious tofu. It is imperative to use firm tofu (often called "pressed tofu"), since the soft variety will disintegrate. For the chickpeas, you can either cook your own or use the canned variety.

Tips

This is excellent served with a salad, steamed rice and a yogurt-based sauce.

For a spicier flavor, substitute cayenne pepper for the chili powder.

Nutrients per serving

Calories	336
Fat	15 g
Carbohydrate	38 g
Fiber	10 g
Protein	15 g
Vitamin A	1270 IU
Vitamin C	37 mg
Iron	4.0 mg
Vitamin E	4 IU
Zinc	1.7 mg
Selenium	3.9 mcg

- **Preheat oven to 375°F (190°C)**
- **6-cup (1.5 L) casserole dish**

1 lb	ripe tomatoes (about 4)	500 g
3 tbsp	olive oil	45 mL
1/2 tsp	salt	2 mL
1/2 tsp	paprika	2 mL
1/2 tsp	cumin seeds	2 mL
1/2 tsp	chili powder	2 mL
2 1/2 cups	thinly sliced onions	625 mL
1/2	green pepper, thinly sliced	1/2
4	cloves garlic, thinly sliced	4
2	bay leaves	2
1 cup	hot water	250 mL
2 tsp	freshly squeezed lime juice	10 mL
2 cups	cooked chickpeas	500 mL
8 oz	firm tofu, cut into 1/2-inch (1 cm) cubes	250 g
1 tsp	olive oil (optional)	5 mL
1/4 cup	finely diced red onion	60 mL
	Few sprigs fresh coriander, chopped	

1. Blanch tomatoes in boiling water for 30 seconds. Over a bowl, peel, core and deseed them. Chop tomatoes into chunks and set aside. Strain any accumulated tomato juices from bowl; add the juices to the tomatoes.

2. In a large frying pan, heat olive oil over high heat for 30 seconds. Add salt, paprika, cumin seeds and chili powder in quick succession. Stir-fry for 30 seconds. Add onions and stir-fry for 1 minute. Add green pepper and stir-fry for 2 to 3 minutes, until soft. Add garlic and stir-fry for 1 minute. Add tomato flesh and juices. Stir-cook for 3 minutes to break up tomato somewhat. Add bay leaves, hot water and lime juice. Cook, stirring often, for 5 minutes.

3. Transfer sauce to casserole dish. Fold chickpeas into the sauce. Distribute tofu cubes evenly over the surface and gently press them down into the sauce.

4. Bake in preheated oven, uncovered, for 25 to 30 minutes, until bubbling and bright. Drizzle with olive oil (if using) and garnish with red onion and coriander.

Fish and Seafood

Simple Grilled Fish

MAKES 4 SERVINGS

The best-tasting food often comes from simple ingredients.

Nutrients per serving

Calories	177
Fat	4 g
Carbohydrate	0 g
Fiber	0 g
Protein	33 g
Vitamin A	308 IU
Vitamin C	1 mg
Iron	2.1 mg
Vitamin E	4 IU
Zinc	0.5 mg
Selenium	132.4 mcg

- **Preheat broiler**
- **Rimmed baking sheet, lightly greased**

1 tbsp	chopped fresh parsley	15 mL
1 tbsp	olive oil	15 mL
	Juice of 1 lemon	
4	orange roughy fillets (about 1¾ lbs/ 875 g total)	4

1. In a small bowl, combine parsley, butter and lemon juice.
2. Place fish fillets on prepared baking sheet and baste both sides with oil mixture.
3. Broil for 5 to 10 minutes or until fish is opaque and flakes easily with a fork.

This recipe courtesy of Eileen Campbell.

Variation

Substitute tilapia, sole, haddock or halibut.

Basil and Tomato Fillets

MAKES 4 SERVINGS

Tomato and basil are natural partners. Add fish for a delicious meal.

Nutrients per serving

Calories	227
Fat	12 g
Carbohydrate	1 g
Fiber	0 g
Protein	27 g
Vitamin A	2733 IU
Vitamin C	3 mg
Iron	1.3 mg
Vitamin E	3 IU
Zinc	0.7 mg
Selenium	41.4 mcg

2 tbsp	olive oil, divided	30 mL
1 lb	whitefish, tuna or salmon	500 g
	Salt and freshly ground black pepper	
½ cup	chopped firm tomatoes	125 mL
2 tbsp	chopped fresh basil leaves	30 mL

1. In a nonstick skillet over medium-high heat, heat 1 tbsp (15 mL) oil. Season fish lightly with salt and pepper. Add to skillet.
2. Combine tomatoes, basil and the remaining oil. Top fish with spoonfuls of the mixture. Cover skillet tightly and cook on medium-high heat for 10 minutes or until fish is opaque and flakes easily when tested with a fork.

Advice for Clear Skin

▶ Choose seafood that is wild-caught, sustainable and preferably local.

Baked Fish and Vegetables en Papillote

The term en papillote *refers to steam-baking in parchment paper or foil. It's a fast, easy and healthy way to cook fish with vegetables.*

Tip

Sliced carrots, zucchini and sweet red or green bell peppers are all good choices to cook this way.

Nutrients per serving

Calories	157
Fat	5 g
Carbohydrate	2 g
Fiber	1 g
Protein	25 g
Vitamin A	342 IU
Vitamin C	11 mg
Iron	0.9 mg
Vitamin E	1 IU
Zinc	0.6 mg
Selenium	37.9 mcg

• **Preheat oven to 450°F (230°C)**

	Nonstick cooking spray	
4	fish fillets (each about $1/4$ lb/125 g)	4
4	large white mushrooms, sliced	4
2	green onions, sliced	2
20	snow peas, trimmed	20
	Salt and freshly ground black pepper	

1. Cut four pieces of parchment paper or foil 4 inches (10 cm) larger on all sides than fish fillets. Lightly spray with cooking spray. Place each fillet in center of paper. Top each with 1 sliced mushroom, half an onion and 5 snow peas. Season lightly with salt and pepper.

2. Fold in long sides of paper or foil twice so mixture is tightly enclosed. Lift short ends, bring together on top and fold twice. Place seam side up on baking pan.

3. Bake for 20 minutes or until fish is opaque and flakes easily when tested with a fork and vegetables are tender. Open each package and serve contents on dinner plates.

Advice for Clear Skin

▶ Choose seafood that is wild-caught, sustainable and preferably local.

▶ Select fatty cold-water fish, such as mackerel, trout or salmon, for higher omega-3 fatty acids to help heal your skin.

▶ Use olive oil cooking spray or brush the parchment or foil with olive oil instead.

Cumin-Crusted Halibut Steaks

MAKES 4 SERVINGS

Sea bass, halibut, grouper or any dense white fish are all excellent cooked in this interesting crust. It is preferable to use toasted cumin seeds, as they have more flavor than ground cumin.

• **Preheat oven to 450°F (230°C)**

1 tbsp	cumin seeds	15 mL
½ tsp	salt	2 mL
¼ tsp	freshly ground black pepper	1 mL
1 lb	halibut or other fish steaks	500 g
2 tsp	olive oil	10 mL
	Chopped fresh parsley (optional)	

1. In a nonstick skillet over medium heat, toast cumin seeds, stirring, for 2 minutes or until golden. Place seeds, salt and pepper in a coffee or spice grinder. Pulse until finely ground. Rub mixture into both sides of fish.

2. Heat olive oil in a large nonstick skillet over medium-high heat. Add fish, in batches, if necessary, and cook for 2 minutes per side or until browned.

3. Return all fish to skillet and wrap handle with foil. Bake in preheated oven for 5 minutes or until fish is opaque and flakes easily when tested with a fork. Sprinkle with parsley (if using) and serve.

Advice for Clear Skin

▸ Choose seafood that is wild-caught, sustainable and preferably local.

Nutrients per serving	
Calories	129
Fat	4 g
Carbohydrate	1 g
Fiber	0 g
Protein	21 g
Vitamin A	97 IU
Vitamin C	0 mg
Iron	1.3 mg
Vitamin E	2 IU
Zinc	0.5 mg
Selenium	51.8 mcg

Herb-Roasted Salmon

Salmon has such a marvelous flavor that little else is needed in the way of seasoning. This simple herb-oil mixture makes it easy.

Tip

Whole salmon is best kept in the coldest part of the refrigerator at a temperature of less than 40°F (4°C), lightly covered with a damp towel. Store steaks, fillets and portions wrapped individually in sealed plastic bags, covered with ice.

- **Preheat oven to 450°F (230°C)**
- **Shallow oblong pan, greased**

1	large salmon fillet (about 2 lbs/1 kg)	1
1 tbsp	olive oil	15 mL
2 tbsp	chopped fresh chives	30 mL
1 tbsp	chopped fresh tarragon (or 1 tsp/ 5 mL dried)	15 mL
	Salt and freshly ground black pepper	

1. Place fish, skin side down, in prepared pan.

2. In a small bowl, combine oil, chives and tarragon. Rub half into flesh of salmon.

3. Bake in preheated oven for 10 minutes per inch (2.5 cm) of thickness or until fish is opaque and flakes easily when tested with a fork.

4. Cut salmon in half crosswise. Lift flesh from skin with a spatula. Transfer fish to a platter. Discard skin, and then drizzle fish with the remaining herbs and oil. Season lightly with salt and pepper.

> ### Advice for Clear Skin
> ▶ Choose seafood that is wild-caught, sustainable and preferably local.

Nutrients per serving

Calories	213
Fat	9 g
Carbohydrate	0 g
Fiber	0 g
Protein	31 g
Vitamin A	225 IU
Vitamin C	1 mg
Iron	0.6 mg
Vitamin E	1 IU
Zinc	0.6 mg
Selenium	47.5 mcg

Broiled Cilantro Ginger Salmon

Broiling the fish on only one side keeps it moist, delicious and full of flavor.

Tip

This can also be cooked on a barbecue with two or more burners. Preheat one side to medium, place salmon on the other side and close the lid. This indirect cooking method is great for delicate proteins like fish. There will be enough heat to cook the salmon without burning it or drying it out.

- **Mortar and pestle or food processor**
- **Rimmed baking sheet, greased**

3	cloves garlic, roughly chopped	3
2 tbsp	grated gingerroot	30 mL
1/2 tsp	salt	2 mL
1/2 cup	chopped fresh cilantro	125 mL
2 tbsp	olive oil	30 mL
1/2 tsp	freshly ground black pepper	2 mL
	Grated zest of 2 limes	
6	salmon fillets (about 2 1/4 lbs/ 1.125 kg total)	6

1. Using the mortar and pestle (or food processor), crush garlic, ginger and salt to form a paste. Stir in cilantro, olive oil, pepper and lime zest.

2. Place salmon on a plate and coat top evenly with paste. Cover and refrigerate for at least 30 minutes or for up to 2 hours. Preheat broiler, with rack set 4 inches (10 cm) from the top.

3. Transfer salmon to prepared baking sheet and broil for 7 to 10 minutes or until salmon is opaque and flakes easily with a fork.

This recipe courtesy of Eileen Campbell.

Advice for Clear Skin

▶ Choose seafood that is wild-caught, sustainable and preferably local.

Nutrients per serving

Calories	260
Fat	12 g
Carbohydrate	1 g
Fiber	0 g
Protein	35 g
Vitamin A	209 IU
Vitamin C	1 mg
Iron	0.7 mg
Vitamin E	2 IU
Zinc	0.7 mg
Selenium	53.7 mcg

Salmon with Spinach

MAKES 4 SERVINGS

Salmon will remain moist using this cooking procedure. Layer spinach and mushrooms, then top with salmon. Bake on high heat for the recommended 10 minutes per inch (2.5 cm) thickness of the fish. Because of the extra thickness of fish and vegetables, you may need a few extra minutes of baking time.

Tip

As well as salmon, any white or firm-fleshed fish will do, such as turbot, swordfish, halibut or tuna. For ease of serving fish fillets, cut them into serving-size pieces before baking.

- Preheat oven to 450°F (230°C)
- Shallow oblong pan, greased

1	package (10 oz/300 g) frozen chopped spinach, thawed	1
1 tbsp	grated gingerroot	15 mL
2	large white mushrooms, thickly sliced	2
	Salt and freshly ground black pepper	
4	salmon steaks or fillets	4

1. In a sieve, drain spinach, pressing with a spoon to remove excess liquid. Discard liquid. Spread spinach in bottom of prepared pan to match the size and shape of the fish. Arrange ginger and mushrooms evenly over spinach. Season lightly with salt and pepper. Add fish. Sprinkle lightly with salt and pepper.

2. Cover pan loosely with a tent of foil. Bake for 15 minutes or until fish is opaque and flakes easily when tested with a fork.

Variation

Crusty Layered Salmon: Sprinkle toasted sesame seeds over the fish before baking to give it a crunchy crust.

> ## Advice for Clear Skin
>
> ▶ Choose seafood that is wild-caught, sustainable and preferably local.

Nutrients per serving	
Calories	427
Fat	14 g
Carbohydrate	3 g
Fiber	2 g
Protein	68 g
Vitamin A	8683 IU
Vitamin C	4 mg
Iron	2.6 mg
Vitamin E	5 IU
Zinc	1.7 mg
Selenium	104.6 mcg

Indian-Spiced Salmon with Spinach

If you're fond of salmon but in a bit of a rut about how to prepare it, here's a dish that will jolt you out of the doldrums. Salmon marinated in gentle spices is poached with spinach in a light but flavorful tomato sauce. It's so easy to make, you can serve it on weekdays, although it's tasty enough to serve to guests.

Make Ahead

Complete steps 1 and 2. Cover and refrigerate fish and vegetable mixtures separately overnight. When you're ready to cook, continue with the recipe.

Nutrients per serving

Calories	350
Fat	12 g
Carbohydrate	22 g
Fiber	6 g
Protein	40 g
Vitamin A	4454 IU
Vitamin C	34 mg
Iron	5.2 mg
Vitamin E	3 IU
Zinc	1.5 mg
Selenium	55.8 mcg

- **Medium (about 3½-quart) slow cooker**

2 tbsp	freshly squeezed lemon juice	30 mL
1 tsp	garam masala	5 mL
¼ tsp	cayenne pepper	1 mL
1½ lbs	salmon fillet, skin removed	750 g
1 tbsp	extra virgin olive oil or ghee	15 mL
2	onions, finely chopped	2
4	cloves garlic, minced	4
1 tbsp	minced gingerroot	15 mL
1 tbsp	ground cumin (see tip, page 289)	15 mL
2 tsp	ground coriander	10 mL
1 tsp	salt	5 mL
1 tsp	cracked black peppercorns	5 mL
½ tsp	ground turmeric	2 mL
1	can (28 oz/796 mL) diced tomatoes, with juice	1
4 cups	packed chopped spinach leaves	1 L

1. In a bowl, combine lemon juice, garam masala and cayenne. Stir well. Add salmon and toss until well coated with mixture. Cover and refrigerate until ready to use.

2. In a skillet, heat oil over medium heat. Add onions and cook, stirring, until softened, about 3 minutes. Add garlic, ginger, cumin, coriander, salt, peppercorns and turmeric and cook, stirring, for 1 minute. Add tomatoes and bring to a boil.

3. Transfer to slow cooker stoneware. Cover and cook on Low for 6 hours or on High for 3 hours. Working in batches, stir in spinach. Cover and cook on High for 10 minutes. Add the reserved salmon, with juices. Cover and cook on High about 7 minutes, until fish flakes easily with a fork.

Advice for Clear Skin

▶ Choose seafood that is wild-caught, sustainable and preferably local.

Braised Swordfish

This is a great dish for entertaining because you can assemble it just before your guests arrive and turn the slow cooker on when they arrive. By the time everyone is done enjoying nibbles, the fish will be cooked. Serve with a big platter of sautéed spinach or rapini alongside.

Tip

If you can't find swordfish that is sustainably caught, substitute another firm white fish such as mahi-mahi or grouper. The cooking time depends upon the configuration of the steaks (thickness and width). It may take up to 1½ hours.

- **Medium to large (3- to 5-quart) oval slow cooker**
- **Large sheet of parchment paper**

2	large swordfish steaks (about 2½ lbs/ 1.25 kg) patted dry	2
1	sweet onion, such as Vidalia, very thinly sliced on the vertical	1
½ cup	finely chopped flat-leaf (Italian) parsley	125 mL
1 cup	pitted black olives, preferably kalamata, halved	250 mL
2	cloves garlic, minced	2
1 tsp	mild chile powder such as Aleppo, piment d'Espelette or hot paprika	5 mL
½ tsp	sea salt	2 mL
½ cup	extra virgin olive oil	125 mL
1½ cups	dry white wine	375 mL

1. Place swordfish in slow cooker stoneware. Sprinkle with onion, parsley, olives, garlic, chile powder and salt. Pour in olive oil, tipping the stoneware to ensure fish is coated. Pour wine evenly over fish. Place a large piece of parchment paper over the mixture, pressing it down to touch the food and extending up the sides of the stoneware so it overlaps the rim. (This ensures fish is well basted during the cooking process.) Cover and cook until fish flakes easily when pierced with a knife, about 1 hour (see tip, at left).

2. To serve, lift out the parchment and discard, being careful not to spill the accumulated liquid into the stoneware. Lift out fish and cut in half.

> ## Advice for Clear Skin
>
> ▶ Choose seafood that is wild-caught, sustainable and preferably local.
>
> ▶ Replace the white wine with 1½ cups (375 mL) gluten-free fish stock or ready-to-use vegetable broth and 2 tbsp (30 mL) freshly squeezed lemon juice.

Nutrients per serving	
Calories	772
Fat	50 g
Carbohydrate	7 g
Fiber	2 g
Protein	57 g
Vitamin A	1316 IU
Vitamin C	12 mg
Iron	3.0 mg
Vitamin E	16 IU
Zinc	2.1 mg
Selenium	163.5 mcg

Balsamic Tuna Salad in Avocado Halves

This extremely quick and easy acne-friendly meal provides a good dose of healthy fats from the fish and avocado.

1	can (6 oz/170 g) tuna packed in olive oil, with oil	1
1 tsp	balsamic vinegar	5 mL
1/4 tsp	Dijon mustard	1 mL
1	firm-ripe Hass avocado, peeled, halved and pitted	1

1. Drain tuna, reserving 2 tsp (10 mL) oil. In a small bowl, whisk together the reserved oil, vinegar and mustard. Set aside 1 tsp (5 mL) of the dressing. Add tuna to the remaining dressing, tossing gently to combine.

2. Fill avocado halves with tuna mixture. Drizzle with the reserved dressing.

Advice for Clear Skin

▸ Choose seafood that is wild-caught, sustainable and preferably local.

▸ Substitute canned salmon or sardines for a higher concentration of omega-3 fatty acids.

Nutrients per serving

Calories	332
Fat	22 g
Carbohydrate	9 g
Fiber	7 g
Protein	27 g
Vitamin A	212 IU
Vitamin C	10 mg
Iron	1.8 mg
Vitamin E	4 IU
Zinc	1.4 mg
Selenium	65.0 mcg

Tuna and White Bean Salad

This easy-to-prepare, high-protein, low-carbohydrate meal is packed with flavor and nutrients that will improve your skin.

1	can (6 oz/170 g) tuna packed in olive oil, with oil	1
1 tbsp	red wine vinegar	15 mL
1/2 tsp	Dijon mustard	2 mL
1	can (14 to 19 oz/398 to 540 mL) white beans, drained and rinsed	1
1/2 cup	finely chopped celery	125 mL
1/4 cup	finely chopped red onion	60 mL
1/3 cup	packed fresh flat-leaf (Italian) parsley leaves, chopped	75 mL
1 tsp	dried rosemary (optional)	5 mL

1. Drain tuna, reserving 1 tbsp (15 mL) oil. In a small bowl, whisk together the reserved oil, vinegar and mustard.

2. In a medium bowl, combine tuna, beans, celery, red onion, parsley and rosemary (if using). Add dressing and gently toss to coat.

Advice for Clear Skin

▶ Choose seafood that is wild-caught, sustainable and preferably local.

▶ Substitute canned salmon or sardines for a higher concentration of omega-3 fatty acids.

Nutrients per serving	
Calories	413
Fat	8 g
Carbohydrate	46 g
Fiber	11 g
Protein	40 g
Vitamin A	1033 IU
Vitamin C	16 mg
Iron	7.9 mg
Vitamin E	4 IU
Zinc	3.2 mg
Selenium	68.0 mcg

Caribbean Fish Stew

The allspice and the Scotch bonnet peppers add an island tang to this tasty stew. For a distinctive and delicious finish, be sure to include the dill.

Tip

One Scotch bonnet pepper is probably enough for most people, but if you're a heat-seeker, use two. You can also use habanero peppers instead.

Make Ahead

This dish can be partially prepared before it is cooked. Complete steps 1 and 2. Cover and refrigerate overnight or for up to 2 days. When you're ready to cook, continue with step 3.

Nutrients per serving	
Calories	191
Fat	4 g
Carbohydrate	13 g
Fiber	3 g
Protein	27 g
Vitamin A	1048 IU
Vitamin C	25 mg
Iron	3.1 mg
Vitamin E	2 IU
Zinc	1.4 mg
Selenium	46.8 mcg

- **Medium to large (3$\frac{1}{2}$- to 6-quart) slow cooker**

2 tsp	cumin seeds	10 mL
6	whole allspice	6
1 tbsp	olive oil	15 mL
2	onions, finely chopped	2
4	cloves garlic, minced	4
2 tsp	dried thyme leaves, crumbled	10 mL
1 tsp	ground turmeric	5 mL
1 tbsp	grated orange or lime zest	15 mL
$\frac{1}{2}$ tsp	cracked black peppercorns	2 mL
1	can (28 oz/796 mL) tomatoes, with juice, coarsely chopped	1
2 cups	fish stock	500 mL
	Salt	
1 to 2	Scotch bonnet peppers, minced	1 to 2
2 cups	sliced okra ($\frac{1}{4}$ inch/0.5 cm)	500 mL
1$\frac{1}{2}$ lbs	skinless grouper fillets, cut into bite-size pieces	750 g
8 oz	shrimp, cooked, peeled and deveined	250 g
$\frac{1}{2}$ cup	finely chopped dill (optional)	125 mL

1. In a large dry skillet over medium heat, toast cumin seeds and allspice, stirring, until fragrant and cumin seeds just begin to brown, about 3 minutes. Immediately transfer to a mortar or a spice grinder and grind. Set aside.

2. In same skillet, heat oil over medium heat for 30 seconds. Add onions and cook, stirring, until softened. Add garlic, thyme, turmeric, orange zest, peppercorns and the reserved cumin and allspice; cook, stirring, for 1 minute. Add tomatoes and stock; bring to a boil. Season with salt to taste. Transfer to slow cooker stoneware.

3. Cover and cook on Low for 6 hours or on High for 3 hours. Add chile peppers, okra, fish and shrimp. Cover and cook on High for 20 minutes, until fish flakes easily with a fork and okra is tender. Stir in dill, if using.

Advice for Clear Skin

▶ Choose seafood that is wild-caught, sustainable and preferably local.

Fragrant Goan-Style Clams

This stir-fried version of a shellfish dish from India's southwestern coast is fragrant and tasty with roasted cauliflower or over kelp noodles. If you have freshly grated coconut on hand, toss some over this dish along with the cilantro at serving time for a luscious finishing touch.

2 tbsp	water or clam juice	30 mL
1 tbsp	white vinegar	15 mL
1 tbsp	curry powder	15 mL
1 tsp	salt (or to taste)	5 mL
1/2 tsp	ground cumin	2 mL
2 tbsp	vegetable oil	30 mL
2 tbsp	chopped garlic	30 mL
2 tbsp	chopped gingerroot	30 mL
2 tsp	chopped serrano or jalapeño pepper (optional)	10 mL
1 cup	chopped onion	250 mL
1	can (12 oz/375 g) clams, drained	1
1/2 cup	chopped fresh cilantro	125 mL
2 tbsp	chopped green onions	30 mL
1 tbsp	freshly squeezed lemon juice	15 mL

1. In a small bowl, combine water, vinegar, curry powder, salt and cumin and stir well. Set aside.

2. Heat a wok or a large, deep skillet over high heat. Add oil and swirl to coat pan. Add garlic and ginger and toss well, until fragrant, about 15 seconds.

3. Add serrano pepper (if using) and onion and cook, tossing often, until fragrant and softened, about 1 minute.

4. Add clams and toss well. Cook, tossing often, until they are heated through, about 1 minute.

5. Add curry mixture, pouring in around sides of pan, and toss well. Cook, tossing often, until clams are evenly seasoned, about 1 minute more.

6. Remove from heat and add cilantro, green onions and lemon juice and toss well. Transfer to a serving plate. Serve hot.

Advice for Clear Skin

▶ Substitute extra virgin olive oil for the vegetable oil.

▶ Choose seafood that is wild-caught, sustainable and preferably local.

Nutrients per serving	
Calories	216
Fat	9 g
Carbohydrate	12 g
Fiber	2 g
Protein	22 g
Vitamin A	484 IU
Vitamin C	7 mg
Iron	3.0 mg
Vitamin E	4 IU
Zinc	0.9 mg
Selenium	44.1 mcg

Stir-Fried Scallops with Curried Sweet Peppers

This is an easy, elegant dish with just a few ingredients. Be careful not to overcook the scallops, as they are delicate and can easily turn rubbery.

2 tbsp	curry powder (or 2 tsp/10 mL mild curry paste)	30 mL
1 tbsp	olive oil, divided	15 mL
Pinch	salt	Pinch
1 lb	sea scallops, halved horizontally	500 g
1	red bell pepper, julienned	1
1	green bell pepper, julienned	1
1	yellow bell pepper, julienned	1
½ cup	white wine, apple juice or water	125 mL
1 tsp	dark sesame oil	5 mL
1 tbsp	chopped fresh cilantro	15 mL

1. In a large bowl, combine curry powder, 1 tsp (5 mL) oil and salt. Add scallops and toss to coat.

2. In a wok or a large skillet, heat the remaining oil over medium-high heat. Add scallops and stir-fry for 1 minute. Add red, green and yellow peppers; stir-fry for 1 minute. Add wine and cook, stirring, for 3 to 4 minutes or until scallops are firm and opaque. Stir in sesame oil.

3. Using a slotted spoon, remove scallops and vegetables to a serving bowl. Boil sauce, uncovered, for 3 to 5 minutes, or until thickened. Taste and add salt, if needed.

4. Pour sauce over scallops and vegetables and sprinkle with cilantro. Serve immediately.

This recipe courtesy of dietitian Edie Shaw-Ewald.

Advice for Clear Skin

▶ Choose seafood that is wild-caught, sustainable and preferably local.

▶ Choose water instead of white wine or apple juice.

Nutrients per serving

Calories	180
Fat	6 g
Carbohydrate	12 g
Fiber	3 g
Protein	15 g
Vitamin A	1169 IU
Vitamin C	148 mg
Iron	1.8 mg
Vitamin E	3 IU
Zinc	1.4 mg
Selenium	15.2 mcg

Poached Jumbo Shrimp

Serve shrimp with freshly made salsa as a dipping sauce. A crunchy chopped vegetable salad will complete the menu.

$1/2$ cup	dry white wine	125 mL
$1/2$ cup	water	125 mL
2	sprigs fresh parsley	2
2	shallots, sliced	2
36	jumbo shrimp	36

1. In a large saucepan, bring wine, water, parsley and shallots to a boil. Add shrimp. Reduce heat to medium and cook slowly for 4 minutes or until shrimp turn pink.

Advice for Clear Skin

▶ Choose seafood that is wild-caught, sustainable and preferably local.

▶ Replace the white wine with $1/2$ cup (175 mL) gluten-free fish stock or ready-to-use vegetable broth and 2 tbsp (30 mL) freshly squeezed lemon juice.

Nutrients per serving

Calories	47
Fat	0 g
Carbohydrate	1 g
Fiber	0 g
Protein	6 g
Vitamin A	116 IU
Vitamin C	1 mg
Iron	0.1 mg
Vitamin E	1 IU
Zinc	0.4 mg
Selenium	12.4 mcg

Sicilian-Style Shrimp Stir-Fry with Fennel

This Italian-inspired dish is a window into the kitchens of Sicily, where sunshine is abundant and fennel grows wild.

Tip

Toasting nuts heightens their flavor and aroma. To toast them on top of the stove, heat a wok or large skillet on medium-low heat. When hot, add nuts and toss until fragrant and barely toasted, 15 to 30 seconds. Or toast them in the oven or a toaster oven, spread out on a baking pan, at 300°F (150°C), until fragrant and just beginning to brown, about 5 minutes.

½ cup	ready-to-use chicken broth, clam juice or water	125 mL
1 tbsp	zante currants or raisins	15 mL
½ tsp	hot pepper flakes	2 mL
Pinch	saffron threads (optional)	Pinch
3 tbsp	olive oil or vegetable oil	45 mL
1 tbsp	chopped garlic	15 mL
½ cup	thinly sliced onion	125 mL
1½ cups	finely chopped fennel (about ½ medium bulb)	375 mL
12 oz	medium shrimp, peeled and deveined	375 g
½ tsp	freshly ground pepper	2 mL
1 tbsp	slivered almonds or pine nuts, toasted, if desired (see tip, at left)	15 mL

1. In a small bowl, combine broth, currants, hot pepper flakes and saffron threads (if using) and stir well. Set aside for 10 minutes.

2. Heat a wok or a large, deep skillet over medium-high heat. Add oil and swirl to coat pan. Add garlic and toss well until fragrant, about 30 seconds.

3. Add onion and fennel and cook, tossing occasionally, until softened and fragrant, 1 to 2 minutes. Add shrimp and cook, tossing occasionally, until pink all over, about 2 minutes.

4. Add broth mixture and cook, tossing often, until shrimp are cooked through and fennel is tender-crisp, about 1 minute more.

5. Remove from heat. Add pepper and almonds and toss well. Transfer to a serving plate. Serve hot or warm.

Advice for Clear Skin

▶ Omit the dried currants or raisins.

▶ Use olive oil instead of vegetable oil.

▶ Choose seafood that is wild-caught, sustainable and preferably local.

Nutrients per serving

Calories	188
Fat	11 g
Carbohydrate	8 g
Fiber	2 g
Protein	13 g
Vitamin A	294 IU
Vitamin C	6 mg
Iron	0.8 mg
Vitamin E	5 IU
Zinc	1.0 mg
Selenium	26.5 mcg

Chicken and Turkey

Brined and Tender Lemon Roast Chicken

Brining chicken in a mild salt solution produces delightfully tender meat. Do not brine the chicken for longer than 8 hours. Over-brining may adversely affect the texture of the cooked chicken. Tenting the chicken with foil and letting it rest before carving allows the juices to redistribute throughout the meat, creating a much moister chicken.

Advice for Clear Skin

▶ Choose organic, pastured chicken.

Nutrients per serving

Calories	270
Fat	8 g
Carbohydrate	1 g
Fiber	0 g
Protein	46 g
Vitamin A	105 IU
Vitamin C	7 mg
Iron	2.4 mg
Vitamin E	1 IU
Zinc	2.8 mg
Selenium	38.4 mcg

- **Roasting pan**

3 to 4 lb	whole roasting chicken	1.5 to 2 kg
3 tbsp	kosher salt	45 mL
12 cups	water	3 L
1	lemon	1
2 tsp	canola or olive oil	10 mL
½ tsp	salt	2 mL

1. Trim excess fat from chicken. Rinse inside and out under cold running water.

2. In a large pot, combine kosher salt and water, stirring to dissolve salt. Add chicken, breast side down, making sure it is fully submerged. Cover and refrigerate for at least 4 hours or for up to 8 hours.

3. About 30 minutes before cooking, drain brine from chicken and discard. Rinse chicken under running water and pat dry. Place on a clean plate and let stand at room temperature.

4. Place oven rack in center of oven, place empty roasting pan on rack and preheat oven to 425°F (220°C).

5. Meanwhile, place whole lemon in a small saucepan and add water to cover. Bring to a boil over high heat. Reduce heat and simmer for 5 minutes. Remove from heat and leave lemon in hot water until ready to use.

6. Rub chicken all over with oil and sprinkle with ½ tsp (2 mL) salt. Remove the lemon from the hot water, discarding water. Poke several holes in the lemon and insert it into the cavity of the chicken.

7. Carefully remove the hot roasting pan from the oven, place chicken, breast side up, in pan, and roast for 30 minutes. Reduce heat to 400°F (200°C). Roast chicken for 60 minutes or until skin is dark golden and crispy, drumsticks wiggle when touched and a meat thermometer inserted in the thickest part of a thigh registers 165°F (74°C). Transfer chicken to a cutting board, tent with foil and let rest for 10 to 15 minutes before carving.

8. Using kitchen tongs, remove lemon from the chicken. Cut lemon in half and squeeze juice over hot chicken pieces.

This recipe courtesy of dietitian Joanne Rankin.

Roast Chicken with Leeks

MAKES 6 SERVINGS

Fresh leeks roasted with the meat are simply marvelous. Leeks contain ample amounts of carotenoids, which are converted to vitamin A in your body and are an important component of skin rejuvenation.

- Preheat oven to 325°F (160°C)
- Roasting pan

1	roasting chicken (about 3 lbs/1.5 kg)	1
1	lemon, quartered	1
6	cloves garlic, sliced	6
2	large leeks, trimmed and washed	2
	Salt and freshly ground black pepper	
¾ cup	water	175 mL

1. Rinse and wipe chicken with paper towels. Place breast side down in a roasting pan. Stuff cavity with lemon and garlic.

2. Slice leeks in half lengthwise. Place cut side down in roasting pan alongside chicken. Sprinkle with salt and pepper. Pour in water. Cover tightly.

3. Roast in preheated oven for 40 minutes. Remove from oven and transfer leeks to a dish and keep warm. Return chicken to oven. Continue roasting, uncovered, for about 1½ hours or until meat thermometer registers 165°F (74°C). Remove chicken from oven. Let stand for 5 minutes before carving. Serve with leeks and any pan juices.

Advice for Clear Skin

▶ Choose organic, pastured chicken.

Nutrients per serving

Calories	278
Fat	6 g
Carbohydrate	7 g
Fiber	1 g
Protein	47 g
Vitamin A	600 IU
Vitamin C	12 mg
Iron	3.1 mg
Vitamin E	1 IU
Zinc	2.8 mg
Selenium	39.1 mcg

Grilled Whole Chicken with Lime or Lemon Butter

This may not be an under-30-minute recipe, but it's a good way to have chicken on hand for speedy recipes such as salads, soups and the like throughout the week. Grill 2 chickens — one to enjoy on Sunday and the other one for leftovers. Or grill one while you have the barbecue on for something else.

• **Grease barbecue grill and preheat to medium-high**

1	chicken (about 4 lbs/2 kg), patted dry	1
1	lime or lemon, halved	1
1 tsp	dried thyme	5 mL
1/4 cup	butter, softened	60 mL
1 tsp	grated lime or lemon zest	5 mL
1/4 cup	freshly squeezed lime or lemon juice	60 mL

1. Rub chicken all over, inside and out, with cut sides of lime. Sprinkle with thyme.

2. Place chicken, breast side up, on grill; cook, turning often, for 10 to 15 minutes or until browned. Turn off one burner and place the chicken over the turned-off burner. Increase heat to high on the remaining burner; cook, covered, for 1 hour, turning halfway through.

3. Meanwhile, whisk together the butter, lime zest and lime juice. Brush chicken with mixture. Cook, turning and basting occasionally, for 30 minutes to 1 hour longer or until meat thermometer registers 165°F (74°C).

Advice for Clear Skin

▶ Choose organic, pastured chicken.

▶ Substitute extra virgin olive oil for the butter.

Nutrients per serving

Calories	251
Fat	12 g
Carbohydrate	2 g
Fiber	0 g
Protein	33 g
Vitamin A	325 IU
Vitamin C	7 mg
Iron	1.9 mg
Vitamin E	1 IU
Zinc	1.9 mg
Selenium	27.0 mcg

Basque Drumsticks

If you happen to have prosciutto or ham on hand, it adds an extra traditional flavor to this one-dish supper.

Make Ahead

The stew can be entirely made ahead, cooled, covered and refrigerated for up to 1 day. Reheat slowly to serve.

2 tbsp	olive oil	30 mL
8	chicken drumsticks	8
	Salt and freshly ground black pepper	
2	onions, thickly sliced	2
1	can (28 oz/796 mL) diced tomatoes	1
2	red or yellow bell peppers, sliced	2
1 cup	coarsely chopped prosciutto or ham (optional)	250 mL
8	cloves garlic, thinly sliced	8
1 tsp	dried thyme	5 mL
1 tsp	paprika	5 mL
1/4 tsp	hot pepper flakes	1 mL
1	orange	1

1. In a deep skillet or shallow saucepan, heat oil. Add chicken and sauté until browned. Season to taste with salt and pepper. Transfer chicken to a plate.

2. Add onions to the skillet and cook for 3 minutes. Stir in tomatoes, peppers, prosciutto, garlic, thyme, paprika and hot pepper flakes. Add reserved chicken and any juices. Bring to a boil, stirring up any bits from the bottom. Grate zest from orange into stew. Peel orange and coarsely chop fruit; add to stew. Cover and simmer for 20 minutes or until the chicken is no longer pink inside.

Advice for Clear Skin

▶ Choose organic, pastured chicken.

Nutrients per serving	
Calories	338
Fat	12 g
Carbohydrate	30 g
Fiber	7 g
Protein	31 g
Vitamin A	3736 IU
Vitamin C	122 mg
Iron	4.8 mg
Vitamin E	4 IU
Zinc	3.7 mg
Selenium	19.3 mcg

Braised Chicken with Eggplant and Chickpeas

If you wish, substitute 4 boneless skinless chicken breasts for the drumsticks in this hearty one-dish supper. Chickpeas are a good source of iron, vitamin B$_6$ and protein, which help support healing and recovery from acne.

2	small eggplants	2
3 tbsp	olive oil (approx.), divided	45 mL
8	chicken drumsticks	8
2	onions, sliced	2
2	cloves garlic, minced	2
½ tsp	ground cumin	2 mL
½ tsp	ground allspice	2 mL
1	can (28 oz/796 mL) diced tomatoes, with juice	1
1	can (19 oz/540 mL) chickpeas, drained and rinsed	1
3 tbsp	freshly squeezed lemon juice	45 mL
	Salt and freshly ground black pepper	
2 tbsp	chopped fresh parsley	30 mL

1. Trim eggplants, cut in half lengthwise and slice across. In a very large, deep skillet, heat 2 tbsp (30 mL) oil over medium-high heat. Add eggplant and cook, stirring often, until golden brown. Remove with a slotted spoon to drain on paper towels.

2. Add 1 tbsp (15 mL) oil to the pan and brown chicken on all sides; push to one side of pan.

3. Add onions and cook 3 minutes, adding more oil if necessary. Stir in garlic, cumin and allspice, arranging chicken pieces evenly around pan. Add tomatoes, chickpeas, lemon juice, and ¼ tsp (1 mL) each salt and pepper. Bring to a boil; reduce heat, cover and simmer for 15 minutes. Add browned eggplant and simmer about 10 minutes longer or until chicken is no longer pink inside. Taste and adjust seasoning. Sprinkle with parsley to serve.

Advice for Clear Skin

▶ Choose organic, pastured chicken.

Nutrients per serving

Calories	556
Fat	17 g
Carbohydrate	67 g
Fiber	20 g
Protein	39 g
Vitamin A	1727 IU
Vitamin C	45 mg
Iron	6.9 mg
Vitamin E	4 IU
Zinc	5.3 mg
Selenium	23.0 mcg

Broiled Rosemary Chicken Thighs

This very simple recipe creates wonderfully moist and delicious chicken. Chicken, besides being a high-protein food, contains selenium, a nutrient that supports detoxification pathways in your body, thereby taking the edge off the inflammation of skin conditions.

Make Ahead

The chicken can be marinated, covered and refrigerated, for up to 4 hours. Bring to room temperature for 30 minutes before cooking.

- **Preheat broiler**
- **Broiler pan, lined with foil**

8	bone-in skin-on chicken thighs	8
1/2 tsp	grated lemon zest	2 mL
3 tbsp	freshly squeezed lemon juice	45 mL
3 tbsp	olive oil	45 mL
1 tbsp	chopped fresh rosemary (or 1 tsp/5 mL crumbled dried)	15 mL
	Salt and freshly ground black pepper	

1. Place chicken thighs in a glass dish just big enough to hold them in a single layer. In a bowl, whisk together lemon zest, lemon juice, olive oil and rosemary. Pour over chicken and turn to coat well. Cover and let stand at room temperature for 30 minutes.

2. Reserving the marinade, arrange chicken thighs, skin side down, on prepared pan; sprinkle with salt and pepper. Broil 4 inches (10 cm) from heat for 7 minutes, basting occasionally.

3. Turn, baste and broil 5 to 8 minutes longer, or until chicken is no longer pink inside.

> ## Advice for Clear Skin
> ▶ Choose organic, pastured chicken.

Nutrients per serving

Calories	347
Fat	26 g
Carbohydrate	1 g
Fiber	0 g
Protein	27 g
Vitamin A	106 IU
Vitamin C	5 mg
Iron	1.6 mg
Vitamin E	5 IU
Zinc	2.7 mg
Selenium	18.6 mcg

Mexican-Style Chicken with Cilantro and Lemon

With a sauce of pumpkin seeds, cumin, oregano and cilantro, this dish is reminiscent of a warm evening dinner in the courtyard of a charming Mexican hacienda. Mexicans have been thickening sauces with pumpkin seeds since long before the Spanish arrived, and, today, every cook has their own recipe for mole, one of the world's great culinary concoctions.

Tip

If you choose to halve this recipe, use a small (2- to 3-quart) slow cooker.

Nutrients per serving

Calories	331
Fat	17 g
Carbohydrate	8 g
Fiber	2 g
Protein	35 g
Vitamin A	231 IU
Vitamin C	9 mg
Iron	3.1 mg
Vitamin E	1 IU
Zinc	3.8 mg
Selenium	25.8 mcg

- **Medium to large (3$\frac{1}{2}$- to 5-quart) slow cooker**
- **Food processor**

$\frac{1}{4}$ cup	green pumpkin seeds (pepitas)	60 mL
2 tsp	cumin seeds	10 mL
1 tbsp	extra virgin olive oil	15 mL
2	onions, thinly sliced	2
4	cloves garlic, minced	4
2 tbsp	tomato paste	30 mL
1 tsp	cracked black peppercorns	5 mL
1 tsp	dried oregano	5 mL
$\frac{1}{2}$ tsp	sea salt	2 mL
$\frac{1}{4}$ tsp	ground cinnamon	1 mL
2 cups	cilantro, leaves and some stems, chopped	500 mL
1 tbsp	grated lemon zest	15 mL
2 tbsp	freshly squeezed lemon juice	30 mL
1 cup	ready-to-use chicken broth	250 mL
3 lbs	skinless bone-in chicken thighs (about 12 thighs)	1.5 kg
1 to 2	jalapeño peppers, minced	1 to 2
	Finely chopped cilantro and green onion	
	Grated lemon zest	

1. In a dry skillet over medium heat, toast pumpkin and cumin seeds, until pumpkin seeds are popping and cumin has released its flavor. Transfer to a mortar or spice grinder and grind. Set aside.

2. In same skillet, heat oil over medium heat. Add onions and cook, stirring, until softened, about 3 minutes. Add garlic, tomato paste, peppercorns, oregano, salt, cinnamon and cilantro and cook, stirring, for 1 minute. Transfer contents of pan to food processor. Add lemon zest and juice, broth, and the reserved ground pumpkin and cumin seeds and process until smooth.

Tip

Buy seeds and nuts at a natural foods or bulk food store with high turnover, as they are likely to be much fresher than those in packages.

Make Ahead

Complete steps 1 and 2. Cover and refrigerate puréed sauce for up to 2 days. When you're ready to cook, complete the recipe.

3. Arrange chicken evenly over bottom of slow cooker stoneware. Pour sauce over chicken. Cover and cook on Low for 6 hours or on High for 3 hours, until juices run clear when chicken is pierced with a fork. Stir in jalapeño pepper to taste. When ready to serve, garnish with cilantro, green onion and lemon zest.

> ### Advice for Clear Skin
>
> ▸ Choose gluten-free broth until the reintroduction phase of the diet plan, when you can test to see if gluten-containing products are safe for your skin.
>
> ▸ Choose organic, pastured chicken.

Indian-Style Chicken

MAKES 8 SERVINGS

Serve this tantalizing dish as the centerpiece of a meal, accompanied with sides of fresh salads. Chicken contains B vitamins to support your metabolism and immune system, while spinach provides a good supply of iron. These nutrients help improve the healing of your skin.

Tips

If using fresh spinach, be sure to remove the stems, and if it has not been prewashed, rinse it thoroughly in a basin of lukewarm water.

One chile produces a medium-hot result. Add a second chile only if you're a true heat-seeker.

Nutrients per serving	
Calories	247
Fat	9 g
Carbohydrate	9 g
Fiber	3 g
Protein	31 g
Vitamin A	6853 IU
Vitamin C	37 mg
Iron	4.5 mg
Vitamin E	4 IU
Zinc	3.2 mg
Selenium	19.7 mcg

- **Large (about 5-quart) oval slow cooker**
- **Food processor or blender**

4 lbs	skinless bone-in chicken thighs	2 kg
1/4 cup	freshly squeezed lemon juice	60 mL
2 tbsp	olive oil	30 mL
2	onions, thinly sliced on the vertical	2
1 tbsp	minced gingerroot	15 mL
1 tbsp	minced garlic	15 mL
1 tbsp	ground cumin	15 mL
2 tsp	ground coriander	10 mL
1 tsp	cracked black peppercorns	5 mL
1 tsp	sea salt (or to taste)	5 mL
1	can (14 oz/398 mL) diced tomatoes, with juice	1
1 tsp	ground turmeric	5 mL
	Juice of 1 lime or lemon	
2	packages (each 10 oz/300 g) fresh or frozen spinach (see tip, at left)	2
1 to 2	long red or green chiles, chopped	1 to 2
1 cup	ready-to-use chicken broth	250 mL

1. Rinse chicken under cold running water and pat dry. In a bowl, combine chicken and lemon juice. Toss well and set aside for 20 to 30 minutes.

2. In a skillet, heat oil over medium-high heat. Add onions and cook, stirring, until they begin to color. Reduce heat to medium and cook, stirring, until golden, about 12 minutes. Add ginger, garlic, cumin, coriander, peppercorns and salt; cook, stirring, for 1 minute. Stir in tomatoes and bring to a boil. Remove from heat.

3. Arrange marinated chicken evenly over the bottom of slow cooker stoneware. Pour tomato mixture over top. Cover and cook on Low for 6 hours or on High for 3 hours, until juices run clear when chicken is pierced with a fork.

4. In a small bowl, combine turmeric and lime juice.

5. In food processor, combine spinach, chile(s) and broth. Pulse until spinach is puréed. Add to chicken along with turmeric mixture and stir well. Cover and cook on High for 20 minutes, until mixture is bubbly.

Gremolata Grilled Chicken

MAKES 2 SERVINGS

Gremolata is usually a final garnish for veal stew, but it makes a delicious addition to grilled chicken as well. This recipe also works well for chicken breasts.

- **Grease barbecue grill and preheat to medium-high**

2	cloves garlic, minced	2
2 tbsp	minced fresh parsley	30 mL
1 tbsp	grated lemon zest	15 mL
2 tbsp	freshly squeezed lemon juice	30 mL
1 tbsp	vegetable oil	15 mL
4	boneless skinless chicken thighs	4

1. In a small bowl, combine garlic, parsley and lemon zest. Set aside 1 tbsp (15 mL) of the mixture and combine remainder of the mixture with lemon juice and oil. Press mixture into both sides of the thighs.

2. Grill for about 12 minutes, turning once, until the chicken is no longer pink inside. Sprinkle with the reserved gremolata and serve.

Advice for Clear Skin

▶ Substitute extra virgin olive oil for the vegetable oil.

▶ Choose organic, pastured chicken.

Nutrients per serving

Calories	237
Fat	12 g
Carbohydrate	3 g
Fiber	1 g
Protein	28 g
Vitamin A	413 IU
Vitamin C	16 mg
Iron	1.8 mg
Vitamin E	3 IU
Zinc	2.7 mg
Selenium	19.1 mcg

Burmese Chicken Thighs

MAKES 2 SERVINGS

This simple dish is loaded with flavor.

Tip

Bottled lemongrass is available in well-stocked supermarkets if fresh lemongrass is not. If you have fresh, use only the bottom 6 inches (15 cm) of the stalk, trimming off the root end and straw-like top. Cut into lengths and crush slightly with a chef's knife or mallet.

1 tbsp	vegetable oil	15 mL
4	boneless skinless chicken thighs, patted dry	4
2	onions, sliced	2
2	cloves garlic, minced	2
3	2-inch (5 cm) pieces lemongrass, crushed	3
1 tbsp	minced gingerroot	15 mL
¼ cup	water (approx.)	60 mL
2 tsp	curry powder	10 mL
2 tbsp	soy sauce	30 mL

1. In a wok, heat oil over high heat. Add the chicken and cook until browned on both sides. Remove with a slotted spoon.

2. Add onions to wok; reduce the heat to medium-high and stir-fry for 3 minutes. Add the garlic, lemongrass and ginger; stir-fry for 1 minute, adding water if the mixture sticks. Stir in curry powder; cook for 1 minute. Stir in the soy sauce and add the reserved chicken, along with any juice. Cover and simmer for 10 to 12 minutes or until the chicken is no longer pink inside. Remove and discard lemongrass.

Advice for Clear Skin

▶ Substitute extra virgin olive oil for the vegetable oil.

▶ Choose organic, pastured chicken.

▶ Use organic, non-GMO, gluten-free soy sauce.

Nutrients per serving

Calories	299
Fat	13 g
Carbohydrate	16 g
Fiber	3 g
Protein	30 g
Vitamin A	112 IU
Vitamin C	10 mg
Iron	3.3 mg
Vitamin E	3 IU
Zinc	3.2 mg
Selenium	20.2 mcg

Chicken Breasts with Chili Butter

This simple but delicious recipe produces moist chicken with nice crisp skin and is easily halved or doubled. Chicken is high in protein and this recipe is low in carbohydrates, which is a great nutritional combination to support acne repair.

- **Preheat oven to 400°F (200°C)**
- **Large, shallow roasting pan with rack**

1/4 cup	unsalted butter, softened	60 mL
1 tbsp	chili powder	15 mL
1/2 tsp	salt	2 mL
1/4 tsp	hot pepper flakes	1 mL
2	cloves garlic, minced	2
4	bone-in skin-on chicken breasts	4

1. In a small bowl, cream together butter, chili powder, salt, hot pepper flakes and garlic, until well blended. Divide into 4 portions.

2. Gently poke your fingers under the skin of each breast and lift the skin slightly. Being careful not to tear the membrane that connects the skin to the chicken, gently stuff one portion of the chili butter under the skin, massaging to even it out.

3. Arrange chicken, skin side up, on rack in roasting pan. Roast in preheated oven for 30 minutes or until chicken is no longer pink inside, brushing once or twice with melted butter from the bottom of the pan.

Advice for Clear Skin

▶ Choose organic, pastured chicken.

▶ Substitute 3 tbsp (15 mL) olive oil for the butter.

Nutrients per serving

Calories	244
Fat	15 g
Carbohydrate	2 g
Fiber	1 g
Protein	26 g
Vitamin A	1004 IU
Vitamin C	2 mg
Iron	0.8 mg
Vitamin E	2 IU
Zinc	0.8 mg
Selenium	38.5 mcg

Lemon Garlic Chicken

MAKES 4 SERVINGS

This nicely balanced chicken dish can be prepared ahead of time and left to marinate until your guests arrive, then popped in the oven while they snack on hors d'oeuvres and refreshments.

Tips

Chicken can be marinated at room temperature for up to 30 minutes if you are short of time. Any longer, make sure it is refrigerated. Throw out the plastic bag used for marinating.

Can't find the cover that fits your casserole? Cover it with foil, dull side out. Press around the rim with your fingers to be sure the foil forms a tight seal.

- **8-cup (2 L) covered casserole dish**

1	clove garlic, minced	1
2 tbsp	freshly squeezed lemon juice	30 mL
1 tbsp	extra virgin olive oil	15 mL
1 tsp	dried thyme	5 mL
¼ tsp	salt	1 mL
Pinch	ground nutmeg	Pinch
Pinch	paprika	Pinch
Pinch	freshly ground white pepper	Pinch
4	boneless skinless chicken breasts	4

1. In a resealable plastic freezer bag set in a bowl, combine garlic, lemon juice, olive oil, thyme, salt, nutmeg, paprika and white pepper. Add chicken breasts to marinade, seal bag and refrigerate for 1 hour.

2. Preheat oven to 375°F (190°C). Place chicken breasts, with marinade, in the casserole dish, and cover tightly. Bake for 45 minutes or until juices run clear and meat thermometer registers 165°F (74°C).

Variations

Rather than baking the chicken, barbecue or grill it for 5 to 8 minutes per side.

Substitute an equal amount of oregano for the thyme. Or use 1 tbsp (15 mL) snipped fresh thyme or oregano.

> ### Advice for Clear Skin
> ▶ Choose organic, pastured chicken.

Nutrients per serving	
Calories	170
Fat	7 g
Carbohydrate	1 g
Fiber	0 g
Protein	25 g
Vitamin A	81 IU
Vitamin C	5 mg
Iron	1.0 mg
Vitamin E	1 IU
Zinc	0.7 mg
Selenium	37.9 mcg

Quick Chicken Chili

A short cooking time gives freshness and crunch to the vegetables in this easy, light version of an old favorite.

Make Ahead

The chili can be made up to 2 days ahead and reheated gently (add the remaining green pepper just before serving).

1 tbsp	vegetable oil	15 mL
1	onion, chopped	1
2	cloves garlic, crushed	2
1	green bell pepper, chopped, divided	1
2 tbsp	chili powder	30 mL
1 tsp	ground cumin	5 mL
1 tsp	dried oregano	5 mL
Pinch	hot pepper flakes	Pinch
1 lb	lean ground chicken	500 g
1	can (28 oz/796 mL) diced tomatoes, with juice	1
1	can (19 oz/540 mL) white kidney beans, rinsed and drained	1
1	stalk celery, sliced	1

1. In a large saucepan, heat oil over medium heat. Add onion, garlic and half the green pepper; cook for 3 minutes. Add chili powder, cumin, oregano and hot pepper flakes; cook, stirring, for 2 minutes or until fragrant. Add chicken, increase heat and cook, breaking up with a spoon, for 5 minutes, until chicken changes color.

2. Stir in tomatoes, beans and celery. Cook, covered, for 15 minutes, stirring occasionally. Mash some of the beans against the side of the pan to thicken chili slightly. Stir in the remaining green pepper.

> ### Advice for Clear Skin
> ▶ Substitute extra virgin olive oil for the vegetable oil.
> ▶ Choose organic, pastured chicken.

Nutrients per serving

Calories	405
Fat	15 g
Carbohydrate	41 g
Fiber	14 g
Protein	31 g
Vitamin A	2758 IU
Vitamin C	47 mg
Iron	6.5 mg
Vitamin E	4 IU
Zinc	3.2 mg
Selenium	15.2 mcg

Turkey Chili with Black-Eyed Peas

This delicious chili is lighter than those made with red meat. This is a generous serving, so you don't need much, if anything, to complete the meal. The Avocado Topping contributes healthy fats and additional nutrients, as well as lip-smacking flavor.

Tip

For this quantity of peas, use 1½ cans (14 to 19 oz/398 to 540 mL) drained and rinsed black-eyed peas with no salt added, or soak and cook 1½ cups (375 mL) dried black-eyed peas.

- **Medium to large (3½- to 5-quart) slow cooker**

1 tbsp	olive oil	15 mL
2	onions, finely chopped	2
3	cloves garlic, minced	3
2 tsp	dried oregano	10 mL
2 tsp	ground coriander	10 mL
2 tsp	ground cumin	10 mL
1 tsp	cracked black peppercorns	5 mL
	Sea salt	
1	can (28 oz/796 mL) no-salt-added diced tomatoes, with juice	1
2 cups	ready-to-use chicken broth	500 mL
2 lbs	boneless skinless turkey breast or thighs, cut into 1-inch (2.5 cm) cubes	1 kg
3 cups	cooked black-eyed peas (see tip, at left)	750 mL
2	green bell peppers, seeded and cut into thin strips	2
2	jalapeño peppers, finely chopped	2
2 tbsp	chili powder	30 mL
	Avocado Topping (optional; see recipe, opposite)	

1. In a skillet, heat oil over medium heat. Add onions and garlic and cook, stirring, until softened, about 3 minutes. Add oregano, coriander, cumin, peppercorns, and salt to taste, and cook, stirring, for 1 minute. Add tomatoes and broth and bring to a boil.

2. Transfer to slow cooker stoneware. Add turkey and peas and stir to combine. Cover and cook on Low for 6 to 8 hours or on High for 3 to 4 hours, until turkey is no longer pink inside.

Nutrients per serving	
Calories	279
Fat	4 g
Carbohydrate	20 g
Fiber	4 g
Protein	42 g
Vitamin A	1804 IU
Vitamin C	61 mg
Iron	4.8 mg
Vitamin E	1 IU
Zinc	2.5 mg
Selenium	40.2 mcg

Make Ahead

Slice bell peppers, cover and refrigerate. Complete step 1. Cover and refrigerate mixture for up to 2 days. When you're ready to cook, complete the recipe.

3. Stir in bell peppers, jalapeño peppers and chili powder. Cover and cook for 20 to 25 minutes, until peppers are tender. Spoon into individual bowls and, if desired, top each with a healthy dollop of Avocado Topping.

> ### Advice for Clear Skin
>
> ▸ Choose gluten-free broth until the reintroduction phase of the diet plan, when you can test to see if gluten-containing products are safe for your skin.
>
> ▸ Choose organic, pastured turkey.

Avocado Topping

MAKES ABOUT 1 CUP (250 ML)

1	avocado, cut into $1/2$-inch (1 cm) cubes	1
2 tbsp	finely chopped red onion	30 mL
2 tbsp	finely chopped cilantro leaves	30 mL
1 tbsp	freshly squeezed lime juice	15 mL
	Sea salt and freshly ground black pepper	

1. In a bowl, combine avocado, red onion, cilantro and lime juice. Mix well. Season to taste with salt and pepper.

Nutrients per 2 tbsp (30 mL)

Calories	42
Fat	4 g
Carbohydrate	3 g
Fiber	2 g
Protein	1 g
Vitamin A	39 IU
Vitamin C	3 mg
Iron	0.2 mg
Vitamin E	1 IU
Zinc	0.2 mg
Selenium	0.1 mcg

Turkey Mole

In Mexico, no special occasion is complete without turkey cooked in mole poblano. The authentic version is quite a production. This mole has been greatly simplified but is still very good. Unsweetened chocolate packs an acne-healing antioxidant punch!

Tips

Tomatillos are available in the Mexican food section of supermarkets.

Serrano chiles are much milder than jalapeños, so choose according to your preference for heat.

- **Medium to large (3½- to 5-quart) slow cooker**
- **Food processor**
- **Blender**

1 tbsp	extra virgin olive oil or pure lard	15 mL
1	turkey breast, skin on, about 2 to 3 lbs (1 to 1.5 kg), patted dry	1
2	onions, sliced	2
3	cloves garlic, sliced	3
4	whole cloves	4
1	2-inch (5 cm) cinnamon stick	1
1 tsp	cracked black peppercorns	5 mL
½ tsp	sea salt	2 mL
1	can (28 oz/796 mL) tomatillos, drained	1
½ cup	whole blanched almonds	125 mL
½ oz	unsweetened chocolate, broken in pieces	15 g
1 cup	ready-to-use chicken broth or turkey stock, divided	250 mL
2	dried ancho chiles	2
½ cup	coarsely chopped cilantro, stems and leaves	125 mL
1 tbsp	chili powder	15 mL
1 to 2	jalapeño or serrano chile peppers, chopped	1 to 2

1. In a skillet, heat oil over medium heat. Add turkey, skin side down, and brown well, about 4 minutes. Transfer to slow cooker stoneware.

2. Add onions to pan and cook, stirring, until softened, about 3 minutes. Add garlic, cloves, cinnamon, pepper and salt and cook, stirring, for 1 minute. Transfer to food processor. Add tomatillos, almonds, chocolate and ½ cup (125 mL) broth and process until smooth.

3. Pour sauce over turkey, cover and cook on Low for 6 hours or on High for 3 hours, until juices run clear when turkey is pierced with a fork or an instant-read thermometer reads 165°F (74°C).

Nutrients per serving	
Calories	447
Fat	22 g
Carbohydrate	24 g
Fiber	5 g
Protein	41 g
Vitamin A	1599 IU
Vitamin C	3 mg
Iron	3.8 mg
Vitamin E	6 IU
Zinc	3.2 mg
Selenium	35.2 mcg

Make Ahead

Complete steps 2 and 4, heating 1 tbsp (15 mL) oil in pan before softening onions. Cover and refrigerate puréed sauces separately for up to 2 days, being aware that the chile mixture will lose some of its vibrancy if held for this long. When you're ready to cook, brown the turkey (step 1) or remove skin from turkey, omit browning and place directly in stoneware. Continue with recipe.

4. About an hour before turkey has finished cooking, in a heatproof bowl, soak dried chiles in boiling water for 30 minutes, weighing down with a cup to ensure they remain submerged. Drain, discarding soaking liquid and stems, and chop coarsely. Transfer to blender. Add cilantro, the remaining broth, chili powder and jalapeño pepper to taste and purée.

5. Add to stoneware and stir gently to combine. Cover and cook on High for 30 minutes, until flavors meld.

Variation

Chicken Mole: Substitute 3 lbs (1.5 kg) skinless bone-in chicken thighs (about 12 thighs) for the turkey.

Advice for Clear Skin

▶ Choose organic, pastured turkey.

▶ Choose gluten-free broth until the reintroduction phase of the diet plan, when you can test to see if gluten-containing products are safe for your skin.

BBQ Tarragon Mustard Turkey

*Grilling is a handy
way to enjoy turkey
in the summertime.
Serve with a tomato-
cucumber salad.*

Tip

Do not overcook
the turkey or it may
become dry. Check
the temperature after
35 minutes, as barbecue
temperatures can vary.

• **Preheat greased barbecue grill to medium**

2	cloves garlic, finely minced	2
2 tsp	dried tarragon	10 mL
1/2 tsp	salt (optional)	2 mL
1/2 tsp	freshly ground black pepper	2 mL
2 tbsp	Dijon mustard	30 mL
2 tbsp	ready-to-use chicken broth	30 mL
1 tbsp	canola oil, divided	15 mL
1	bone-in skin-on turkey breast (about 2 lbs/1 kg)	1

1. In a small bowl, combine garlic, tarragon, salt (if using), pepper, mustard, broth and 2 tsp (10 mL) oil.

2. Gently loosen and raise the skin of the turkey breast, but do not remove it. Spread the garlic mixture evenly on the meat under the skin and replace the skin. Spread the remaining oil over the skin.

3. Place turkey, skin side down, on preheated grill. Close lid and grill for 10 minutes. Turn breast over so skin side is up, close lid and grill for 40 to 45 minutes or until no longer pink inside and a meat thermometer inserted in the thickest part registers 165°F (74°C). Transfer to a cutting board, tent with foil and let rest for 10 minutes before slicing.

This recipe courtesy of dietitian Jessie Kear.

Advice for Clear Skin

▶ Choose gluten-free broth until the reintroduction phase of the diet plan, when you can test to see if gluten-containing products are safe for your skin.

▶ Substitute olive oil for the canola oil.

▶ Choose organic, pastured turkey.

Nutrients per serving

Calories	147
Fat	3 g
Carbohydrate	1 g
Fiber	0 g
Protein	28 g
Vitamin A	7 IU
Vitamin C	0 mg
Iron	1.4 mg
Vitamin E	1 IU
Zinc	1.4 mg
Selenium	27.9 mcg

Pork, Beef and Lamb

Baked Pork Chops with Vegetable Rice

Advice for Clear Skin

▶ Substitute extra virgin olive oil for the vegetable oil.

▶ Choose naturally raised, organic pork.

▶ Replace the white rice with brown rice. Divided over 6 servings, this amount of rice is not a concern from a carbohydrate perspective.

▶ Choose gluten-free broth until the reintroduction phase of the diet plan, when you can test to see if gluten-containing products are safe for your skin.

Nutrients per serving	
Calories	460
Fat	16 g
Carbohydrate	33 g
Fiber	3 g
Protein	45 g
Vitamin A	1253 IU
Vitamin C	47 mg
Iron	3.2 mg
Vitamin E	2 IU
Zinc	3.6 mg
Selenium	66.2 mcg

- **Preheat oven to 350°F (180°C)**
- **13- by 9-inch (33 by 23 cm) baking dish with cover**

2 tsp	vegetable oil	10 mL
6	boneless pork loin chops, trimmed	6
1	onion, chopped	1
1	clove garlic, minced	1
1 cup	long-grain white rice	250 mL
1 tsp	curry powder	5 mL
1 tsp	ground cumin	5 mL
1 tsp	dried oregano	5 mL
2 cups	diced or sliced zucchini	500 mL
2 cups	ready-to-use chicken broth	500 mL
1½ cups	chopped plum (Roma) tomatoes	375 mL
1 cup	finely chopped bell pepper (red or yellow)	250 mL
½ tsp	salt	2 mL
¼ tsp	freshly ground black pepper	1 mL
1	bay leaf	1

1. In a large skillet, heat oil over medium-high heat. Brown chops on both sides, about 4 minutes per side. Remove to a plate.

2. Add onion and garlic to skillet and sauté for about 5 minutes or until softened. Add rice, curry powder, cumin and oregano; stir to coat rice. Add zucchini, broth, tomatoes, bell pepper, salt, pepper and bay leaf; bring to a boil. Reduce heat, cover and simmer for 10 minutes. Transfer to baking dish.

3. Nestle pork chops into rice mixture in baking dish and pour any juices from meat over top.

4. Cover and bake in preheated oven for 30 to 35 minutes or until rice is tender, liquid is absorbed and just a hint of pink remains in pork and it has reached an internal temperature of 160°F (71°C). Discard bay leaf.

This recipe courtesy of dietitian Patti Thomson.

Thai-Style Pork Slices with Oyster Mushrooms

With a side of peas or a salad of apples, toasted walnuts and crispy greens, this makes a fine meal.

Advice for Clear Skin

▶ Choose gluten-free broth until the reintroduction phase of the diet plan, when you can test to see if gluten-containing products are safe for your skin.

▶ Substitute extra virgin olive oil for the vegetable oil.

▶ Choose naturally raised, organic pork.

2 tbsp	fish sauce	30 mL
3 tbsp	ready-to-use chicken broth or water	45 mL
1/2 tsp	freshly ground pepper	2 mL
8 oz	fresh oyster or button mushrooms	250 g
2 tbsp	vegetable oil	30 mL
2 tbsp	chopped garlic	30 mL
2 tbsp	chopped shallots or green onions	30 mL
1/2 cup	thinly sliced onion	125 mL
8 oz	boneless pork (such as loin or tenderloin), thinly sliced	250 g
2 tbsp	chopped cilantro leaves	30 mL

1. In a small bowl, combine fish sauce, broth and pepper and stir well. Set aside.

2. Cut oyster mushrooms in half lengthwise. (Cut into thirds if very large and leave whole if very small.) Thinly slice button mushrooms lengthwise as well. Set aside.

3. Heat a wok or a large skillet over medium-high heat. Add oil and swirl to coat pan. Add garlic and toss well, until fragrant, about 15 seconds. Add shallots and onion and cook, tossing occasionally, until softened, about 1 minute.

4. Add pork and spread out in a single layer. Cook, undisturbed, until edges change color, about 1 minute. Toss well. Cook, tossing occasionally, until no longer pink, about 1 minute more.

5. Add mushrooms and toss well. Cook, tossing occasionally, until beginning to soften, about 1 minute.

6. Add fish sauce mixture, pouring in around sides of pan, and toss well. Cook, tossing occasionally, until mushrooms are tender and pork is cooked through, about 1 minute more. Add cilantro and toss well. Transfer to a serving plate. Serve hot or warm.

Nutrients per serving

Calories	156
Fat	8 g
Carbohydrate	6 g
Fiber	1 g
Protein	15 g
Vitamin A	66 IU
Vitamin C	4 mg
Iron	1.1 mg
Vitamin E	2 IU
Zinc	1.5 mg
Selenium	24.5 mcg

Pork with Escarole, Cherry Tomatoes and Pine Nuts

Escarole is a sturdy and delicious cruciferous vegetable that walks a fine line between being a lettuce and a cabbage. It contains compounds that help support metabolism of hormones, making it an ally on your path to clear skin.

Tip

To prepare escarole, halve or quarter a head lengthwise and then chop it crosswise into approximately 2-inch (5 cm) chunks.

2 tbsp	vegetable oil	30 mL
2 tbsp	chopped garlic	30 mL
8 oz	boneless pork (such as loin or tenderloin), thinly sliced	250 g
1	head escarole, cut into 2-inch (5 cm) chunks (about 7 cups/1.75 L)	1
1 tsp	salt (or to taste)	5 mL
1/2 tsp	freshly ground pepper	2 mL
3/4 cup	halved cherry tomatoes	175 mL
1/4 cup	pine nuts	60 mL

1. Heat a wok or large skillet over high heat. Add oil and swirl to coat the pan. Add garlic and toss well, until fragrant, about 15 seconds.

2. Add pork and spread out in a single layer. Cook, undisturbed, until edges change color, about 30 seconds.

3. Add escarole and toss again. Add salt and pepper. Continue cooking, tossing occasionally, until escarole is softened but still retains a pleasing crunch, 2 to 3 minutes.

4. Add cherry tomatoes and pine nuts and toss well. Cook, tossing occasionally, until tomatoes are beginning to wilt, about 1 minute. Transfer to a serving plate. Serve hot or warm.

Advice for Clear Skin

▶ Substitute extra virgin olive oil for the vegetable oil.

▶ Choose naturally raised, organic pork.

Nutrients per serving	
Calories	214
Fat	14 g
Carbohydrate	8 g
Fiber	5 g
Protein	15 g
Vitamin A	3016 IU
Vitamin C	14 mg
Iron	2.3 mg
Vitamin E	4 IU
Zinc	2.7 mg
Selenium	18.4 mcg

Marinated Pork Kebabs

Beer makes a wonderful marinade for meats, especially pork kebabs. Add an assortment of vegetables to the skewers when you are grilling the meat, if desired.

Tips

Flat beer is preferable because it is less foamy.

Thread meat and vegetables on skewers with sufficient separation to allow even cooking.

The remaining one-quarter of the marinade may be used to marinate any vegetables you are using. Any marinade in which raw meats have marinated should either be discarded or boiled for 5 minutes before further use, to kill harmful bacteria.

- **Wooden skewers**

1	pork tenderloin (about 1 lb/500 g), cut into large cubes	1
1	bottle (12 oz/341 mL) beer (see tip, at left)	1
2	cloves garlic, minced	2
1 tbsp	dry mustard	15 mL
	Salt and freshly ground black pepper	

1. In a non-metallic dish, arrange pork cubes in a single layer. Whisk together beer, garlic and mustard. Pour three-quarters of the mixture over the pork. Cover and let stand for 30 minutes at room temperature or overnight in the refrigerator.

2. Preheat barbecue. Soak wooden skewers in cold water for at least 10 minutes to prevent charring during cooking.

3. Remove pork and discard marinade. Thread meat (and vegetables, if using) onto skewers. Grill on preheated barbecue, turning occasionally, for 12 minutes or until a hint of pink remains inside. Brush meat and any vegetables with the remaining marinade during grilling (see tip, at left).

Advice for Clear Skin

▶ Choose naturally raised, organic pork.

▶ Replace the beer with 1⅓ cups (325 mL) gluten-free ready-to-use chicken broth (for a lighter taste) or beef broth (for a stronger taste).

Nutrients per serving	
Calories	168
Fat	3 g
Carbohydrate	3 g
Fiber	0 g
Protein	25 g
Vitamin A	1 IU
Vitamin C	1 mg
Iron	1.3 mg
Vitamin E	1 IU
Zinc	2.3 mg
Selenium	38.3 mcg

Chipotle Pork "Tacos"

Liberally garnished, these yummy tacos are a meal in themselves.

Tips

Chipotle peppers pack quite a wallop, so only add the second one if you're a real heat-seeker. Check the label to make sure the brand you are using is gluten-free. If you prefer, substitute 2 minced jalapeño peppers.

This recipe makes slightly too much sauce for the pork, so spoon it over the shredded pork in a quantity that suits your taste, then refrigerate the excess. When you're ready for lunch, heat it to the boiling point and serve it over napa cabbage.

Nutrients per serving

Calories	487
Fat	35 g
Carbohydrate	16 g
Fiber	4 g
Protein	28 g
Vitamin A	1168 IU
Vitamin C	20 mg
Iron	4.4 mg
Vitamin E	1 IU
Zinc	4.1 mg
Selenium	38.4 mcg

- **Medium to large ($3\frac{1}{2}$- to 5-quart) slow cooker**

2 tbsp	clarified butter or pure lard, divided	30 mL
2 lbs	trimmed boneless pork shoulder or blade (butt), patted dry	1 kg
2	onions, thinly sliced on the vertical	2
2	stalks celery, diced	2
4	cloves garlic, minced	4
1 tbsp	each ground cumin and dried oregano	15 mL
1 tsp	cracked black peppercorns	5 mL
$\frac{1}{2}$ tsp	sea salt	2 mL
1	2-inch (5 cm) cinnamon stick	1
2	bay leaves	2
1	can (28 oz/796 mL) tomatoes, with juice, coarsely chopped	1
1 to 2	chipotle pepper(s) in adobo sauce, minced	1 to 2
	Hearts of romaine lettuce or napa cabbage leaves	
	Diced avocado tossed in fresh lime juice	
	Finely chopped green or red onion	

1. In a skillet, heat 1 tbsp (15 mL) butter over medium-high heat. Add pork and brown well, about 3 minutes per side. Transfer to slow cooker stoneware.

2. Add the remaining butter to pan. Add onions and celery and cook, stirring, until softened, about 5 minutes. Add garlic, cumin, oregano, peppercorns, sea salt, cinnamon stick and bay leaves and cook, stirring, for 1 minute. Add tomatoes and bring to a boil, scraping up brown bits.

3. Transfer to stoneware. Cover and cook on Low for 8 hours or on High for 4 hours, until pork is very tender. Add chipotle pepper to taste, stir well, cover and cook on High for 10 minutes. Discard cinnamon stick and bay leaves.

4. Transfer pork to a cutting board and, using 2 forks, shred. To serve, spoon pork onto lettuce and spoon sauce to taste over it (see tip, at left). Garnish with avocado and onion.

Advice for Clear Skin

▶ Substitute extra virgin olive oil for the clarified butter.

▶ Choose naturally raised, organic pork.

Italian Sausage Patties

MAKES 12 PATTIES

Serve these spicy meat patties over pasta, in a pesto sauce or with a mild tomato sauce. Make ahead and freeze for up to 3 months for a last-minute supper or snack. Fennel seeds help to dampen the effect of androgens in the body, which may reduce the development of acne.

Tips

If you use an indoor contact grill, there is no need to turn the patties. Cooking time will be much shorter; check the manufacturer's instructions.

For a stronger flavor, substitute caraway or anise seeds for the fennel.

Nutrients per patty

Calories	50
Fat	2 g
Carbohydrate	1 g
Fiber	0 g
Protein	8 g
Vitamin A	1 IU
Vitamin C	0 mg
Iron	0.8 mg
Vitamin E	0 IU
Zinc	1.7 mg
Selenium	0.1 mcg

• **Preheat barbecue grill or broiler**

1 lb	lean ground beef	500 g
3	cloves garlic, minced	3
2 tsp	fennel seeds	10 mL
1 tsp	hot pepper flakes	5 mL
3/4 tsp	salt	3 mL
1/2 tsp	freshly ground black pepper	2 mL
1/4 tsp	cayenne pepper (optional)	1 mL

1. In a medium bowl, using a fork, gently combine beef, garlic, fennel seeds, hot pepper flakes, salt, pepper and cayenne pepper, if using. Form into 12 patties, 2 inches (5 cm) in diameter.

2. On preheated barbecue, grill patties for 2 to 3 minutes, turning only once, until meat thermometer registers 160°F (71°C) and patties are no longer pink inside.

Variations

Substitute ground veal, pork, chicken or turkey for the ground beef.

Make into meatballs. Bake on a baking sheet at 400°F (200°C) for 15 to 20 minutes, or until no longer pink in the center.

Advice for Clear Skin

▸ Choose naturally raised, grass-fed, organic beef.

Classic Beef Stew

MAKES 6 SERVINGS

This hearty homemade stew can be accentuated with a dollop of slow-roasted garlic (see Variations, page 341). Garlic contains compounds that have strong antimicrobial properties, making them an ideal addition to your acne-fighting arsenal.

Tip

If you choose to halve this recipe, use a small (2- to 3-quart) slow cooker.

• **Medium to large (3^1/$_2$- to 5-quart) slow cooker**

2 tbsp	extra virgin olive oil	30 mL
2 lbs	stewing beef, cut into 1-inch (2.5 cm) cubes and patted dry	1 kg
2	onions, finely chopped	2
4	stalks celery, thinly sliced	4
2	large carrots, peeled and diced	2
2	cloves garlic, minced	2
1 tsp	dried thyme	5 mL
1 tsp	sea salt	5 mL
^{1}/$_2$ tsp	cracked black peppercorns	2 mL
2	bay leaves	2
^{1}/$_2$ cup	dry red wine or additional ready-to-use beef broth	125 mL
1 cup	ready-to-use beef broth	250 mL
1 tbsp	beef demi-glace (see tip, page 341)	15 mL
	Finely chopped flat-leaf (Italian) parsley	

1. In a skillet, heat oil over medium heat. Add beef, in batches, and brown, about 4 minutes per batch. Using a slotted spoon, transfer to slow cooker stoneware.

2. Add onions, celery and carrots and cook, stirring, until vegetables are softened, about 7 minutes. Add garlic, thyme, sea salt, peppercorns and bay leaves and cook, stirring, for 1 minute. Add wine and cook, stirring and scraping brown bits up from the bottom of the pan, for 1 minute. Add broth and bring to a boil. Add demi-glace.

3. Transfer to stoneware and stir well. Cover and cook on Low for 6 to 8 hours or on High for 3 to 4 hours, until beef is very tender. Discard bay leaves. Just before serving, garnish liberally with parsley.

Nutrients per serving	
Calories	307
Fat	13 g
Carbohydrate	8 g
Fiber	2 g
Protein	34 g
Vitamin A	4141 IU
Vitamin C	5 mg
Iron	3.0 mg
Vitamin E	2 IU
Zinc	6.2 mg
Selenium	40.4 mcg

Tip

Demi-glace is intensely flavored stock that has been reduced to a state of concentration. It is useful for adding a burst of flavor to dishes. After making stock, transfer about 2 cups (500 mL) to a saucepan, bring to a boil, reduce the heat and simmer until syrupy, about 1½ hours. Let cool, then transfer to a shallow dish and refrigerate. After it has solidified, lift it out in 1 piece, place on a cutting board and then cut it into squares (each containing a volume of about 1 tbsp/15 mL). Wrap individually in plastic and freeze. When frozen, place in resealable bags and label.

Variations

Beef Stew with Madeira Mushrooms: In a skillet, melt 2 tbsp (30 mL) butter over medium-high heat. Add 12 oz (375 g) sliced button mushrooms and sauté until mushrooms release their liquid, about 7 minutes. Season with salt and pepper to taste. Stir in ¼ cup (60 mL) Madeira or port wine and bring to a boil. Cook for 2 minutes. Just before serving, stir into stew, then garnish with parsley.

Beef Stew with Roasted Garlic: Mash 6 cloves roasted garlic and stir into stew before garnishing with parsley. To roast garlic, peel the cloves, remove the pith (the center part that often sprouts) and then place the cloves on a piece of foil. Drizzle about ½ tsp (2 mL) extra virgin olive oil over the garlic, then fold up the foil to make a tight packet. Bake in 400°F (200°C) oven for 20 minutes.

Advice for Clear Skin

▶ Choose naturally raised, grass-fed, organic beef.

▶ Use the broth rather than the red wine.

▶ Choose gluten-free broth until the reintroduction phase of the diet plan, when you can test to see if gluten-containing products are safe for your skin.

Moroccan-Spiced Beef Stew

MAKES 6 SERVINGS

This delicious mélange is easy to make and so good you'll want to share it with friends. All you need to add is a simple green vegetable such as steamed beans.

Advice for Clear Skin

▸ Opt for beef tallow rather than clarified butter. Or substitute olive oil or virgin coconut oil.

▸ Choose naturally raised, grass-fed, organic beef.

Nutrients per serving	
Calories	346
Fat	16 g
Carbohydrate	15 g
Fiber	4 g
Protein	36 g
Vitamin A	7819 IU
Vitamin C	19 mg
Iron	4.7 mg
Vitamin E	2 IU
Zinc	6.2 mg
Selenium	37.2 mcg

• **Medium to large (3½- to 5-quart) slow cooker**

1 tbsp	cumin seeds	15 mL
2 tbsp	clarified butter or beef tallow, divided	30 mL
2 lbs	stewing beef, cut into 1-inch (2.5 cm) cubes	1 kg
2	onions, thinly sliced on the vertical	2
4	cloves garlic, minced	4
1 tbsp	minced gingerroot	15 mL
1	2-inch (5 cm) cinnamon stick	1
½ tsp	freshly grated nutmeg	2 mL
½ tsp	cracked black peppercorns	2 mL
4	whole cloves	4
1	can (14 oz/398 mL) diced tomatoes, with juice	1
2 cups	ready-to-use beef broth	500 mL
2 cups	sliced peeled carrots	500 mL
½ cup	finely chopped flat-leaf (Italian) parsley	125 mL
1 to 3 tsp	harissa (optional)	5 to 15 mL

1. In a skillet over medium heat, cook cumin seeds, stirring, until fragrant and seeds just begin to brown, about 3 minutes. Using a mortar and pestle or a spice grinder, pound or grind as finely as you can. Set aside.

2. In same skillet, heat 1 tbsp (15 mL) clarified butter over medium-high heat. Add beef, in batches, and cook, stirring, until lightly browned on all sides, about 4 minutes per batch. Transfer to slow cooker stoneware as completed.

3. Reduce heat to medium. Add the remaining butter to pan. Add onions and cook, stirring, until softened, about 3 minutes. Add garlic, ginger, cinnamon stick, nutmeg, peppercorns, cloves and the reserved cumin and cook, stirring, for 1 minute. Add tomatoes, broth and carrots. Bring to a boil and cook, stirring and scraping up brown bits from bottom of pan, for 2 minutes.

4. Transfer to stoneware. Cover and cook on Low for 8 hours or on High for 4 hours, until beef and carrots are tender. Stir in harissa (if using), 1 tsp (5 mL) at a time, tasting after each addition, until desired spiciness is achieved. Cover and cook on High for 10 minutes, until flavors meld.

Slow-Cooked Chili Flank Steak or Brisket

MAKES 8 SERVINGS

Advice for Clear Skin

▶ Choose naturally raised, grass-fed, organic beef.

▶ Substitute extra virgin olive oil for the vegetable oil.

▶ Choose gluten-free broth until the reintroduction phase of the diet plan, when you can test to see if gluten-containing products are safe for your skin.

Nutrients per serving

Calories	229
Fat	10 g
Carbohydrate	8 g
Fiber	2 g
Protein	26 g
Vitamin A	192 IU
Vitamin C	8 mg
Iron	3.0 mg
Vitamin E	2 IU
Zinc	4.5 mg
Selenium	27.9 mcg

• **Large (5- to 6-quart) slow cooker**

2 lbs	flank steak or beef brisket	1 kg
1/2 tsp	freshly ground black pepper	2 mL
1 tbsp	vegetable oil	15 mL
3	stalks celery, with leaves, cut into chunks and leaves chopped	3
2	cloves garlic, minced	2
1	onion, cut into chunks	1
1 cup	ready-to-use reduced-sodium beef broth	250 mL
1	can (19 oz/540 mL) chili-flavored or regular stewed tomatoes, with juice (about 2 1/3 cups/575 mL)	1
1	large carrot, cut into chunks	1
1	bay leaf	1
1/2 tsp	dried thyme	2 mL
2 tsp	chili powder	10 mL

1. Cut beef into large pieces that will comfortably fit in your slow cooker. Season with pepper.

2. In a large skillet, heat oil over medium-high heat. Cook beef for 3 to 4 minutes per side or until browned on all sides. Transfer beef to slow cooker.

3. In the fat remaining in the skillet, sauté celery (including leaves), garlic and onion until lightly browned, about 5 minutes. Add to slow cooker.

4. Add broth to skillet and scrape up any brown bits from the bottom. Pour liquid into slow cooker.

5. To the slow cooker, add tomatoes and juice, carrot, bay leaf, thyme and chili powder; stir to combine. Cover and cook on Low for 6 to 8 hours or until beef is fork-tender. Discard bay leaf.

6. Slice beef across the grain and arrange on a platter. Skim fat from sauce, pour over meat and serve.

This recipe courtesy of Eileen Campbell.

Coconut Beef Curry

This aromatic curry borrows from both Indian and Thai cuisines. The multitude of culinary spices provides an ample dose of skin-healing antioxidants.

Tip

If your meat is not completely covered by liquid, stir it once or twice during cooking.

Advice for Clear Skin

▶ Choose naturally raised, grass-fed, organic beef.

Nutrients per serving

Calories	383
Fat	23 g
Carbohydrate	9 g
Fiber	2 g
Protein	35 g
Vitamin A	151 IU
Vitamin C	26 mg
Iron	5.3 mg
Vitamin E	1 IU
Zinc	6.5 mg
Selenium	51.9 mcg

• **Medium (3½- to 4-quart) slow cooker**

2 tbsp	virgin coconut oil, divided	30 mL
2 lbs	trimmed stewing beef, cut into ½-inch (1 cm) cubes and patted dry	1 kg
2	onions, finely chopped	2
4	cloves garlic, minced	4
2 tbsp	minced gingerroot	30 mL
2 tsp	ground coriander (see tip, page 289)	10 mL
1 tsp	ground cumin	5 mL
1 tsp	ground turmeric	5 mL
1 tsp	sea salt	5 mL
1 tsp	cracked black peppercorns	5 mL
2	black cardamom pods, crushed	2
1	3-inch (7.5 cm) cinnamon stick	1
1 cup	ready-to-use beef, chicken or vegetable broth or water	250 mL
2	long red chiles, seeded and minced	2
1 tsp	Dijon mustard	5 mL
1 cup	coconut milk	250 mL
	Finely chopped cilantro	

1. In a skillet, heat 1 tbsp (15 mL) oil over medium-high heat. Add beef, in batches, and cook, stirring, until lightly browned on all sides, about 4 minutes per batch. Transfer to slow cooker stoneware as completed.

2. Add the remaining oil to pan. Add onions and cook, stirring, until they begin to turn golden, about 5 minutes. Add garlic, ginger, coriander, cumin, turmeric, sea salt, peppercorns, cardamom and cinnamon stick and cook, stirring, for 1 minute. Add broth and bring to a boil.

3. Transfer to stoneware and stir well. Cover and cook on Low for 8 hours or on High for 4 hours, until meat is very tender.

4. In a small bowl, combine chiles, mustard and coconut milk, stirring well to combine. Stir into meat. Cover and cook on High for 30 minutes, until flavors meld. Garnish with cilantro.

Beef and Chickpea Curry with Spinach

MAKES 4 SERVINGS

This combination of beef and chickpeas in an Indian-inspired sauce is particularly delicious.

Advice for Clear Skin

▶ Choose naturally raised, grass-fed, organic beef.

▶ Choose gluten-free broth until the reintroduction phase of the diet plan, when you can test to see if gluten-containing products are safe for your skin.

Nutrients **per serving**	
Calories	392
Fat	13 g
Carbohydrate	34 g
Fiber	10 g
Protein	37 g
Vitamin A	10,667 IU
Vitamin C	38 mg
Iron	8.9 mg
Vitamin E	5 IU
Zinc	6.6 mg
Selenium	41.6 mcg

- **Medium to large (3¹/₂- to 5-quart) slow cooker**

1 tbsp	olive oil	15 mL
1 lb	trimmed stewing beef, cut into ¹/₂-inch (1 cm) cubes	500 g
2	onions, finely chopped	2
4	cloves garlic, minced	4
1 tbsp	minced gingerroot	15 mL
¹/₂ tsp	cracked black peppercorns	2 mL
1	1-inch (2.5 cm) cinnamon stick	1
1	bay leaf	1
1 cup	ready-to-use beef broth	250 mL
2 cups	cooked chickpeas, drained	500 mL
1 tsp	curry powder, dissolved in 2 tsp (10 mL) freshly squeezed lemon juice	5 mL
1 lb	fresh spinach, stems removed, or 1 package (10 oz/300 g) spinach leaves, thawed if frozen	500 g

1. In a skillet, heat oil over medium-high heat. Add beef, in batches, and cook, stirring, adding additional oil if necessary, until browned, about 4 minutes per batch. Transfer to slow cooker stoneware.

2. Reduce heat to medium. Add onions to pan and cook, stirring, until softened, about 3 minutes. Add garlic, ginger, peppercorns, cinnamon stick and bay leaf and cook, stirring, for 1 minute. Add broth and bring to a boil.

3. Transfer to stoneware. Add chickpeas and stir well. Cover and cook on Low for 8 hours or on High for 4 hours, until beef is tender. Add curry powder solution and stir well. Add spinach, in batches, stirring until each batch is submerged in the curry. Cover and cook on High for 20 minutes, until spinach is wilted. Discard cinnamon stick and bay leaf.

Roman-Style Oxtails with Celery

The sauce in this oxtail recipe is much lighter than most and the abundance of blanched celery adds beautiful flavor.

Advice for Clear Skin

▶ Opt for beef tallow or lard rather than clarified butter. Or substitute olive oil or virgin coconut oil.

▶ Choose naturally raised, grass-fed, organic beef.

▶ Substitute an extra cup (250 mL) of ready-to-use chicken broth plus 1 tbsp (15 mL) lemon juice for the white wine.

Nutrients per serving

Calories	513
Fat	27 g
Carbohydrate	9 g
Fiber	2 g
Protein	54 g
Vitamin A	1225 IU
Vitamin C	14 mg
Iron	7.0 mg
Vitamin E	1 IU
Zinc	13.6 mg
Selenium	8.1 mcg

• **Large (about 5-quart) slow cooker**

2 tbsp	clarified butter, beef tallow or pure lard (approx.), divided	30 mL
4 oz	pancetta, diced	125 g
4 lbs	oxtails, cut into 2-inch (5 cm) pieces and patted dry	2 kg
1	onion, diced	1
2	stalks celery, diced	2
2	cloves garlic, minced	2
1 tsp	sea salt	5 mL
1 tsp	cracked black peppercorns	5 mL
1 cup	dry white wine	250 mL
1/4 cup	tomato paste or 1/2 cup (125 mL) crushed tomatoes	60 mL
2 cups	ready-to-use chicken broth	500 mL
6 cups	sliced celery (cut into 1-inch/2.5 cm pieces)	1.5 L
1/2 cup	finely chopped parsley leaves	125 mL

1. In a skillet, heat 1 tbsp (15 mL) clarified butter over medium-high heat. Add pancetta and cook, stirring, until nicely browned, about 4 minutes. Transfer to slow cooker stoneware.

2. Add oxtails, in batches, and brown on all sides, about 4 minutes per batch, adding more butter if necessary. Transfer to stoneware as completed. Drain off all the fat from pan.

3. Reduce heat to medium. Add the remaining butter to pan. Add onion, diced celery, garlic, sea salt and peppercorns and cook, stirring, until onions begin to turn golden, about 8 minutes. Add wine, bring to a boil and cook, stirring and scraping up brown bits from bottom of pan, for 2 minutes. Stir in tomato paste and broth.

4. Transfer to stoneware. Cover and cook on Low for 8 to 10 hours or on High for 4 to 5 hours, until meat is falling off the bone.

5. When oxtails are almost cooked, bring a large pot of salted water to a boil. Add sliced celery and return to a boil. Reduce heat and simmer until celery is tender, about 5 minutes. Drain and add to oxtails. Cover and cook on High for 10 minutes, until flavors meld. Garnish with parsley and serve immediately.

Braised Lamb Shanks with Lemon Gremolata

Braised in a light tomato sauce and finished with lemon gremolata, these lamb shanks have Mediterranean overtones.

Advice for Clear Skin

▶ Substitute beef tallow, pure lard, olive oil or virgin coconut oil for the clarified butter.

▶ Choose naturally raised, grass-fed, organic lamb.

▶ Substitute an extra cup (250 mL) of ready-to-use chicken broth plus 1 tbsp (15 mL) lemon juice for the white wine.

Nutrients per serving

Calories	817
Fat	27 g
Carbohydrate	30 g
Fiber	7 g
Protein	100 g
Vitamin A	8042 IU
Vitamin C	49 mg
Iron	11.1 mg
Vitamin E	2 IU
Zinc	28.6 mg
Selenium	40.2 mcg

• **Large (about 5-quart) slow cooker**

2 tbsp	clarified butter, divided	30 mL
4	large lamb shanks (about 4 lbs/2 kg)	4
3	onions, finely chopped	3
2	stalks celery, diced	2
2	carrots, peeled and diced	2
6	cloves garlic, minced	6
1 tsp	dried thyme	5 mL
1 tsp	sea salt	5 mL
1 tsp	cracked black peppercorns	5 mL
1 cup	dry white wine	250 mL
1 cup	ready-to-use chicken broth	250 mL
1	can (28 oz/796 mL) tomatoes, with juice, coarsely chopped	1

LEMON GREMOLATA

2	cloves garlic, minced	2
1 cup	finely chopped flat-leaf (Italian) parsley	250 mL
	Grated zest of 1 lemon	
1 tbsp	extra virgin olive oil	15 mL

1. In a large skillet, heat 1 tbsp (15 mL) clarified butter over medium-high heat. Add lamb, in batches, and brown on all sides, about 8 minutes per batch. Transfer to slow cooker stoneware as completed. Drain off fat from pan.

2. Reduce heat to medium. Add the remaining butter to pan. Add onions, celery and carrots and cook, stirring, until vegetables are softened, about 7 minutes. Add garlic, thyme, sea salt and peppercorns and cook, stirring, for 1 minute. Add wine, bring to a boil and boil for 2 minutes, scraping up brown bits from bottom of pan. Stir in broth and tomatoes.

3. Transfer to stoneware. Cover and cook on Low for 10 to 12 hours or on High for 5 to 6 hours, until meat is falling off the bone.

4. *Lemon Gremolata:* About half an hour before serving, in a small serving bowl, combine garlic, parsley, lemon zest and olive oil. Pass around the table, allowing guests to individually garnish their meat.

Souvlaki

Everybody loves this traditional Greek dish of marinated lamb chunks cooked on a skewer. It combines well with a tomato and cucumber salad. Lamb supplies your body with selenium, zinc and vitamins B_{12} and B_3, all important nutrients that improve your skin by supporting immunity, metabolism and detoxification.

Tips

If desired, prepare the marinade, add the lamb and freeze for up to 1 month. Defrost in the refrigerator for at least 24 hours before cooking.

For faster, more even cooking, leave a space between the meat cubes when threading on the wooden skewers.

Nutrients per serving	
Calories	450
Fat	33 g
Carbohydrate	2 g
Fiber	1 g
Protein	35 g
Vitamin A	30 IU
Vitamin C	8 mg
Iron	3.3 mg
Vitamin E	2 IU
Zinc	7.1 mg
Selenium	39.7 mcg

- **Preheat barbecue grill or broiler**
- **12-inch (30 cm) wooden skewers**

1	clove garlic, coarsely chopped	1
1/3 cup	freshly squeezed lemon juice	75 mL
2 tbsp	extra virgin olive oil	30 mL
1 tbsp	dried oregano	15 mL
1 tbsp	chopped fresh rosemary	15 mL
1/4 tsp	freshly ground black pepper	1 mL
1 1/2 lb	boneless shoulder or leg of lamb, trimmed and cut into 1-inch (2.5 cm) cubes	750 g

1. In a resealable plastic freezer bag set in a bowl, combine garlic, lemon juice, olive oil, oregano, rosemary and pepper. Add lamb to marinade, seal bag and refrigerate for at least 4 hours or overnight.

2. Meanwhile, soak wooden skewers in water for 30 minutes. Thread lamb cubes evenly on skewers. Barbecue, turning frequently, for 8 to 10 minutes, or until medium-rare or desired doneness.

Variations

Substitute pork tenderloin or chicken breast for the lamb.

If you're in a hurry, drain marinade and place cubes in an 8-inch (20 cm) square baking pan. Bake in a 350°F (180°C) oven for 30 minutes, or until meat is tender.

Alternate green pepper and onions with the meat on the skewer before grilling.

> ### Advice for Clear Skin
> ▶ Choose naturally raised, grass-fed, organic lamb.

Side Dishes

Pan-Fried Baby Bok Choy with Sesame Oil and Ginger

Bok choy, a juicy and refreshing Chinese white cabbage, is also packed with vitamins and nutrients. For additional flavor, cook this dish in the same pan in which your meat or fish has been cooked.

1 lb	baby bok choy	500 g
1 tbsp	vegetable oil	15 mL
1 tbsp	minced gingerroot	15 mL
3 tbsp	water or ready-to-use chicken broth	45 mL
1 tsp	sesame oil	5 mL
	Salt and freshly ground black pepper	

1. With a heavy knife, cut bok choy across the bottom to separate stems. Cut each stem in half lengthwise and wash thoroughly.

2. In a nonstick pan, heat oil for 30 seconds. Add ginger and sauté until fragrant, about 1 minute. Add bok choy and cook until it begins to color and the leaves turn bright green, about 2 to 3 minutes. Add water and sesame oil; cook until all the liquid has evaporated.

3. Transfer to a platter, season to taste with salt and pepper and serve immediately.

Advice for Clear Skin

▶ Substitute extra virgin olive oil for the vegetable oil.

▶ Choose gluten-free broth until the reintroduction phase of the diet plan, when you can test to see if gluten-containing products are safe for your skin.

Nutrients per serving	
Calories	57
Fat	5 g
Carbohydrate	3 g
Fiber	1 g
Protein	2 g
Vitamin A	5067 IU
Vitamin C	51 mg
Iron	0.9 mg
Vitamin E	1 IU
Zinc	0.2 mg
Selenium	0.6 mcg

Shanghai-Style Bok Choy

Baby bok choy is a cousin of regular bok choy. It has soft green stems and smooth, oval leaves, and it is often sold in sets of three or four plump little stalks. It cooks quickly and can be quartered lengthwise, with stalks left intact, for an elegant presentation. Bok choy contains compounds that help regulate hormones.

1 lb	baby bok choy (about 3 small stalks)	500 g
2 tbsp	vegetable oil	30 mL
1 tbsp	chopped garlic	15 mL
1 tbsp	chopped gingerroot	15 mL
1 tsp	salt or to taste	5 mL
2 tbsp	water	30 mL

1. Trim each bok choy stalk, cutting away about $\frac{3}{4}$ inches (2 cm) from the base of each. Then slice crosswise on the diagonal into $1\frac{1}{2}$-inch (4 cm) pieces. Keep stems and leaves in separate piles.

2. Heat a wok or a large, deep skillet over high heat. Add oil and swirl to coat pan. Add garlic and ginger and toss well, until fragrant, about 15 seconds.

3. Add bok choy stems and spread out in a single layer. Cook for 1 minute. Toss well and add leaves. Cook, undisturbed, for 1 minute. Toss once.

4. Add salt and water, pouring in slowly around sides of pan. Cook, tossing occasionally, until bok choy is tender-crisp, 1 to 2 minutes more. Transfer to a serving plate. Serve hot or warm.

Advice for Clear Skin

▶ Substitute extra virgin olive oil for the vegetable oil.

Nutrients per serving

Calories	81
Fat	7 g
Carbohydrate	3 g
Fiber	1 g
Protein	2 g
Vitamin A	5067 IU
Vitamin C	52 mg
Iron	1.0 mg
Vitamin E	2 IU
Zinc	0.3 mg
Selenium	0.9 mcg

Gailan in Anchovy Garlic Butter

Commonly known as Chinese broccoli, gailan has a rich, almost nutty flavor, with a slight hint of bitterness. Its dull, waxy jade-green stems and leaves turn an attractive deep green when cooked. Look for stems that are ¼ to ¾ inch (5 mm to 1.5 cm) in diameter and about 6 to 8 inches (15 cm to 20 cm) in length, with healthy-looking bud clusters or white flowers at the top.

1 lb	gailan or broccoli	500 g
2 tbsp	butter	30 mL
2 or 3	anchovy fillets, finely chopped	2 or 3
2 tsp	minced garlic	10 mL
1 tbsp	ready-to-use chicken broth	15 mL
	Salt and freshly ground black pepper	
1 tbsp	toasted sesame seeds	15 mL

1. With a sharp knife, cut gailan horizontally into 2-inch (5 cm) segments. If stem is too thick, cut lengthwise in half before cutting into segments. If using broccoli, cut into bite-size florets.

2. In a nonstick wok or skillet, melt butter over medium heat. Add anchovies and garlic; stir-fry for 15 seconds. Add gailan or broccoli; stir until well coated. Add broth; cover and cook until tender-crisp, about 2 minutes. Season to taste with salt and pepper. Transfer to serving platter; sprinkle with sesame seeds and serve.

Advice for Clear Skin

▶ Substitute olive oil for the butter.

▶ Choose gluten-free broth until the reintroduction phase of the diet plan, when you can test to see if gluten-containing products are safe for your skin.

Nutrients per serving	
Calories	99
Fat	7 g
Carbohydrate	7 g
Fiber	4 g
Protein	4 g
Vitamin A	3580 IU
Vitamin C	106 mg
Iron	1.4 mg
Vitamin E	0 IU
Zinc	0.7 mg
Selenium	5.0 mcg

Cauliflower "Mashed Potatoes"

This delicious, dairy-free alternative to mashed potatoes is certain to please. Nutritional yeast is packed with B vitamins and provides a good dose of zinc — a great combination of nutrients to help you recover from acne.

Tips

Remove the tougher stems from the cauliflower; they will not blend as well as the florets.

Chopping the ingredients in a food processor before blending creates a smooth purée with very little liquid, ensuring a creamy result.

- **Food processor**
- **Blender**

1 cup	whole raw cashews	250 mL
3 tbsp	nutritional yeast	45 mL
1 tsp	fine sea salt	5 mL
3 cups	chopped cauliflower (see tip, at left)	750 mL
3 tbsp	cold-pressed (extra virgin) olive oil	45 mL
1 tbsp	freshly squeezed lemon juice	15 mL

1. In food processor, process cashews, nutritional yeast and salt until flour-like in consistency. Add cauliflower, olive oil and lemon juice. Process at high speed until finely chopped, stopping motor to scrape down sides of work bowl as necessary.

2. Transfer mixture to blender and blend on high speed until smooth and creamy. Transfer to a bowl. Serve immediately or cover and refrigerate for up to 4 days.

Variations

For an even creamier dish, soak 2 cups (500 mL) whole raw cashews in 4 cups (1 L) warm water for 15 minutes. Drain, then add to ingredients in step 2, along with an additional 1 cup (250 mL) chopped cauliflower florets and ½ cup (125 mL) filtered water.

Herbed Cauliflower "Mashed Potatoes": In step 2, add 1 tbsp (15 mL) chopped chives, 1 tsp (5 mL) chopped fresh rosemary and ½ tsp (2 mL) chopped fresh thyme leaves.

Nutrients per serving	
Calories	328
Fat	26 g
Carbohydrate	17 g
Fiber	3 g
Protein	11 g
Vitamin A	0 IU
Vitamin C	40 mg
Iron	3.0 mg
Vitamin E	3 IU
Zinc	2.4 mg
Selenium	6.9 mcg

Stuffed Cucumber Cups

These little stuffed cups balance the slightly sweet taste and creamy texture of cashews with fresh cucumber. Cucumber contains vitamin C, an important cofactor for the production of collagen in the skin.

Tips

A medium lemon will yield about 3 tbsp (45 mL) fresh juice.

If you can, use an English cucumber to make the cups, as they do not contain seeds. If you are using a field cucumber, be sure to peel off the skin and scoop out all the seeds — they are tough and bitter.

Nutrients per 1 of 12 cups

Calories	56
Fat	4 g
Carbohydrate	4 g
Fiber	1 g
Protein	2 g
Vitamin A	400 IU
Vitamin C	10 mg
Iron	0.7 mg
Vitamin E	1 IU
Zinc	0.6 mg
Selenium	1.1 mcg

- **Food processor**

³/₄ cup	whole raw cashews	175 mL
¹/₂ cup	chopped red bell pepper	125 mL
¹/₄ cup	filtered water	60 mL
2 tbsp	freshly squeezed lemon juice	30 mL
2 tsp	smoked paprika	10 mL
³/₄ tsp	fine sea salt	3 mL
1	clove garlic	1
1	large English or field cucumber (see tip, at left)	1

1. In food processor, combine cashews, red pepper, water, lemon juice, paprika, salt and garlic. Process until smooth. Transfer to a bowl and set aside.

2. Cut the ends off the cucumber, then cut it crosswise into 10 to 12 equal pieces. Using a melon baller, scoop out the seeds and pulp from each piece, hollowing it out to make a ring.

3. Place the cucumber cups on a serving plate. Fill each with 1 tbsp (15 mL) of the cashew mixture. Serve immediately or cover and refrigerate for up to 2 days.

Asian Eggplant with Peppers and Peas

Asian eggplants are smaller in size, with a more tender texture, compared to eggplants used in Western cooking, so they do not need to be salted or peeled before cooking. Eggplants contain chlorogenic acid, a potent antioxidant that has also been shown to exhibit antimicrobial properties.

Tip

Frozen tiny peas are also referred to as "petite" or "baby." You can also use regular-size frozen peas, if you allow a little extra cooking time to heat them through.

1 lb	Asian eggplants (about 3)	500 g
2 tbsp	vegetable oil, divided	30 mL
1/2 cup	thinly sliced red bell pepper	125 mL
1/3 cup	frozen tiny peas (see tip, at left)	75 mL
1 tsp	salt (or to taste)	5 mL
1 tsp	Asian sesame oil	5 mL

1. Trim both ends from each eggplant and slice crosswise into thin rounds.

2. Heat a wok or a large, deep skillet over high heat. Add 1 tbsp (15 mL) vegetable oil and swirl to coat pan. Add eggplant and spread out in an even layer. Cook, tossing often, for 2 minutes.

3. Push eggplant aside and add the remaining vegetable oil to center of pan. When hot, add red pepper and peas. Toss well. Cook, tossing occasionally, until eggplant is tender and red pepper and peas are tender-crisp, about 2 minutes more. Add salt and sesame oil and toss well. Transfer to a serving plate. Serve hot or warm.

Advice for Clear Skin

▶ Substitute extra virgin olive oil for the vegetable oil.

Nutrients per serving

Calories	113
Fat	8 g
Carbohydrate	9 g
Fiber	5 g
Protein	2 g
Vitamin A	844 IU
Vitamin C	28 mg
Iron	0.5 mg
Vitamin E	3 IU
Zinc	0.3 mg
Selenium	0.6 mcg

Creamed Greens with Pumpkin Seeds and Lemon

MAKES 2 SERVINGS

The combination of tahini, hemp oil, olive oil and pumpkin seeds provides a good supply of skin-restoring omega-3s.

Tips

Before slicing the chard, remove the long stem that runs up through the leaf almost to the top of the plant. Use only the leafy green parts.

You can make this recipe without a dehydrator. Complete step 1, then cover spinach and set aside at room temperature for 1 hour or until soft. However, be aware that the dehydrator creates the mouthfeel of a sautéed food, which marinating can't duplicate.

Nutrients per serving	
Calories	591
Fat	58 g
Carbohydrate	14 g
Fiber	3 g
Protein	12 g
Vitamin A	3633 IU
Vitamin C	30 mg
Iron	4.0 mg
Vitamin E	10 IU
Zinc	2.9 mg
Selenium	13.0 mcg

- **Electric food dehydrator**
- **Blender**

2 cups	Swiss chard, trimmed and cut into 1-inch (2.5 cm) slices	500 mL
1 cup	baby spinach	250 mL
3	cloves garlic, divided, minced	3
3 tbsp	cold-pressed (extra virgin) olive oil	45 mL
1/4 cup	freshly squeezed lemon juice, divided	60 mL
1 tsp	fine sea salt, divided	5 mL
1/2 cup	filtered water	125 mL
1/4 cup	tahini	60 mL
2 tbsp	cold-pressed hemp oil	30 mL
1/4 cup	raw pumpkin seeds	60 mL

1. In a bowl, toss chard, spinach, 2 cloves minced garlic, olive oil, 2 tbsp (30 mL) lemon juice and 1/2 tsp (2 mL) salt.

2. Transfer to a nonstick dehydrator sheet, spreading evenly. Dehydrate at 105°F (41°C) for 30 to 45 minutes or until soft and slightly wilted.

3. In blender, combine water, tahini, the remaining garlic and lemon juice and salt, and hemp oil. Blend at high speed until emulsified.

4. Pour tahini sauce over wilted greens. Add pumpkin seeds and toss well. Serve immediately.

Tangy Green Beans

A robust citrus vinaigrette combined with subtle-tasting green beans makes for a great combination of flavors.

1 tbsp	grated orange zest	15 mL
1/3 cup	freshly squeezed orange juice	75 mL
1/3 cup	rice vinegar	75 mL
1/4 cup	vegetable oil	60 mL
1/4 tsp	Dijon mustard	1 mL
2	cloves garlic, minced (about 2 tsp/10 mL)	2
1/4 tsp	grated gingerroot	1 mL
1 tbsp	sesame oil	15 mL
3 cups	chopped trimmed green beans (1-inch/2.5 cm pieces)	750 mL

1. In a serving bowl, whisk together orange zest and juice, rice vinegar, oil, mustard, garlic and ginger. Set aside.

2. In a nonstick skillet, heat sesame oil over medium heat for 1 minute. Add green beans, reduce heat to low and cook, stirring, for 3 to 4 minutes or until coated and bright green. Add to vinaigrette and toss well. Let stand for 5 minutes or until flavors are blended. Serve immediately.

Variations

To add taste and texture, sprinkle with slivered almonds just before serving.

If you're trying to reduce your dietary fat intake, steam the beans for 3 to 4 minutes instead of frying them, and omit the sesame oil. Toss with vinaigrette as directed.

Advice for Clear Skin

▶ Substitute extra virgin olive oil for the vegetable oil.

▶ The small quantity of fresh orange juice in the vinaigrette is insignificant enough to be of no concern.

Nutrients per serving	
Calories	191
Fat	18 g
Carbohydrate	8 g
Fiber	2 g
Protein	2 g
Vitamin A	565 IU
Vitamin C	22 mg
Iron	0.9 mg
Vitamin E	4 IU
Zinc	0.2 mg
Selenium	0.7 mcg

Green Beans with Cashews

The simple addition of cashews and red onions to this dish transforms ordinary green beans into a formidable companion to any gourmet main course. Green beans contain vitamin C and carotenoids to help reduce inflammation in your skin.

1 lb	green beans, trimmed	500 g
2 tbsp	olive oil	30 mL
1/2 cup	slivered red onion	125 mL
1/3 cup	raw cashews	75 mL
1/4 tsp	salt	1 mL
1/4 tsp	freshly ground black pepper	1 mL
	Few sprigs fresh parsley, chopped	

1. Blanch green beans in a pot of boiling water for 5 minutes. Drain and immediately refresh in a bowl of ice-cold water. Drain and set aside.

2. In a large frying pan, heat olive oil over medium-high heat for 30 seconds. Add onion, cashews, salt and pepper and stir-fry for 2 to 3 minutes, until the onion is softened. Add cooked green beans, increase heat to high, and stir-fry actively for 2 to 3 minutes, until the beans feel hot to the touch. (Take care that you don't burn any cashews in the process.) Transfer to a serving plate and garnish with chopped parsley. Serve immediately.

Nutrients per serving

Calories	167
Fat	12 g
Carbohydrate	13 g
Fiber	4 g
Protein	4 g
Vitamin A	784 IU
Vitamin C	15 mg
Iron	1.9 mg
Vitamin E	2 IU
Zinc	0.9 mg
Selenium	2.1 mcg

Marinated Mushrooms

This is a refreshing and meaningful appetizer or side vegetable that requires next to no cooking. It can sit nicely in the fridge for up to 2 days while waiting to be eaten, improving its flavor all the while. Mushrooms contain iron and vitamin D, which are important for supporting your mood and energy levels.

5 cups	mushrooms, washed and trimmed	1.25 L
1/4 cup	slivered red onion	60 mL
3	cloves garlic, minced	3
1/4 cup	walnut pieces	60 mL
1 tsp	olive oil	5 mL
6 tbsp	extra virgin olive oil	90 mL
2 tbsp	white wine vinegar	30 mL
1 tbsp	soy sauce	15 mL
Pinch	cayenne pepper (optional)	Pinch
	Salt and freshly ground black pepper	
	Few sprigs fresh parsley and/or basil, chopped	

1. In a bowl, toss mushrooms, red onion and garlic until well mixed.

2. In a small frying pan over medium heat, stir-fry walnut pieces in 1 tsp (5 mL) olive oil for 1 to 2 minutes, being careful not to let them burn. Add to mushroom mixture.

3. In a small bowl, whisk together 6 tbsp (90 mL) olive oil, vinegar, soy sauce, cayenne (if using), and salt and pepper to taste, until emulsified. Add dressing to mushrooms and fold gently until the vegetables are well coated. Season to taste with salt and pepper. Leave uncovered for at least 1 hour, gently folding every 15 minutes or so. Transfer to a serving bowl and garnish liberally with the herb(s). Serve immediately or keep for up to 1 hour more, covered and unrefrigerated.

> ## Advice for Clear Skin
> ▶ Use organic, non-GMO, gluten-free soy sauce.

Nutrients per serving

Calories	264
Fat	26 g
Carbohydrate	6 g
Fiber	2 g
Protein	4 g
Vitamin A	2 IU
Vitamin C	3 mg
Iron	0.9 mg
Vitamin E	5 IU
Zinc	0.7 mg
Selenium	8.9 mcg

Stewed Okra

A staple of Southern cooking, okra is the magical ingredient that can be used to thicken gumbo or, when breaded and deep-fried, served as a crunchy snack. This okra recipe concentrates on the sweet-tart taste of okra itself. Okra provides vitamin C and vitamin A, both important for skin rejuvenation.

2	tomatoes	2
1 lb	okra	500 g
2 tbsp	butter (optional)	30 mL
1 tbsp	olive oil	15 mL
1/2 tsp	hot pepper flakes	2 mL
4	cloves garlic, thinly sliced	4
1/2 tsp	freshly ground black pepper	2 mL
1 cup	water	250 mL
1 tbsp	freshly squeezed lime juice	15 mL
1/2 tsp	salt	2 mL
	Few sprigs fresh coriander, chopped	

1. Blanch tomatoes in boiling water for 30 seconds. Over a bowl, peel, core and deseed them. Chop tomatoes into chunks and set aside. Strain any accumulated tomato juices from bowl; add the juices to the tomatoes.

2. With a sharp knife, trim 1/4 inch (0.5 cm) from the okra stems. Cut a vertical slit, 1 inch (2.5 cm) long, through the bellies of the okra, taking care not to slice them in half.

3. In a large frying pan, heat butter (if using) and oil over high heat until sizzling. Add hot pepper flakes and stir-fry for 30 seconds. Add okra and fry, actively tossing and turning, for about 5 minutes, until they are scorched on both sides. Add garlic and black pepper; toss-fry for just under 1 minute, until the garlic is sizzling (but before it burns).

4. Immediately add the reserved tomatoes and tomato juice. Stir-fry for 1 minute until the tomatoes are beginning to fry. Add water and stir until it begins to boil around the okra. Reduce heat and simmer for 20 minutes, gently folding and stirring every few minutes. (The okra will become increasingly tender and the sauce will thicken.)

5. Sprinkle okra with lime juice and salt. Gently fold and stir for under a minute and remove from heat. Transfer to a serving dish and garnish with chopped coriander. The okra can be served immediately but will improve if allowed to rest for about 30 minutes.

Advice for Clear Skin

▸ Omit the optional butter in this recipe.

Nutrients per serving

Calories	83
Fat	4 g
Carbohydrate	12 g
Fiber	5 g
Protein	3 g
Vitamin A	1035 IU
Vitamin C	35 mg
Iron	1.2 mg
Vitamin E	2 IU
Zinc	0.8 mg
Selenium	1.3 mcg

Pea Tops with Pancetta and Tofu

Pea tops are the shoots of snow pea plants. They're now available almost year round in Asian markets. They are tasty in salads and have a subtle nutty flavor when cooked. However, they are quite perishable and won't last much longer than a couple of days in your refrigerator. Pea tops help support the healing of acne, thanks to their folate, vitamin C and vitamin A content.

1	3-inch (7.5 cm) square medium tofu	1
2 tbsp	vegetable oil, divided	30 mL
	Salt and freshly ground black pepper	
1 tsp	sesame oil	5 mL
2	slices pancetta or prosciutto, finely chopped	2
2 tsp	minced garlic	10 mL
8 oz	pea tops or arugula	250 g
2 tbsp	ready-to-use chicken or vegetable broth	30 mL

1. Slice tofu into pieces $\frac{1}{2}$ inch (1 cm) thick by $1\frac{1}{2}$ inches (3.5 cm) square.

2. In a nonstick skillet, heat 1 tbsp (15 mL) oil over medium-high heat for 30 seconds. Add tofu and season lightly with salt, pepper and sesame oil; fry until golden, about 1 minute per side. Remove from skillet; arrange on a platter and keep warm.

3. Add the remaining oil to skillet and heat for 30 seconds. Add pancetta and garlic; fry briefly until fragrant, about 20 to 30 seconds. Add pea tops and broth; stir-fry until pea tops are just wilted. Arrange evenly over tofu and serve.

Advice for Clear Skin

▶ Substitute extra virgin olive oil for the vegetable oil.

▶ Choose gluten-free broth until the reintroduction phase of the diet plan, when you can test to see if gluten-containing products are safe for your skin.

Nutrients per serving

Calories	124
Fat	10 g
Carbohydrate	3 g
Fiber	1 g
Protein	6 g
Vitamin A	1346 IU
Vitamin C	9 mg
Iron	1.3 mg
Vitamin E	2 IU
Zinc	0.3 mg
Selenium	0.5 mcg

Peppery Red Onions

Red onions contain vitamin C, the antioxidant quercetin, and allicin, a compound with antimicrobial properties. These nutrients help to make red onions an acne-fighting food.

Tips

Use your favorite hot sauce, such as Tabasco or Louisiana Hot Sauce, or try other, more exotic brands to vary the flavors in this recipe.

If you choose to halve this recipe, use a small (1½- to 2-quart) slow cooker.

Make Ahead

Complete step 1. Cover and refrigerate overnight. The next day, complete the recipe.

Nutrients per serving

Calories	91
Fat	4 g
Carbohydrate	14 g
Fiber	3 g
Protein	2 g
Vitamin A	7 IU
Vitamin C	11 mg
Iron	0.4 mg
Vitamin E	1 IU
Zinc	0.3 mg
Selenium	0.8 mcg

- **Small to medium (2- to 4-quart) slow cooker**

4	large red onions, quartered	4
1 tbsp	olive oil	15 mL
1 tsp	dried oregano	5 mL
¼ cup	water or ready-to-use vegetable broth	60 mL
	Salt and freshly ground black pepper	
	Hot pepper sauce (see tip, at left)	

1. In slow cooker stoneware, combine onions, olive oil, oregano, water, and salt and pepper, to taste. Stir thoroughly.

2. Cover and cook on Low for 6 hours or on High for 3 hours, until onions are tender. Add hot sauce to taste, toss well and serve.

Advice for Clear Skin

▶ Choose gluten-free broth until the reintroduction phase of the diet plan, when you can test to see if gluten-containing products are safe for your skin.

Spinach, Sunflower Seed and Garlic Sauté

MAKES 4 SERVINGS

Spinach is high in both iron and calcium — and it is full of wholesome flavor. Cook spinach just until leaves begin to wilt but are still bright green.

1 tbsp	vegetable oil	15 mL
1 tbsp	minced garlic	15 mL
8 oz	spinach, trimmed and washed	250 g
2 tbsp	water	30 mL
1 tsp	sesame oil	5 mL
	Salt and freshly ground black pepper	
1 cup	toasted sunflower seeds	250 mL

1. In a nonstick pan, heat oil for 30 seconds. Add garlic and sauté until soft and beginning to color, about 2 minutes. Add spinach and sauté until it begins to soften and wilt, about 1 minute. Add water and continue to cook until it evaporates.

2. Drizzle spinach with sesame oil and season to taste with salt and pepper. Add sunflower seeds; toss well. Transfer spinach to a warm platter and serve immediately.

Advice for Clear Skin

▶ Substitute extra virgin olive oil for the vegetable oil.

Nutrients per serving	
Calories	243
Fat	21 g
Carbohydrate	10 g
Fiber	5 g
Protein	8 g
Vitamin A	5320 IU
Vitamin C	17 mg
Iron	2.8 mg
Vitamin E	15 IU
Zinc	2.0 mg
Selenium	26.2 mcg

Slow-Cooked Sunchokes

MAKES 6 SERVINGS

Sunchokes, also known as Jerusalem artichokes, are knobby-looking tubers native to North America. They are crunchy and sweet-tasting and are reminiscent of water chestnuts, although they are often mashed and served as a replacement for potatoes.

Tip

If you prefer, peel the chokes before cooking, placing them in a bowl of lemon water as they are peeled, to prevent browning.

- **Small (1¹/₂- to 3-quart) slow cooker**

4 cups	cubed (about 2 inches/5 cm) sunchokes (see tips, at left)	1 L
2 tbsp	extra virgin olive oil	30 mL
	Salt and freshly ground pepper	
	Finely chopped fresh parsley or chives	

1. In slow cooker stoneware, combine sunchokes and olive oil. Toss to coat sunchokes well. Cover and cook on High for 3 hours, until chokes are just tender. Season to taste with salt and pepper and garnish liberally with parsley.

Nutrients per serving	
Calories	113
Fat	5 g
Carbohydrate	17 g
Fiber	2 g
Protein	2 g
Vitamin A	20 IU
Vitamin C	4 mg
Iron	3.4 mg
Vitamin E	1 IU
Zinc	0.1 mg
Selenium	0.7 mcg

Summer Zucchini

MAKES 4 SERVINGS

This is an ideal recipe for lush, juicy zucchini. The mix of colors means the recipe provides a good range of various carotenoid compounds to support your skin.

4	young zucchini, preferably 2 each of green and yellow, less than 6 inches (15 cm) in length	4
3 tbsp	olive oil	45 mL
$\frac{1}{4}$ tsp	salt	1 mL
$\frac{1}{4}$ tsp	freshly ground black pepper	1 mL
1	red bell pepper, cut into thick strips	1
3	green onions, chopped	3
1 tbsp	freshly squeezed lemon juice	15 mL
	Few sprigs fresh basil and/or parsley, chopped	

1. Trim ends of zucchini and cut into $\frac{3}{4}$-inch (2 cm) chunks. Set aside.

2. In a large frying pan, heat olive oil over high heat for 30 seconds. Add salt and pepper and stir. Add zucchini chunks and red pepper strips. Stir-fry for 4 to 6 minutes, until the zucchini have browned on both sides and the red pepper has softened. Add green onions and stir-fry for 30 seconds. Transfer to a serving dish and drizzle evenly with lemon juice. Garnish with basil and/or parsley and serve immediately.

Nutrients per serving

Calories	121
Fat	11 g
Carbohydrate	6 g
Fiber	2 g
Protein	2 g
Vitamin A	1206 IU
Vitamin C	61 mg
Iron	0.7 mg
Vitamin E	3 IU
Zinc	0.5 mg
Selenium	0.3 mcg

Curried Zucchini Strips

Fast, easy and delicious, these zucchini strips go well with any meal. They can also be eaten cold as a snack. Zucchini has good amounts of vitamin C and vitamin B$_6$, which both contribute to the health of your immune system, metabolism and skin repair.

Tip

Leftovers of this dish are delicious. Eat them on their own or cut them into chunks and add to a salad or stir-fry.

3	zucchini	3
1 tbsp	vegetable oil	15 mL
1/4 tsp	curry powder	1 mL
	Salt	

1. Cut ends off zucchini. Cut in half lengthwise, then cut each half in half crosswise. Cut each quarter lengthwise into two or three strips of equal size. These will vary depending on the size of your zucchini.

2. In a large nonstick skillet, heat oil over medium-high heat until hot but not smoking. Add zucchini and cook, stirring occasionally, for 5 minutes or until soft.

3. Sprinkle with curry powder and salt to taste, and mix well. Cover and cook for 2 minutes or until tender and fragrant.

Advice for Clear Skin

▸ Substitute extra virgin olive oil for the vegetable oil.

Nutrients per serving

Calories	33
Fat	4 g
Carbohydrate	0 g
Fiber	0 g
Protein	0 g
Vitamin A	42 IU
Vitamin C	3 mg
Iron	0.1 mg
Vitamin E	1 IU
Zinc	0.1 mg
Selenium	0.1 mcg

Veggie Kabobs

In summer and early fall, when fresh vegetables are in season, these kabobs are a standby. They are equally delicious served hot or at room temperature.

Tips

The longer the marinating time, the deeper the flavors.

Any leftover veggies from these kabobs make a perfect beginning for tasty pasta dishes or salads.

Vary the flavor by replacing the oregano with the same quantity of thyme, basil or rosemary.

Nutrients per serving

Calories	99
Fat	7 g
Carbohydrate	8 g
Fiber	2 g
Protein	2 g
Vitamin A	1355 IU
Vitamin C	58 mg
Iron	0.7 mg
Vitamin E	3 IU
Zinc	0.4 mg
Selenium	1.9 mcg

- **Preheat barbecue grill or broiler**
- **16 bamboo or metal skewers**

1/3 cup	freshly squeezed lemon juice	75 mL
1/4 cup	olive oil	60 mL
1	clove garlic, minced (about 1 tsp/5 mL)	1
2 tsp	dried oregano (or 2 tbsp/30 mL finely chopped fresh)	10 mL
	Salt and freshly ground black pepper	
2	bell peppers (any color), cut into 1-inch (2.5 cm) strips	2
2	small zucchini and/or yellow summer squash, cut into 1-inch (2.5 cm) thick slices	2
2 cups	grape tomatoes or cherry tomatoes (about 16)	500 mL
2 cups	whole button mushrooms (about 16)	500 mL
1	large onion, cut into 8 wedges and halved crosswise, separated into single layers	1
1	yellow summer squash (such as golden zucchini), cut into 1-inch (2.5 cm) cubes	1

1. In a large bowl or sealable plastic bag, combine lemon juice, olive oil, garlic, oregano and salt and pepper to taste. Add peppers, zucchini, tomatoes, mushrooms, onion and squash and stir to evenly coat. Marinate at room temperature for 15 to 20 minutes or in the refrigerator for up to 12 hours.

2. Thread vegetables onto skewers, alternating to form an attractive pattern and leaving a bit of space between the pieces to allow air to circulate.

3. Grill or broil, turning and basting often with the remaining marinade, for 8 to 10 minutes or until vegetables are browned on all sides and tender. While cooking, rotate location of the skewers on the grill or under the broiler to ensure even cooking.

Variations

The vegetables (unskewered) can also be spread in a single layer on two greased rimmed baking sheets and baked in a preheated 400°F (200°C) oven for 30 to 35 minutes. Turn the vegetables and rotate the pans after 20 minutes.

Contributing Authors

Byron Ayanoglu with contributions from Algis Kemezys
125 Best Vegetarian Recipes
Recipes from this book are found on pages 268, 296, 358–60 and 365.

Pat Crocker
The Healing Herbs Cookbook
Recipes from this book are found on pages 258 and 292.

Pat Crocker
The Smoothies Bible, Second Edition
Recipes from this book are found on pages 216–20 and 255.

Pat Crocker
The Vegan Cook's Bible
Recipes from this book are found on pages 235, 249, 287 and 293.

Dietitians of Canada
Simply Great Food
Recipes from this book are found on pages 252, 253, 259, 273, 295, 298 (top), 302, 310, 334 and 343.

Maxine Effenson-Chuck and Beth Gurney
125 Best Vegan Recipes
Recipes from this book are found on pages 227, 232, 357, 366 and 367.

Judith Finlayson
The 163 Best Paleo Slow Cooker Recipes
Recipes from this book are found on pages 304, 305, 320, 330, 338, 340–42, 344, 346 and 347.

Judith Finlayson
The Healthy Slow Cooker, Second Edition
Recipes from this book are found on pages 229, 230, 242–44, 308, 322, 328 and 345.

Judith Finlayson
The Vegetarian Slow Cooker
Recipes from this book are found on pages 256, 286, 288–91, 294, 362 and 364.

Margaret Howard
The 250 Best 4-Ingredient Recipes
Recipes from this book are found on pages 250, 254, 298 (bottom), 299–301, 303, 311, 315 and 337.

Bill Jones and Stephen Wong
125 Best Chinese Recipes
Recipes from this book are found on pages 257, 350, 352, 361 and 363.

Nancie McDermott
300 Best Stir-Fry Recipes
Recipes from this book are found on pages 251, 309, 312, 335, 336, 351 and 355.

Douglas McNish
Eat Raw, Eat Well
Recipes from this book are found on pages 223, 233, 234, 237, 241, 265, 266 (top), 278, 283 and 356.

Douglas McNish
Raw, Quick & Delicious!
Recipes from this book are found on pages 222, 224, 274, 279, 282, 284, 285, 353 and 354.

Rose Murray
125 Best Chicken Recipes
Recipes from this book are found on pages 260, 316–19, 323–25 and 327.

Deb Roussou
350 Best Vegan Recipes
Recipes from this book are found on pages 213, 226, 238, 240, 271, 276 and 280.

Camilla V. Saulsbury
5 Easy Steps to Healthy Cooking
Recipes from this book are found on pages 247, 263, 267, 269, 270, 275, 306 and 307.

Camilla V. Saulsbury
Complete Coconut Cookbook
Recipes from this book are found on pages 210–12, 214, 215, 231, 246, 264, 266 (bottom) and 272.

Mary Sue Waisman
Dietitians of Canada Cook!
Recipes from this book are found on pages 225, 228, 236, 239, 248, 262, 314 and 332.

Donna Washburn & Heather Butt
Easy Everyday Gluten-Free Cooking
Recipes from this book are found on pages 326, 339 and 348.

References

Abulnaja KO. Oxidant/antioxidant status in obese adolescent females with acne vulgaris. *Indian J Dermatol*, 2009; 54 (1): 36–40. doi: 10.4103/0019-5154.48984.

Adebamowo CA, Spiegelman D, Berkey CS, et al. Milk consumption and acne in adolescent girls. *Dermatol Online J*, 2006 May 30; 12 (4): 1.

Adityan B, Kumari R, Thappa DM. Scoring systems in acne vulgaris. *Indian J Dermatol Venereol Leprol*, 2009 May–Jun; 75 (3): 323–6. doi: 10.4103/0378-6323.51258.

Akdoğan M, Tamer MN, Cüre E, et al. Effect of spearmint (*Mentha spicata* Labiatae) teas on androgen levels in women with hirsutism. *Phytother Res*, 2007 May; 21 (5): 444–7.

Al-Shobaili HA. Oxidants and anti-oxidants status in acne vulgaris patients with varying severity. *Ann Clin Lab Sci*, 2014 Spring; 44 (2): 202–7.

Al-Shobaili HA, Alzolibani AA, Al Robaee AA, et al. Biochemical markers of oxidative and nitrosative stress in acne vulgaris: Correlation with disease activity. *J Clin Lab Anal*, 2013 Jan; 27 (1): 45–52. doi: 10.1002/jcla.21560.

Anderson KE, Rosner W, Khan MS, et al. Diet-hormone interactions: Protein/carbohydrate ratio alters reciprocally the plasma levels of testosterone and cortisol and their respective binding globulins in man. *Life Sci*, 1987 May 4; 40 (18): 1761–8.

Anderson ML. Evaluation of Resettin® on serum hormone levels in sedentary males. *J Int Soc Sports Nutr*, 2014 Aug 23; 11: 43. doi: 10.1186/s12970-014-0043-x. eCollection 2014.

Arck P, Handjiski B, Hagen E, et al. Is there a "gut-brain-skin axis"? *Exp Dermatol*, 2010 May; 19 (5): 401–5. doi: 10.1111/j.1600-0625.2009.01060.x. Epub 2010 Jan 25.

Ashat M, Kochhar R. Non-celiac gluten hypersensitivity. *Trop Gastroenterol*, 2014 Apr–Jun; 35 (2): 71–8.

Aziz I, Lewis NR, Hadjivassiliou M, et al. A UK study assessing the population prevalence of self-reported gluten sensitivity and referral characteristics to secondary care. *Eur J Gastroenterol Hepatol*, 2014 Jan; 26 (1): 33–9. doi: 10.1097/01.meg.0000435546.87251 f7.

Azzouni F, Godoy A, Li Y, et al. The 5 alpha-reductase isozyme family: A review of basic biology and their role in human diseases. *Adv Urol*, 2012; 2012: 530121. doi: 10.1155/2012/530121. Epub 2011 Dec 25.

Balta I, Ekiz O, Ozuguz P, et al. Nutritional anemia in reproductive age women with postadolescent acne. *Cutan Ocul Toxicol*, 2013 Sep; 32 (3): 200–3. doi: 10.3109/15569527.2012.751393. Epub 2013 Jan 25.

Baquerizo Nole KL, Yim E, Keri JE. Probiotics and prebiotics in dermatology. *J Am Acad Dermatol*, 2014 Oct; 71 (4): 814–21. doi: 10.1016/j.jaad.2014.04.050. Epub 2014 Jun 4.

Başak PY, Cetin ES, Gürses I, et al. The effects of systemic isotretinoin and antibiotic therapy on the microbial floras in patients with acne vulgaris. *J Eur Acad Dermatol Venereol*, 2013 Mar; 27 (3): 332–6. doi: 10.1111/j.1468-3083.2011.04397.x. Epub 2012 Jan 13.

Bataille V, Snieder H, MacGregor AJ, et al. The influence of genetics and environmental factors in the pathogenesis of acne: A twin study of acne in women. *J Invest Dermatol*, 2002 Dec; 119 (6): 1317–22.

Ben-Amitai D, Laron Z. Effect of insulin-like growth factor-1 deficiency or administration on the occurrence of acne. *J Eur Acad Dermatol Venereol*, 2011 Aug; 25 (8): 950–4. doi: 10.1111/j.1468-3083.2010.03896.x. Epub 2010 Nov 4.

Benninghoff AD, Williams DE. The role of estrogen receptor ß in transplacental cancer prevention by indole-3-carbinol. *Cancer Prev Res (Phila)*, 2013 Apr; 6 (4): 339–48. doi: 10.1158/1940-6207.CAPR-12-0311. Epub 2013 Feb 27.

Blasbalg TL, Hibbeln JR, Ramsden CE, et al. Changes in consumption of omega-3 and omega-6 fatty acids in the United States during the 20th century. *Am J Clin Nutr*, 2001 May; 93 (5): 950–62.

Brandt S. The clinical effects of zinc as a topical or oral agent on the clinical response and pathophysiologic mechanisms of acne: A systematic review of the literature. *J Drugs Dermatol*, 2013 May; 12 (5): 542–5.

Buck Louis GM, Kannan K, Sapra KJ, et al. Urinary concentrations of benzophenone-type ultraviolet radiation filters and couples' fecundity. *Am J Epidemiol*, 2014 Dec 15; 180 (12): 1168–75. doi: 10.1093/aje/kwu285. Epub 2014 Nov 13.

Burris J, Rietkerk W, Woolf K. Acne: The role of medical nutrition therapy. *J Acad Nutr Diet*, 2013 Mar; 113 (3): 416–30. doi: 10.1016/j.jand.2012.11.016.

———. Relationships of self-reported dietary factors and perceived acne severity in a cohort of New York young adults. *J Acad Nutr Diet*, 2014 Mar; 114 (3): 384–92. doi: 10.1016/j.jand.2013.11.010. Epub 2014 Jan 9.

Cappuccio FP, D'Elia L, Strazzullo P, Miller MA. Sleep duration and all-cause mortality: A systematic review and meta-analysis of prospective studies. *Sleep*, 2010 May; 33 (5): 585–92.

Cesko E, Korber A, Dissemond J. Smoking and obesity are associated factors in acne inversa: Results of a retrospective investigation in 100 patients. *Eur J Dermatol*, 2009 Sep–Oct; 19 (5): 490–3. doi: 10.1684/ejd.2009.0710. Epub 2009 Jun 15.

Chen M, Rao Y, Zheng Y, et al. Association between soy isoflavone intake and breast cancer risk for pre- and post-menopausal women: A meta-analysis of epidemiological studies. *PLoS One*, 2014 Feb 20; 9 (2): e89288. doi: 10.1371/journal.pone.0089288. eCollection 2014.

Cheng S, Leow YH, Goh CL, et al. Contact sensitivity to preservatives in Singapore: Frequency of sensitization to 11 common preservatives 2006–2011. *Dermatitis*, 2014 Mar–Apr; 25 (2): 77–82. doi: 10.1097/DER.0000000000000031.

Cockayne S, Adamson J, Lanham-New S, et al. Vitamin K and the prevention of fractures: Systematic review and meta-analysis of randomized controlled trials. *Arch Intern Med*, 2006 Jun 26; 166 (12): 1256–61.

Cormia, FE. Food sensitivity as a factor in the etiology of acne vulgaris. *J Allergy*, 1940; 12: 34.

Darbre PD, Harvey PW. Parabens can enable hallmarks and characteristics of cancer in human breast epithelial cells: A review of the literature with reference to new exposure data and regulatory status. *J Appl Toxicol*, 2014 Sep; 34 (9): 925–38. doi: 10.1002/jat.3027. Epub 2014 Jul 22.

de Groot AC, Veenstra M. Formaldehyde-releasers in cosmetics in the USA and in Europe. *Contact Dermatitis*, 2010 Apr; 62 (4): 221–4. doi: 10.1111/j.1600-0536.2009.01623.x. Epub 2010 Mar 3.

Desbois AP, Lawlor KC. Antibacterial activity of long-chain polyunsaturated fatty acids against *Propionibacterium acnes* and *Staphylococcus aureus*. *Mar Drugs*, 2013 Nov 13; 11 (11): 4544–57. doi: 10.3390/md11114544.

Downing DT, Stewart ME, Wertz PW, et al. Skin lipids: An update. *J Invest Dermatol*, 1987 Mar; 88 (3 Suppl): 2s–6s.

Dyer DG, Dunn JA, Thorpe SR, et al. Accumulation of Maillard reaction products in skin collagen in diabetes and aging. *J Clin Invest*, 1993 Jun; 91 (6): 2463–9.

El-Akawi Z, Abdel-Latif N, Abdul-Razzak K. Does the plasma level of vitamins A and E affect acne condition? *Clin Exp Dermatol*, 2006; 31: 430–4.

El-Akawi Z, Abdel-Latif Nemr N, Abdul-Razzak K, et al. Factors believed by Jordanian acne patients to affect their acne condition. *East Mediterr Health J*, 2006 Nov; 12 (6): 840–6.

Felson DT, Zhang Y. Smoking and osteoarthritis: A review of the evidence and its implications. *Osteoarthritis Cartilage*, 2015 Mar; 23 (3): 331–3. doi: 10.1016/j.joca.2014.11.022. Epub 2014 Nov 29.

Ferdowsian HR, Levin S. Does diet really affect acne? *Skin Therapy Lett*, 2010 Mar; 15 (3): 1–2, 5.

Feskanich D, Bischoff-Ferrari HA, Frazier AL, et al. Milk consumption during teenage years and risk of hip fractures in older adults. *JAMA Pediatr*, 2014 Jan; 168 (1): 54–60. doi: 10.1001/jamapediatrics.2013.3821.

Floam S, Simpson N, Nemeth E, et al. Sleep characteristics as predictor variables of stress systems markers in insomnia disorder. *J Sleep Res*, 2014 Dec 18. doi: 10.1111/jsr.12259. [Epub ahead of print]

Food Allergy Research & Education (FARE). *Allergens*. Accessed April 2015, www.foodallergy.org/allergens.

Forsythe P, Kunze WA, Bienenstock J. On communication between gut microbes and the brain. *Curr Opin Gastroenterol*, 2012 Nov; 28 (6): 557–62. doi: 10.1097/MOG.0b013e3283572ffa.

Francis, TE. Diet in the causation of acne and boils. *BMJ*, 1912; 2 (2694): 402.

Grossbart TA, Sherman C. *Skin Deep: A Mind/Body Program for Healthy Skin* (digital edition). Albuquerque, NM: Health Press, 2009.

Grossi E, Cazzaniga S, Crotti S, et al. The constellation of dietary factors in adolescent acne: A semantic connectivity map approach. *J Eur Acad Dermatol Venereol*, 2014 Dec 2. doi: 10.1111/jdv.12878. [Epub ahead of print]

Guo H, Jiang T, Wang J, et al. The value of eliminating foods according to food-specific immunoglobulin G antibodies in irritable bowel syndrome with diarrhoea. *J Int Med Res*, 2012; 40 (1): 204–10.

Harris WS, Klurfeld DM. Twentieth-century trends in essential fatty acid intakes and the predicted omega-3 index: Evidence versus estimates. *Am J Clin Nutr*, 2011 May; 93 (5): 907–8. doi:10.3945/ajcn.111.014365.

Hayashi S, Hamada T, Zaidi SF, et al. Nicotine suppresses acute colitis and colonic tumorigenesis associated with chronic colitis in mice. *Am J Physiol Gastrointest Liver Physiol*, 2014 Nov 15; 307 (10): G968–78. doi: 10.1152/ajpgi.00346.2013. Epub 2014 Sep 25.

He L, Wu WJ, Yang JK, et al. Two new susceptibility loci 1q24.2 and 11p11.2 confer risk to severe acne. *Nat Commun*, 2014; 5: 2870. doi: 10.1038/ncomms3870.

Higgins EM, du Vivier AW. Cutaneous disease and alcohol misuse. *Br Med Bull*, 1994 Jan; 50 (1): 85–98.

Hitch JM, Greenburg BG. Adolescent acne and dietary iodine. *Arch Dermatol*, 1961; 84 (6): 898–911. doi:10.1001/archderm.1961.01580180014002.

Holt SH, Miller JC, Petocz P. An insulin index of foods: The insulin demand generated by 1000-kJ portions of common foods. *Am J Clin Nutr*, 1997 Nov; 66 (5): 1264–76.

Horton R, Pasupuletti V, Antonipillai I. Androgen induction of steroid 5 alpha-reductase may be mediated via insulin-like growth factor-I. *Endocrinology*, 1993 Aug; 133 (2): 447–51.

ISAAA. ISAAA brief 49-2014: Top ten facts. *International Service for the Acquisition of Agri-Biotech Applications*. Accessed Apr 2015, www.isaaa.org/resources/publications/briefs/49/toptenfacts/default.asp.

Ismail NH, Manaf ZA, Azizan NZ. High glycemic load diet, milk and ice cream consumption are related to acne vulgaris in Malaysian young adults: A case control study. *BMC Dermatol*, 2012 Aug 16; 12: 13. doi: 10.1186/1471-5945-12-13.

Iurassich S, Trotta C, Palagiano A, et al. Correlations between acne and polycystic ovary: A study of 60 cases. *Minerva Ginecol*, 2001 Apr; 53 (2): 107–11. [Article in Italian]

Jansson T, Lodén M. Strategy to decrease the risk of adverse effects of fragrance ingredients in cosmetic products. *Am J Contact Dermat*, 2001 Sep; 12 (3): 166–9.

Javidnia K, Dastgheib L, Mohammadi Samani S, et al. Antihirsutism activity of fennel (fruits of *Foeniculum vulgare*) extract: A double-blind placebo controlled study. *Phytomedicine*, 2003; 10 (6–7): 455–8.

Jones, JM. In U.S., 40% get less than recommended amount of sleep. *Gallup*. 2013 Dec 19, accessed Apr 2015, www.gallup.com/poll/166553/less-recommended-amount-sleep.aspx.

Jung GW, Tse JE, Guiha I, et al. Prospective, randomized, open-label trial comparing the safety, efficacy, and tolerability of an acne treatment regimen with and without a probiotic supplement and minocycline in subjects with mild to moderate acne. *J Cutan Med Surg*, 2013 Mar–Apr; 17 (2): 114–22.

Jung JY, Yoon MY, Min SU, et al. The influence of dietary patterns on acne vulgaris in Koreans. *Eur J Dermatol*, 2010 Nov–Dec; 20 (6): 768–72. doi: 10.1684/ejd.2010.1053. Epub 2010 Sep 7.

Kabbani TA, Vanga RR, Leffler DA, et al. Celiac disease or non-celiac gluten sensitivity? An approach to clinical differential diagnosis. *Am J Gastroenterol*, 2014 May; 109 (5): 741–6; quiz 747. doi: 10.1038/ajg.2014.41. Epub 2014 Mar 11.

Karakuła-Juchnowicz H, Szachta P, Opolska A, et al. The role of IgG hypersensitivity in the pathogenesis and therapy of depressive disorders. *Nutr Neurosci*, 2014 Sep 30. [Epub ahead of print]

Kennedy PJ, Cryan JF, Dinan TG, et al. Irritable bowel syndrome: A microbiome-gut-brain axis disorder? *World J Gastroenterol*, 2014 Oct 21; 20 (39): 14105–25. doi: 10.3748/wjg.v20.i39.14105.

Khayef G, Young J, Burns-Whitmore B, et al. Effects of fish oil supplementation on inflammatory acne. *Lipids Health Dis*, 2012 Dec 3; 11: 165. doi: 10.1186/1476-511X-11-165.

Klaschka U. The hazard communication of fragrance allergens must be improved. *Integr Environ Assess Manag*, 2013 Jul; 9 (3): 358–62. doi: 10.1002/ieam.1397. Epub 2013 Apr 18.

Klaz I, Kochba I, Shohat T, et al. Severe acne vulgaris and tobacco smoking in young men. *J Invest Dermatol*, 2006 Aug; 126 (8): 1749–52. Epub 2006 Apr 27.

Kobylewski S, Jacobson MF. Toxicology of food dyes. *Int J Occup Environ Health*, 2012 Jul–Sep; 18 (3): 220–46. doi: 10.1179/1077352512Z.00000000034.

Kohler C, Tschumi K, Bodmer C, et al. Effect of finasteride 5 mg (Proscar) on acne and alopecia in female patients with normal serum levels of free testosterone. *Gynecol Endocrinol*, 2007 Mar; 23 (3): 142–5.

Kraus AL, Munro IC, Orr JC, et al. Benzoyl peroxide: An integrated human safety assessment for carcinogenicity. *Regul Toxicol Pharmacol*, 1995 Feb; 21 (1): 87–107.

Krowchuk DP, Stancin T, Keskinen R, et al. The psychosocial effects of acne on adolescents. *Pediatr Dermatol*, 1991 Dec; 8 (4): 332–8.

Kurokawa I, Danby FW, Ju Q, et al. New developments in our understanding of acne pathogenesis and treatment. *Exp Dermatol*, 2009 Oct; 18 (10): 821–32. doi: 10.1111/j.1600-0625.2009.00890.x. Epub 2009 Jun 23.

Kwon HH, Yoon JY, Hong JS, et al. Clinical and histological effect of a low glycaemic load diet in treatment of acne vulgaris in Korean patients: A randomized, controlled trial. *Acta Derm Venereol*, 2012 May; 92 (3): 241–6. doi: 10.2340/00015555-1346.

Lands, WEM. *Fish, Omega 3 and Human Health*. Urbana, IL: American Oil Chemists' Society, 2005.

Lane AR, Duke JW, Hackney AC. Influence of dietary carbohydrate intake on the free testosterone: cortisol ratio responses to short-term intensive exercise training. *Eur J Appl Physiol*, 2010 Apr; 108 (6): 1125–31. doi: 10.1007/s00421-009-1220-5. Epub 2009 Dec 20.

Library of Congress. Restrictions on genetically modified organisms: Japan. Accessed April 2015, http://www.loc.gov/law/help/restrictions-on-gmos/japan.php.

Liepa GU, Sengupta A, Karsies D. Polycystic ovary syndrome (PCOS) and other androgen excess–related conditions: Can changes in dietary intake make a difference? *Nutr Clin Pract*, 2008 Feb; 23 (1): 63–71.

Liu J, Kurashiki K, Shimizu K, et al. Structure–activity relationship for inhibition of 5 alpha-reductase by triterpenoids isolated from *Ganoderma lucidum*. *Bioorg Med Chem*, 2006 Dec 15; 14 (24): 8654–60. Epub 2006 Sep 8.

Liu SY, Wrosch C, Miller GE, et al. Self-esteem change and diurnal cortisol secretion in older adulthood. *Psychoneuroendocrinology*, 2014 Mar; 41: 111–20. doi: 10.1016/j.psyneuen.2013.12.010. Epub 2013 Dec 22.

Liu XJ, Zhu TT, Zeng R, et al. An epidemiological study of food intolerance in 2434 children. *Zhongguo Dang Dai Er Ke Za Zhi*, 2013 Jul; 15 (7): 550–4. [Article in Chinese]

Lyons TJ, Bailie KE, Dyer DG, et al. Decrease in skin collagen glycation with improved glycemic control in patients with insulin-dependent diabetes mellitus. *J Clin Invest*, 1991 Jun; 87 (6): 1910–5.

Magin P, Adams J, Heading G, et al. Psychological sequelae of acne vulgaris: Results of a qualitative study. *Can Fam Physician*, 2006 Aug; 52: 978–9.

Mahmood SN, Bowe WP. Diet and acne update: Carbohydrates emerge as the main culprit. *J Drugs Dermatol*, 2014 Apr; 13 (4): 428–35.

Matthews CE, Chen KY, Freedson PS, et al. Amount of time spent in sedentary behaviors in the United States, 2003–2004. *Am J Epidemiol*, 2008 Apr 1; 167 (7): 875–81.

Mayer EA. Gut feelings: The emerging biology of gut–brain communication. *Nat Rev Neurosci*, 2011 Jul 13; 12 (8): 453–66. doi: 10.1038/nrn3071.

Melnik B. Dietary intervention in acne: Attenuation of increased mTORC1 signaling promoted by Western diet. *Dermatoendocrinol,* 2012 Jan 1; 4 (1): 20–32. doi: 10.4161/derm.19828.

Melnik BC. Evidence for acne-promoting effects of milk and other insulinotropic dairy products. *Nestle Nutr Workshop Ser Pediatr Program*, 2011; 67: 131–45. doi: 10.1159/000325580. Epub 2011 Feb 16.

Melnik BC, John SM, Plewig G. Acne: Risk indicator for increased body mass index and insulin resistance. *Acta Derm Venereol*, 2013 Nov; 93 (6): 644–9. doi: 10.2340/00015555-1677.

Melnik BC, Schmitz G. Role of insulin, insulin-like growth factor-1, hyperglycaemic food and milk consumption in the pathogenesis of acne vulgaris. *Exp Dermatol*, 2009 Oct; 18 (10): 833–41. doi: 10.1111/j.1600-0625.2009.00924.x. Epub 2009 Aug 25.

Michaëlsson K, Wolk A, Langenskiöld S, et al. Milk intake and risk of mortality and fractures in women and men: Cohort studies. *BMJ*, 2014 Oct 28; 349: g6015. doi: 10.1136/bmj.g6015.

Mills CM, Peters TJ, Finlay AY. Does smoking influence acne? *Clin Exp Dermatol*, 1993 Mar; 18 (2): 100–1.

Minkley N, Westerholt DM, Kirchner WH. Academic self-concept of ability and cortisol reactivity. *Anxiety Stress Coping*, 2014 May; 27 (3): 303–16. doi: 10.1080/10615806.2013.848273. Epub 2013 Nov 13.

Monteleone P, Fuschino A, Nolfe G, et al. Temporal relationship between melatonin and cortisol responses to nighttime physical stress in humans. *Psychoneuroendocrinology*, 1992; 17 (1): 81–6.

Mooney T. Preventing psychological distress in patients with acne. *Nurs Stand*, 2014 Jan 29–Feb 4; 28 (22): 42–8. doi: 10.7748/ns2014.01.28.22.42.e8166.

Morimoto Y, Maskarinec G, Park SY, et al. Dietary isoflavone intake is not statistically significantly associated with breast cancer risk in the Multiethnic Cohort. *Br J Nutr*, 2014 Sep 28; 112 (6): 976–83. doi: 10.1017/S0007114514001780.

Mouritsen A, Aksglaede L, Sørensen K, et al. Hypothesis: Exposure to endocrine-disrupting chemicals may interfere with timing of puberty. *Int J Androl*, 33 (2): 346–59.

Munday MR, Brush MG, Taylor RW. Correlations between progesterone, oestradiol and aldosterone levels in the premenstrual syndrome. *Clin Endocrinol* (Oxf), 1981 Jan (1): 1–9.

Nagata C, Mizoue T, Tanaka K, et al; Research Group for the Development and Evaluation of Cancer Prevention Strategies in Japan. Soy intake and breast cancer risk: An evaluation based on a systematic review of epidemiologic evidence among the Japanese population. *Jpn J Clin Oncol*, 2014 Mar; 44 (3): 282–95. doi: 10.1093/jjco/hyt203. Epub 2014 Jan 22.

Nakayama O, Yagi M, Kiyoto S, et al. Riboflavin, a testosterone 5α-reductase inhibitor. *Antibiot* (Tokyo), 1990 Dec; 43 (12): 1615–6.

Navarini AA, Simpson MA, Weale M, et al. Genome-wide association study identifies three novel susceptibility loci for severe acne vulgaris. *Nat Commun*, 2014 Jun 13; 5: 4020. doi: 10.1038/ncomms5020.

O'Connell JF, Klein-Szanto AJ, DiGiovanni DM, et al. Enhanced malignant progression of mouse skin tumors by the free-radical generator benzoyl peroxide. *Cancer Res*, 1986 Jun; 46 (6): 2863–5.

Parish LC, Fine E. Alcoholism and skin disease. *Int J Dermatol*, 1985 Jun; 24 (5): 300–1.

Pavlovic S, Daniltchenko M, Tobin DJ, et al. Further exploring the brain–skin connection: Stress worsens dermatitis via substance P-dependent neurogenic inflammation in mice. *J Invest Dermatol*, 2008 Feb; 128 (2): 434–46. Epub 2007 Oct 4.

Peterson CK, Harmon-Jones E. Anger and testosterone: Evidence that situationally-induced anger relates to situationally-induced testosterone. *Emotion*, 2012 Oct; 12 (5): 899–902. doi: 10.1037/a0025300. Epub 2011 Sep 12.

Pruthi GK, Babu N. Physical and psychosocial impact of acne in adult females. *Indian J Dermatol*, 2012 Jan; 57 (1): 26–9. doi: 10.4103/0019-5154.92672.

Pusztai A, Grant G. Assessment of lectin inactivation by heat and digestion. *Methods Mol Med*, 1998; 9: 505–14. doi: 10.1385/0-89603-396-1:505.

Qureshi N, Lowenstein EJ. The role of nutrition in acne pathogenesis: YouTube as a reflection of current popular thought. *Skinmed*, 2011 Sep–Oct; 9 (5): 279–80.

Ramos-e-Silva M, Ramos-e-Silva S, Carneiro S. Acne in women. *Br J Dermatol*, 2015 Jan 17. doi: 10.1111/bjd.13638. [Epub ahead of print]

Ramsay B, Alaghband-Zadeh J, Carter G, et al. Raised serum androgens and increased responsiveness to luteinizing hormone in men with acne vulgaris. *Acta Derm Venereol*, 1995 Jul; 75 (4): 293–6.

Rapp DA, Brenes GA, Feldman SR, et al. Anger and acne: Implications for quality of life, patient satisfaction and clinical care. *Br J Dermatol*, 2004 Jul; 151 (1): 183–9.

Raudrant D, Rabe T. Progestogens with antiandrogenic properties. *Drugs*, 2003; 63 (5): 463–92.

Rhodes JM, Campbell BJ, Yu LG. Lectin-epithelial interactions in the human colon. *Biochem Soc Trans*, 2008 Dec; 36 (Pt 6): 1482–6. doi: 10.1042/BST0361482.

Roos N, Sørensen JC, Sørensen H, et al. Screening for anti-nutritional compounds in complementary foods and food aid products for infants and young children. *Matern Child Nutr*, 2013 Jan; 9 Suppl 1: 47–71. doi: 10.1111/j.1740-8709.2012.00449.x.

Rostami Mogaddam M, Safavi Ardabili N, Maleki N, et al. Correlation between the severity and type of acne lesions with serum zinc levels in patients with acne vulgaris. *Biomed Res Int*, 2014; 2014: 474108. doi: 10.1155/2014/474108. Epub 2014 Jul 24.

Roudsari MR, Karimi R, Mortazavian AM. Health effects of probiotics on the skin. *Crit Rev Food Sci Nutr*, 2015 Jul 29; 55 (9): 1219–40.

Sakamoto S, Sato K, Maitani T, et al. Analysis of components in natural food additive "grapefruit seed extract" by HPLC and LC/MS. *Eisei Shikenjo Hokoku*, 1996; 114: 38–42. [Article in Japanese]

Sarici G, Cinar S, Armutcu F, et al. Oxidative stress in acne vulgaris. *J Eur Acad Dermatol Venereol*, 2010 Jul; 24 (7): 763–7. doi: 10.1111/j.1468-3083.2009.03505.x. Epub 2009 Nov 23.

Savelkoul FH, van der Poel AF, Tamminga S. The presence and inactivation of trypsin inhibitors, tannins, lectins and amylase inhibitors in legume seeds during germination: A review. *Plant Foods for Hum Nutr*, 1992 Jan; 42 (1): 71–85.

Schäfer T, Nienhaus A, Vieluf D, et al. Epidemiology of acne in the general population: The risk of smoking. *Br J Dermatol*, 2001 Jul; 145 (1): 100–4.

Sestak K, Fortgang I. Celiac and non-celiac forms of gluten sensitivity: Shifting paradigms of an old disease. *Br Microbiol Res J*, 2013 Oct; 3 (4): 585–9.

Shelley, WB. Generalized pustular psoriasis induced by potassium iodide: A postulated role for dihydrofolic reductase. *JAMA*, 1967; 201 (13): 1009–14. doi:10.1001/jama.1967.03130130035009.

Shen Y, Wang T, Zhou C, et al. Prevalence of acne vulgaris in Chinese adolescents and adults: A community-based study of 17,345 subjects in six cities. *Acta Derm Venereol*, 2012 Jan; 92 (1): 40–4. doi: 10.2340/00015555-1164.

Short RW, Agredano YZ, Choi JM, et al. A single-blinded, randomized pilot study to evaluate the effect of exercise-induced sweat on truncal acne. *Pediatr Dermatol*, 2008 Jan–Feb; 25 (1): 126–8. doi: 10.1111/j.1525-1470.2007.00604.x.

Siegle RJ, Fekety R, Sarbone PD, et al. Effects of topical clindamycin on intestinal microflora in patients with acne. *J Am Acad Dermatol*, 1986 Aug; 15 (2 Pt 1): 180–5.

Simopoulos, AP. The importance of the ratio of omega-6/omega-3 essential fatty acids. *Biomed Pharmacoth*, 2002; 56 (8): 365–79.

Siniavskiĭ IuA, Tsoĭ NO. Influence of nutritional patterns on the severity of acne in young adults. *Vopr Pitan*, 2014; 83 (1): 41–7. [Article in Russian]

Smith R, Mann N, Mäkeläinen H, et al. A pilot study to determine the short-term effects of a low glycemic load diet on hormonal markers of acne: A nonrandomized, parallel, controlled feeding trial. *Mol Nutr Food Res*, 2008 Jun; 52 (6): 718–26. doi: 10.1002/mnfr.200700307.

Smith RN, Mann NJ, Braue A, et al. A low-glycemic-load diet improves symptoms in acne vulgaris patients: A randomized controlled trial. *Am J Clin Nutr*, 2007 Jul; 86 (1): 107–15.

Smith S, Sepkovic D, Bradlow HL, et al. 3,3'-diindolylmethane and genistein decrease the adverse effects of estrogen in LNCaP and PC-3 prostate cancer cells. *J Nutr*, 2008 Dec; 138 (12): 2379–85. doi: 10.3945/jn.108.090993.

Stamatiadis D, Bulteau-Portois MC, Mowszowicz I. Inhibition of 5 alpha-reductase activity in human skin by zinc and azelaic acid. *Br J Dermatol*, 1988 Nov; 119 (5): 627–32.

Stokes JH, Pillsbury DM. Effect on the skin of emotional and nervous states: Theoretical and practical consideration of a gastro-intestinal mechanism. *Arch Derm Syphilol*, 1930; 22 (6): 962–93.

Suh DH, Kim BY, Min SU. A multicenter epidemiological study of acne vulgaris in Korea. *Int J Dermatol*, 2011 Jun; 50 (6): 673–81. doi: 10.1111/j.1365-4632.2010.04726.x.

Swanson NL, Leu A, Abrahamson J, et al. Genetically engineered crops, glyphosate and the deterioration of health in the United States of America. *J Organic Systems*, 2014; 9 (2).

Tasoula E, Gregoriou S, Chalikias J, et al. The impact of acne vulgaris on quality of life and psychic health in young adolescents in Greece: Results of a population survey. *An Bras Dermatol*, 2012 Nov–Dec; 87 (6): 862–9.

Troiano RP, Berrigan D, Dodd KW, et al. Physical activity in the United States measured by accelerometer. *Med Sci Sports Exerc*, 2008 Jan; 40 (1): 181–8.

USDA. Water in meat and poultry. *United States Department of Agriculture Food Safety and Inspection Service*. 2011 May, accessed Apr 2015, www.fsis.usda.gov/wps/wcm/connect/42a903e2-451d-40ea-897a-22dc74ef6e1c/Water_in_Meats.pdf?MOD=AJPERES.

U.S. Environmental Protection Agency. *Integrated Risk Information System (IRIS) on Formaldehyde*. Washington, DC: National Center for Environmental Assessment, Office of Research and Development, 1999.

Uygur MC, Arik AI, Altuğ U, et al. Effects of the 5 alpha-reductase inhibitor finasteride on serum levels of gonadal, adrenal, and hypophyseal hormones and its clinical significance: A prospective clinical study. *Steroids*, 1998 Apr; 63 (4): 208–13.

Varma TR. Hormones and electrolytes in premenstrual syndrome. *Int J Gynaecol Obstet*, 1984 Feb; 22 (1): 51–8.

Vermeer C, Shearer MJ, Zittermann A, et al. Beyond deficiency: Potential benefits of increased intakes of vitamin K for bone and vascular health. *Eur J Nutr*, 2004 Dec; 43 (6): 325–35. Epub 2004 Feb 5.

Victor Antony Santiago J, Jayachitra J, Shenbagam M, et al. Dietary d-limonene alleviates insulin resistance and oxidative stress–induced liver injury in high-fat diet and L-NAME-treated rats. *Eur J Nutr*, 2012 Feb; 51 (1): 57–68. doi: 10.1007/s00394-011-0182-7. Epub 2011 Mar 29.

von Woedtke T, Schlüter B, Pflegel P, et al. Aspects of the antimicrobial efficacy of grapefruit seed extract and its relation to preservative substances contained. *Pharmazie*, 1999; 54: 452–6.

Wang RY, Needham LL, Barr DB. Effects of environmental agents on the attainment of puberty: Considerations when assessing exposure to environmental chemicals in the National Children's Study. *Environ Health Perspect*, 2005 Aug; 113 (8): 1100–7.

Wolkenstein P, Misery L, Amici JM, et al. Smoking and dietary factors associated with moderate-to-severe acne in French adolescents and young adults: Results of a survey using a representative sample. *Dermatology*, 2015; 230 (1): 34–9. doi: 10.1159/000366195. Epub 2014 Nov 19.

Wróbel AM, Gregoraszczuk EŁ. Actions of methyl-, propyl- and butylparaben on estrogen receptor-α and -β and the progesterone receptor in MCF-7 cancer cells and non-cancerous MCF-10A cells. *Toxicol Lett*, 2014 Nov 4; 230 (3): 375–81. doi: 10.1016/j.toxlet.2014.08.012. Epub 2014 Aug 13.

Yang CM, Li YQ. The therapeutic effects of eliminating allergic foods according to food-specific IgG antibodies in irritable bowel syndrome. *Zhonghua Nei Ke Za Zhi*, 2007 Aug; 46 (8): 641–3. [Article in Chinese]

Yang YS, Lim HK, Hong KK, et al. Cigarette smoke–induced interleukin-1 alpha may be involved in the pathogenesis of adult acne. *Ann Dermatol*, 2014 Feb; 26 (1): 11–6. doi: 10.5021/ad.2014.26.1.11. Epub 2014 Feb 17.

Yosipovitch G, Tang M, Dawn AG, et al. Study of psychological stress, sebum production and acne vulgaris in adolescents. *Acta Derm Venereol*, 2007; 87 (2): 135–9.

Zhang H, Liao W, Chao W, et al. Risk factors for sebaceous gland diseases and their relationship to gastrointestinal dysfunction in Han adolescents. *J Dermatol*, 2008 Sep; 35 (9): 555–61. doi: 10.1111/j.1346-8138.2008.00523.x.

Zółtaszek R, Hanausek M, Kilińska ZM, et al. The biological role of D-glucaric acid and its derivatives: Potential use in medicine. *Postepy Hig Med Dosw* (online), 2008 Sep 5; 62: 451–62. [Article in Polish]

Zouboulis CC. Acne as a chronic systemic disease. *Clin Dermatol*, 2014 May–Jun; 32 (3): 389–96. doi: 10.1016/j.clindermatol.2013.11.005. Epub 2013 Nov 23.

Other Resources

Environmental Working Group's Skin Deep Cosmetics Database: www.ewg.org/skindeep
Melanoma Education Foundation: www.skincheck.org

Lab Testing

Doctor's Data: www.doctorsdata.com
Rocky Mountain Analytical: www.rmalab.com
US Biotek Laboratories: www.usbiotek.com

Index

A

Absorica (isotretinoin), 60–61
Accutane (isotretinoin), 60–61
acne
  adult, 26, 38
  associated conditions, 28–30
  bacteria responsible, 26, 184
  causative factors, 24–28, 31
  conventional treatments, 56–68, 134
  cystic, 14
  diet as trigger, 39, 43, 81–93
  emotional effects, 122–32
  genetics and, 24–25
  hormonal, 94, 180–81
  managing (quick guide), 10
  nodulocystic, 16
  non-pharmaceutical treatments, 24, 76–80
  pigmentation changes, 21, 67
  premenstrual, 94
  psychological effects, 13, 21–22
  rebound, 56, 59–60, 61
  scarring from, 19–21, 67
  severe, 14, 16
  stages of, 17
  stress as trigger, 30–37, 106
  types, 14–16
acne mechanica, 15, 108
adapalene (Differin), 63, 65
adrenal glands, 29, 36
AGEs (advanced glycation end products), 46–47
alcohol. See also wine and beer
  as beverage, 34, 112, 159
  isopropyl, 74
allergies (food), 50, 51, 52, 88
almonds
  Mushroom Tart, 282
  Salty Almonds with Thyme, 229
  Spicy Tamari Almonds, 230
  "Steak and Potatoes," 279
  Tangy Green Beans (variation), 357
  Turkey Mole, 330
amino acids, 165
Amnesteen (isotretinoin), 60–61
amylase, 85
androgens. See also testosterone
  birth control pills and, 59–60
  elevated levels, 26, 29, 48–49, 104
  mTORC1 and, 45
  prescribed, 29
  reducing levels, 61, 181

andropause, 29
anger, 122–27
  awareness log, 125–26, 127
antibiotics, 57–58, 183
  topical, 58, 65
anti-nutrients, 93, 170
antioxidants, 34, 114
  sources, 175, 181–82
anxiety, 12, 37, 50. See also self-criticism; sleep
appetizers, 222–27
apples, 151, 167
  Apple Cinnamon Hemp Porridge, 211
  Avocado Melissa Sue Anderson, 268
  Creamy Fennel, 218
  Fennel, Apple and Coconut Salad, 266
  Flaming Antibiotic, 218
  Kale, Apple and Walnut Slaw, 263
  Rustproofer, 220
Asian Eggplant with Peppers and Peas, 355
Asian-Style Baked Tofu, 227
asparagus
  Gingered Greens, 219
  Portobello Pot-au-Feu, 249
avobenzone, 67–68
avocado, 175
  Avocado Cucumber Hand Rolls, 224
  Avocado Melissa Sue Anderson, 268
  Avocado Topping, 329
  Balsamic Tuna Salad in Avocado Halves, 306
  Caprese Salad with Tomatoes, Basil and Avocado, 276
  Chilled Avocado, Mint and Coconut Soup, 246
  Chipotle Pork "Tacos," 338
  Creamy Cherry Tomato Salad, 274
  Garden Patch Spinach Salad, 273
  Guacamole, Perfect, 234
  Nori Hand Rolls (variation), 223

B

bacteria. See also microbiome
  as acne cause, 26
  beneficial, 184
  in skin-care products, 72

Balsamic Tuna Salad in Avocado Halves, 306
bananas, 151
basil. See also herbs
  Basil and Tomato Fillets, 298
  Caprese Salad with Tomatoes, Basil and Avocado, 276
  Cucumber and Mint Coconut Water (variation), 215
  Pesto-Stuffed Tomatoes, 225
  Sardine Pesto Spread, 239
  Sea Gumbo, 258
  Tomato Basil Soup, 250
Basque Drumsticks, 317
BBQ Tarragon Mustard Turkey, 332
beans, dried
  Black Bean Chili, 292
  Bok Choy, Mushroom and Black Bean Stir-Fry, 293
  Country Lentil Soup (variation), 253
  Piquant White Bean and Parsley Dip, 236
  Quick Chicken Chili, 327
  Tuna and White Bean Salad, 307
beans, green
  Green Bean Salad with Toasted Hazelnuts, 270
  Green Beans with Cashews, 358
  Portobello Pot-au-Feu, 249
  Tangy Green Beans, 357
beef
  Beef and Chickpea Curry with Spinach, 345
  Bolognese Sauce, Best-Ever, 242
  Classic Beef Stew, 340
  Coconut Beef Curry, 344
  Italian Sausage Patties, 339
  Moroccan-Spiced Beef Stew, 342
  Roman-Style Oxtails with Celery, 346
  Slow-Cooked Chili Flank Steak or Brisket, 343
benzophenones, 68
benzoyl peroxide, 65
berries, 114, 151, 167, 178
  Green Tea and Blueberries, 216
beverages
  alcohol, 34, 112, 159
  recipes for, 215–20
  as snacks, 142

Library and Archives Canada Cataloguing in Publication

Trotter, Makoto, 1977–, author
   The complete acne health & diet guide : naturally clear skin without antibiotics / Dr. Makoto Trotter, BSc (Hons), ND.

Includes index.
ISBN 978-0-7788-0512-0 (paperback)

1. Acne—Diet therapy. 2. Acne—Nutritional aspects. 3. Acne—Treatment.
I. Title. II. Title: Complete acne health and diet guide.

RL131.T76 2015   616.5'3   C2015-903863-4